OXFORD MEDICAL PUBLICATIONS

Oxford Handbook of
Adult Nursing

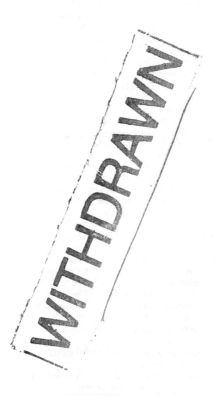

WITHDRAWN

Published and forthcoming Oxford Handbooks in Nursing

Oxford Handbook of Cancer Nursing
Edited by Mike Tadman and Dave Roberts

Oxford Handbook of Cardiac Nursing, 2e
Edited by Kate Olson

Oxford Handbook of Children's and Young People's Nursing, 2e
Edited by Edward Alan Glasper, Gillian McEwing, and Jim Richardson

Oxford Handbook of Clinical Skills for Children's and Young People's Nursing
Paula Dawson, Louise Cook, Laura-Jane Holliday, and Helen Reddy

Oxford Handbook of Clinical Skills in Adult Nursing
Jacqueline Randle, Frank Coffey, and Martyn Bradbury

Oxford Handbook of Critical Care Nursing, 2e
Sheila Adam and Sue Osborne

Oxford Handbook of Dental Nursing
Elizabeth Boon, Rebecca Parr, Dayananda Samarawickrama, and Kevin Seymour

Oxford Handbook of Diabetes Nursing
Lorraine Avery and Sue Beckwith

Oxford Handbook of Emergency Nursing, 2e
Edited by Robert Crouch, Alan Charters, Mary Dawood, and Paula Bennett

Oxford Handbook of Gastrointestinal Nursing
Edited by Christine Norton, Julia Williams, Claire Taylor, Annmarie Nunwa, and Kathy Whayman

Oxford Handbook of Learning and Intellectual Disability Nursing
Edited by Bob Gates and Owen Barr

Oxford Handbook of Mental Health Nursing, 2e
Edited by Patrick Callaghan and Catherine Gamble

Oxford Handbook of Midwifery, 3e
Janet Medforth, Susan Battersby, Maggie Evans, Beverley Marsh, and Angela Walker

Oxford Handbook of Musculoskeletal Nursing
Edited by Susan Oliver

Oxford Handbook of Neuroscience Nursing
Edited by Sue Woodward and Catheryne Waterhouse

Oxford Handbook of Nursing Older People
Beverley Tabernacle, Marie Barnes, and Annette Jinks

Oxford Handbook of Orthopaedic and Trauma Nursing
Rebecca Jester, Julie Santy, and Jean Rogers

Oxford Handbook of Perioperative Practice
Suzanne Hughes and Andy Mardell

Oxford Handbook of Prescribing for Nurses and Allied Health Professionals
Sue Beckwith and Penny Franklin

Oxford Handbook of Primary Care and Community Nursing, 2e
Edited by Vari Drennan and Claire Goodman

Oxford Handbook of Renal Nursing
Edited by Althea Mahon, Karen Jenkins, and Lisa Burnapp

Oxford Handbook of Respiratory Nursing
Terry Robinson and Jane Scullion

Oxford Handbook of Surgical Nursing
Edited by Alison Smith, Maria Kisiel, and Mark Radford

Oxford Handbook of Women's Health Nursing
Edited by Sunanda Gupta, Debra Holloway, and Ali Kubba

Oxford Handbook of
Adult Nursing

Second edition

Edited by

Dr Maria Flynn
Senior Lecturer
Faculty of Health and Life Sciences,
University of Liverpool, UK

Dr Dave Mercer
Lecturer in Nursing
Faculty of Health and Life Sciences,
University of Liverpool, UK

OXFORD
UNIVERSITY PRESS

OXFORD
UNIVERSITY PRESS

Great Clarendon Street, Oxford, OX2 6DP,
United Kingdom

Oxford University Press is a department of the University of Oxford.
It furthers the University's objective of excellence in research, scholarship,
and education by publishing worldwide. Oxford is a registered trade mark of
Oxford University Press in the UK and in certain other countries

Published in the United States of America by Oxford University Press
198 Madison Avenue, New York, NY 10016, United States of America

British Library Cataloguing in Publication Data
Data available

Library of Congress Control Number: 2017953758

ISBN 978–0–19–874347–7

Printed and bound in China by
C&C Offset Printing Co., Ltd.

Foreword

As nurses, it is important we have easy access to information to gain the knowledge we need to underpin our practice and to better understand the context in which we work.

As students and as qualified nurses, we must continue to develop, to keep up-to-date and increase our expertise. As well as learning new things, we also need to remind ourselves of things we may have forgotten or have not encountered for some time.

We all need to learn and remember why we do what we do and explore our own values and our role in leading practice, teams, and our profession. We make important decisions every day with our patients, families, and our colleagues, and have a key role in ensuring a safe and positive practice environment.

Nursing is both a science and an art. We constantly reflect on our practice and question what we have learnt and what we may do better to continually improve the quality of our care. And as we learn, so we pass our knowledge and expertise to others through teaching, supervision, and mentorship.

Increasingly, we are working under pressure, dealing with increased complexity, and can be time-poor, so having a resource such as this handbook enables quick access to a comprehensive range of helpful information.

Janet Davies BSc (Hons) RGN RMN MBA FRCN
Chief Executive & General Secretary
Royal College of Nursing

Preface

Since the publication of the first edition of the *Oxford Handbook of Adult Nursing*, global health priorities, health technology, and international and national politics have had significant impact on the way adult nursing is practised in all care environments. Alongside these cultural drivers, the dominant discourse within the profession has shifted from one of delivering nursing interventions to one which recognizes that caring and compassionate nursing works with people and families in the management of health conditions.

In this context, what we are presenting in this second edition is an entirely new text. The second edition of the *Oxford Handbook of Adult Nursing* reflects how nurses relate to people, engage critically with professional knowledge, and organize and deliver appropriate nursing care and interventions. It also recognizes the inter-relatedness of physical and mental functioning and well-being.

The approach we have taken in the second edition of the handbook is to address the philosophy, principles, and practice of general adult nursing in an accessible and convenient format. We have not tried to compile a text which addresses everything that nurses may encounter in the course of their everyday work. Rather, we have highlighted key information, which we hope will help nurses to draw on their personal and professional values, knowledge, and experience when making practice decisions and organizing care.

Part 1 of the handbook describes key nursing values and standards which frame clinical decision-making and safe nursing practice. The material in Part 2, addressing aspects of communication, is written from a critical perspective to stimulate thought when dealing with diverse clinical populations. At a time when the NHS and the nursing profession are under profound strain, we are reminded daily of the centrality of nursing and healthcare as a political issue. This section therefore reflects our own position in relation to communication and nursing practice.

In Part 3, which deals specifically with clinical nursing practice and decision-making, we have taken a systems approach. Each of the chapters gives a broad introduction and an overview of clinical conditions, investigations, and treatments, including frequently prescribed medicines, and highlights relevant nursing practice considerations. Again, this section is designed to support nurses in their clinical thinking and decision-making. Part 4 provides an overview of nursing leadership, teamwork, professional development, and engagement with external agencies, patients, and service users.

Each chapter of the handbook also lists useful sources of further information. The majority of these are online resources, in recognition of the way most people use information and communication technology in everyday nursing practice, education, and research. Other texts in the *Oxford Nursing Handbook* series provide a wide range of specialist texts to cover the detail of more specialized aspects of nursing, and references to these are included.

We have deliberately excluded details of clinical procedures, as these are expertly addressed in the *Oxford Handbook of Clinical Skills in Adult Nursing*. However, we envisage that, together, these two handbooks will provide nursing students and general adult nurses with a robust framework for thinking about, and practising, safe and compassionate values-based nursing.

In rewriting this important text, we have brought together specialist and generalist clinical nurses, nursing students, educators, and researchers. We have interpreted and edited all the complex information from contributors within the framework of our own substantial experiences in adult nursing practice, education, and research.

We are proud and privileged to be members of the nursing profession and hope that this handbook provides a useful source of information and inspiration to our fellow nurses and future professionals.

Maria Flynn
Dave Mercer

For our families.

Contents

Contributors

Emma Addie
Lecturer in Nursing
Faculty of Health and Life Sciences
University of Liverpool

Vicky Ashworth
Advanced Nurse Practitioner
Royal Liverpool and Broadgreen
University Hospital NHS Trust

Nicola Blair
Diabetic Specialist Nurse
Lancashire Care NHS
Foundation Trust

Rebekah Burton
Staff Nurse
Royal Liverpool and Broadgreen
University Hospital NHS Trust

Lynda Carey
Senior Lecturer
Faculty of Health and Social Care
Edge Hill University

Emma Caton
Consultant Nurse
East Lancashire Hospitals NHS Trust

Dan Cooper
Advanced Nurse Practitioner
Mid Cheshire Hospitals NHS
Foundation Trust

Layla Davies
Policy Officer (Refugee Support)
St Helen's Council

Dr Maria Flynn
Senior Lecturer
Faculty of Health and Life
Sciences
University of Liverpool

Rebecca Flynn
Solicitor
Probation Services consultant

Alison Graham
Lead Practitioner (Diabetes)
Clinic Based Services Business Unit
Lancashire Care NHS
Foundation Trust

Jess Hough
Staff Nurse
University Hospital of South
Manchester NHS Foundation Trust

Julie Hutton
Advanced Nurse Practitioner
Mid Cheshire Hospitals NHS
Foundation Trust

Fran Ion
Clinical Nurse Specialist in Pain
Management
Royal Liverpool and Broadgreen
University Hospital NHS Trust

Stella Kenrick
Advanced Nurse Practitioner
Lancashire Teaching Hospitals NHS
Foundation Trust

Professor Mick McKeown
Professor of Democratic
Mental Health
College of Health and Wellbeing
University of Central Lancashire

Dr Steve McKinnell
Lecturer and TEL academic
Faculty of Health and Life Sciences
University of Liverpool

Dr Dave Mercer
Lecturer in Nursing
Faculty of Health and Life Sciences
University of Liverpool

Justine Monks
Advanced Nurse Practitioner
Liverpool Heart and Chest NHS
Foundation Trust

Sarah Mooney
Staff Nurse
Aintree University Hospital NHS
Foundation Trust

Pete Noon
Staff Nurse
Liverpool Heart and Chest NHS
Foundation Trust

Sharon Phillips
Learning and Teaching Lead
Marie Curie Palliative Care Institute
University of Liverpool

Steven Simpson
Chief Pharmacist
Royal Bolton Hospital NHS
Foundation Trust

Isobel Thompson
Nurse Practitioner
Mid Cheshire Hospitals NHS
Foundation Trust

Dr Vicky Thornton
Lecturer in Nursing
Faculty of Health and Life Sciences
University of Liverpool

Amanda Walthew
Advanced Nurse Practitioner
Liverpool Heart and Chest NHS
Foundation Trust

Phil Whelan
Clinical Nurse Specialist
Royal Liverpool and Broadgreen
University Hospital NHS Trust

Symbols and abbreviations

β	beta
°C	degree Celsius
=	equal to
>	greater than
<	less than
%	per cent
®	registered trademark
™	trademark
ℛ	website
➲	cross-reference
ABG	arterial blood gas
ABPM	ambulatory blood pressure monitoring
ACE	angiotensin-converting enzyme
AChE	acetylcholinesterase (inhibitor drugs)
ACP	advance care planning
ACS	acute coronary syndrome
ADRT	advanced decision to refuse treatment
AED	automatic electrical defibrillator
AFP	alpha fetoprotein
AKI	acute kidney injury
ALF	acute liver failure
ALT	alanine aminotransferase
AMD	acute macular degeneration
ANTT	aseptic non-touch technique
APA	American Psychiatric Association
APD	automated peritoneal dialysis
APTT	activated partial thromboplastin time
ARDS	acute respiratory distress syndrome
AS	ankylosing spondylitis
AV	atrioventricular
AVF	arteriovenous fistula
AVPU	alertness, voice, pain, and unresponsiveness
BAHA	bone-anchored hearing aid
BAI	breath-actuated inhaler
BCG	bacille calmette–Guérin
BiPAP	bi-level positive airway pressure
BJP	Bence–Jones protein

BLS	basic life support
BME	black and minority ethnic
BMI	body mass index
BNF	*British National Formulary* (UK)
BNP	brain natriuretic peptide
BPD	borderline personality disorder
bpm	beat per minute
BSL	British Sign Language
BTS	British Thoracic Society (UK)
CABG	coronary artery bypass graft
CAPD	continuous ambulatory peritoneal dialysis
CAS	computer-assisted surgery
CBT	cognitive behavioural therapy
CD	controlled drug
CF	cystic fibrosis
CHFG	Clinical Human Factors Group
CK	(serum) creatine kinase
CKD	chronic kidney disease
cmH_2O	centimetre of water
CMP	clinical management plan
CNS	central nervous system
CO_2	carbon dioxide
COPD	chronic obstructive pulmonary disease
COSHH	control of substances hazardous to health
COX-2	cyclo-oxygenase 2
CPAP	continuous positive airway pressure
CPD	continuous professional development
CPHVA	Community Practitioners & Health Visitors Association
CPR	cardiopulmonary resuscitation
CPRS	complex regional pain syndrome
CQC	Care Quality Commission (UK)
CRE	controlled radial expansion
CRP	C-reactive protein
C&S	culture and sensitivity
CSF	cerebrospinal fluid
CT	computerized tomography
CVD	cardiovascular disease
CVP	central venous pressure
CXR	chest X-ray
DEXA	dual-energy X-ray absorptiometry

DIC	disseminated intravascular coagulation
DKA	diabetic ketoacidosis
DNA	deoxyribonucleic acid
DOLS	deprivation of liberty safeguards
DPI	dry powder inhaler
DSM	*Diagnostic and Statistical Manual*
DVLA	Driver and Vehicle Licensing Agency (UK)
DVT	deep vein thrombosis
EBP	evidence-based practice
EBUS	endoscopic bronchial ultrasound
ECG	electrocardiogram
EEG	electroencephalogram
eGFR	estimated glomerular filtration rate
EMG	electromyogram
EMR	endoscopic mucosal resection
ENT	ear, nose, and throat
EPAP	expiratory positive airway pressure
EPS	electrophysiological studies
ERAS	enhanced recovery after surgery
ERCP	endoscopic retrograde cholangiopancreatography
ESR	erythrocyte sedimentation rate
ESWL	extracorporeal shock wave lithotripsy
ETT	exercise tolerance test
EUS	endoscopic or endoluminal ultrasound
EWS	early warning scores
FBC	full blood count
FEV1	forced expiratory volume
FES	fat embolism syndrome
FESS	functional endoscopic sinus surgery
FEV1	forced expiratory volume in 1 second
FGM	female genital mutilation
fL	femtolitre
FTD	frontotemporal dementia
g	gram
GFR	glomerular filtration rate
GI	gastrointestinal
GP	general practitioner (UK)
GSL	general sales list (drugs)
GTN	glyceryl trinitrate
h	hour

Hb	haemoglobin
HbA1c	glycated haemoglobin
HCAI	healthcare-associated infection
HCC	hepatocellular carcinoma
HCO$_3$	bicarbonate
HCT	haematocrit
HD	haemodialysis
HDF	haemodiafiltration
HDL	high-density lipoprotein
HDL-C	high-density lipoprotein cholesterol
HDU	high dependency unit
HF	haemofiltration
HHS	hyperosmolar hyperglycaemic state
HIV	human immunodeficiency virus
HRT	hormone replacement therapy
HSE	Health and Safety Executive (UK)
IAD	incontinence-associated dermatitis
IBD	inflammatory bowel disease
IBS	irritable bowel syndrome
ICD	internal cardioverter–defibrillator
ICP	intracranial pressure
ICT	information and communication technology
ICU	intensive care unit
ILR	implantable loop recorder
IM	intramuscular
INR	international normalized ratio
IO	intraosseous
IOP	intraocular pressure
IPAP	inspiratory positive airway pressure
ITU	intensive therapy unit
IU	international unit
IV	intravenous
IVP	intravenous pyelography
IVU	intravenous urography
kg	kilogram
kPa	kilopascal
KWPD	Kausch–Whipple pancreatoduodenectomy
L	litre
LDH	lactate dehydrogenase
LDL	low density lipoprotein

LDL-C	low density lipoprotein cholesterol
LFT	liver function test
LMW	low molecular weight (heparin)
LOC	level of consciousness
LVF	left ventricular failure
m	metre
MCH	mean corpuscular haemoglobin
mcL	microlitre
MCV	mean corpuscular volume
MDI	metered-dose inhaler
MDT	multidisciplinary team
ME	myalgic encephalopathy
mg	milligram
MHNA	Mental Health Nurses Association (UK)
MHRA	Medicine & Healthcare products Regulatory Agency (UK)
MI	myocardial infarction
min	minute
mIU	milli international unit
mm	millimetre
mmHg	millimetre of mercury
mmol	millimole
MMSE	mini mental state examination
MND	motor neuron disease
mol	mole
mOsm	milliosmole
MPT	multi-professional team
MRC	Medical Research Council (UK)
MRI	magnetic resonance imaging
MRSA	meticillin-resistant *Staphylococcus aureus*
MS	multiple sclerosis
MSK	musculoskeletal
MSSA	meticillin-sensitive *Staphylococcus aureus*
MSU	midstream urine
MUST	Malnutrition Universal Screening Tool
NAFLD	non-alcoholic fatty liver disease
NEWS	national early warning system
ng	nanogram
NG	nasogastric
NHS	National Health Service (UK)
NICE	National Institute for Health and Care Excellence (UK)

NIHR	National Institute for Health Research (UK)
NMC	Nursing and Midwifery Council (UK)
nmol	nanomole
NOAC	novel oral anticoagulant
NOMS	National Offender Management System
NPSA	National Patient Safety Agency (UK)
NRES	National Research Ethics Service (UK)
NSAID	non-steroidal anti-inflammatory drug
NSTEMI	non-ST elevation myocardial infarction
NYHA	New York Heart Association
O_2	oxygen
OA	osteoarthritis
OGTT	oral glucose tolerance test
ORIF	open reduction internal fixation
$PaCO_2$	partial pressure of carbon dioxide
PAINAD	Pain Assessment in Advanced Dementia
PaO_2	partial pressure of arterial oxygen
PBC	primary biliary cirrhosis
PCA	patient-controlled analgesia
PCEA	patient-controlled epidural analgesia
PCNL	percutaneous nephrolithotomy
PCO_2	partial pressure of carbon dioxide
PD	peritoneal dialysis
PE	pulmonary embolus/embolism
PEG	percutaneous endoscopic gastrostomy
PET	positron emission tomography
pg	picogram
PGD	patient group direction
PICC	peripherally inserted central catheter
pmol	picomole
PO	orally (*per os*)
PO_2	partial pressure of oxygen
POAG	primary open-angle glaucoma
POM	prescription-only medicine
PPE	personal protective equipment
PPI	patient and public involvement
PPMS	primary progressive multiple sclerosis
PPPD	pylorus-preserving pancreatoduodenectomy
PSA	prostate-specific antigen
PSC	primary sclerosing cirrhosis

PSD	patient-specific direction
PT	prothrombin time
PTFE	polytetrafluoroethylene
PTSD	post-traumatic stress disorder
PTT	partial thromboplastin time
PV	per vagina
RA	rheumatoid arthritis
RCM	Royal College of Midwives (UK)
RCN	Royal College of Nursing (UK)
R&D	research and development
RICE	rest, ice, compression, and elevation
RRMS	relapsing–remitting multiple sclerosis
RVF	right ventricular failure
SA	sinoatrial
SAH	subarachnoid haemorrhage
SaO_2	arterial saturation
SC	subcutaneous
SCS	spinal cord stimulation
SIRS	systemic inflammatory response syndrome
SL	sublingual
SLE	systemic lupus erythematosus
SSRI	selective serotonin reuptake inhibitor
STD	sexually transmitted disease
STEMI	ST elevation myocardial infarction
TAP	transversus abdominis plane
TB	tuberculosis
TEM	transanal endoscopic micro-surgery
TENS	transcutaneous electrical nerve stimulation
TFT	thyroid function test
TIA	transient ischaemic attack
TOE	transoesophageal echocardiography
TSH	thyroid-stimulating hormone
TUC	Trades Union Congress (UK)
TURP	transurethral resection of the prostate
U	unit
UA	unstable angina
U&Es	urea, electrolytes, and creatinine (levels)
UK	United Kingdom
UTI	urinary tract infection
VAS	visual analogue scale

VATS	video-assisted thoracic surgery
VC	vital capacity
VRS	verbal rating scale
VTE	venous thromboembolism
WCC	white cell count
WHO	World Health Organization
WRES	Workforce Race Equality Standard

Part 1

Professional nursing values

Professional nursing values

Introduction

Health policy, legislation, and changing health priorities have always impacted on the way adult nursing is organized and delivered, and in the twenty-first century, the dominant discourse of professional nursing practice has shifted from one of 'delivering nursing care' to 'working with people'. Across all service sectors the way nurses work with people is shaped by professional and legal requirements, by ethical principles, and by their own personal values and beliefs. It is important for all nurses to understand the statutory framework in which they operate, and also the key values and responsibilities which underpin professional nursing practices.

Definition of nursing

The International Council of Nurses (⚕ www.icn.ch) defines nursing as:

> *The autonomous and collaborative care of individuals of all ages,
> families, groups and communities, sick or well and in all settings. Nursing
> includes the promotion of health, prevention of illness, and the care of ill,
> disabled, and dying people. Advocacy, promotion of a safe environment,
> research, participation in shaping health policy and in patient health
> systems, management, and education are also key nursing roles.*

Key characteristics of nursing

Nursing is a vocation and a profession, and the role is a multifaceted blend
of knowledge, skills, and personal characteristics. The practice of nursing
demands a balance of technical and clinical competence, alongside humanistic and caring values. Nurses in any care environment are charged with
maintaining excellent clinical standards and demonstrating compassion and
care to people and their families.

Whilst the concepts of 'care' and 'compassion' are difficult to define, they
are central to the expectations of the public, and the professional and statutory bodies, about what constitutes 'good' nursing. In the United Kingdom
(UK), nursing also has to be practised within the framework of the values
of the National Health Service (NHS) constitution:

- Working together for patients.
- Respect and dignity.
- Commitment to quality of care.
- Compassion.
- Improving lives.
- Everyone counts.

(⚕ www.nhs.uk)

Regulation of nursing practice

With the responsibility which nursing assumes, statutory regulation is
required in order to protect the public, whose safety and well-being remain
at the forefront of nursing practice and decision-making.

In the UK, the Nursing and Midwifery Council (NMC) is the statutory
body responsible for regulating nurses and midwives in England, Wales,
Scotland, and Northern Ireland, with the purpose of safeguarding the public
and ensuring safe and competent practitioners.

The four functions of the NMC are:

- Maintaining the register of members admitted to practice.
- Determining the standards for education and training for admission to
  the different parts of the register.
- Giving guidance about standards of conduct and performance.
- Administering procedures (including making rules) relating to
  misconduct, fitness to practice, and similar matters.

The UK Nursing and Midwifery Council Code

The NMC Code of professional standards of practice and behaviour for nurses and midwives (℘ www.nmc.org.uk) describes the expected competencies and duties commensurate with being a nurse. It reflects the changing roles, responsibilities, and expectations of nurses in the twenty-first century.

Upholding these standards is a commitment each nurse makes on entry to the professional register, and at all subsequent re-registrations and revalidations. The Code contains a series of statements that, taken together, indicate what good nursing and midwifery practice should be. It puts the interests of patients and service users first and promotes trust through professional behaviour. The twenty-five standards of the Code require all nurses to:

- Treat people as individuals and uphold their dignity and human rights at all times.
- Listen to people and respond to their preferences and concerns.
- Make sure that people's physical, social, and psychological needs are assessed and responded to.
- Act in the best interests of people at all times.
- Respect people's right to privacy and confidentiality, even after they have died.
- Always practise in line with the best available evidence.
- Communicate clearly.
- Work cooperatively.
- Share skills, knowledge, and experience with colleagues and for the benefit of people receiving care.
- Keep clear and accurate records relevant to practice.
- Be accountable for decisions to delegate tasks and duties to other people.
- Have in place an indemnity arrangement which provides appropriate cover for any practice as a nurse or midwife in the UK.
- Recognize and work within the limits of competence.
- Be open and candid with all service users about all aspects of care and treatment, including when any mistakes or harm have taken place.
- Always offer help if an emergency arises in a practice setting or anywhere else.
- Act without delay if there is a risk to patient safety or public protection.
- Raise concerns immediately if a person is vulnerable or at risk and needs extra support and protection.
- Advise on, prescribe, supply, dispense, or administer medicines within the limits of training and competence, the law, NMC guidance, and other relevant policies, guidance, and regulations.
- Be aware of, and reduce as far as possible, any potential for harm associated with nursing practice.
- Uphold the reputation of the profession at all times.

- Uphold the position as a registered nurse or midwife.
- Fulfil all registration requirements.
- Cooperate with all investigations and audits.
- Respond to any complaints made relating to the professional role.
- Provide leadership to make sure people's well-being is protected and improve their experiences of the healthcare system.

In promoting the values which complement clinical knowledge, skills, and competence, the Code also describes mechanisms and behaviours by which each of the standards may be met.

The Code outlines appropriate conduct for a professional nurse. These mark a clear distinction between behaviour and acts which may be permissible in lay people but which are not acceptable for nurses.

Nurses and midwives are required to work within the boundaries of this Code, aware of their limitations when working autonomously, and always in accordance with relevant statutory legislation of the country in which they practise. Whilst the Code cannot be enforced in a court of law, if questions regarding professional misconduct or fitness to practice are raised, it is used by the NMC to judge a nurse's actions. Students in training have separate guidance which mirrors the standards represented in the Code.

Professional accountability

Accountability means that each individual nurse is answerable for her/his conduct and actions, and is responsible for the decisions she/he makes and how these affect the people to whom she/he owes a duty of care. Accountability underpins the professional, legal, and ethical aspect of the nursing role. The responsibility that this brings is to ensure that all reasonable actions are taken to ensure patient safety. This implies that all nurses should be:

- Aware of the professional standards described in the regulatory body's Code.
- Confident that all decision-making is appropriately informed.
- Able to justify all clinical actions or omissions.
- Able to communicate appropriately and effectively with people, families, and other members of the healthcare team, whether in verbal, written, digital, or electronic formats.

When considering the nurse's accountability to patients and the public, the nurse must also be aware of the 'duty of candour'. This is a legal requirement on hospital, community, and mental health Trusts to inform and apologize to patients if there have been mistakes in their care or if they have suffered harm. The purpose of this duty of candour is:

- To ensure that people are able to receive timely, accurate, and truthful information from health providers.
- To provide all necessary information regarding an incident if an error occurs in the course of care or treatment provision.
- To furnish an apology when things go wrong.

The duty of candour regulation applies to any registered persons carrying out a regulated activity (see also ➲ Chapter 3, Safety in the clinical environment).

Responsibility

To be responsible means discharging a moral or legal obligation or duty. For nurses, this means ensuring that their approach to work and general conduct can be held to account and conforms to the law at all times.

By following the NMC Code, nurses demonstrate responsibility towards the profession and to people in their care. Nurses must also be responsible towards their employer and act in accordance with the role descriptor of their position and all local policies and procedures.

Duty of care

In the UK, the duty of nursing care has been expressed in terms of six key principles, which reflect the standards described in the NMC Code:
- Care.
- Compassion.
- Competence.
- Communication.
- Courage.
- Commitment.

When exercising a duty of care, a nurse's approach should be informed by these principles and should seek to establish an appropriate working partnership to support and enhance the health and well-being of those people in their care.

The NMC also emphasizes that safe and effective care delivery should revolve around partnership working, in an environment where healthcare professionals are able to share good practice and discuss issues relating to patient safety and care.

Nursing and the law

There is an obligation on professional nurses to always act within the laws of the country in which they are practising (NMC), and should a matter be brought to court, ignorance of the law is not a defence. When considering the legal context of nursing in the UK, it is important to understand the meaning of legal statutes (see Box 1.1).

> **Box 1.1 Statutes and statutory instruments**
> - *Statutes* are described as a general framework of legal rules, from which secondary legislation can be introduced.
> - *Statutory instruments* provide a more detailed set of regulations which often govern practice more closely than the primary legislation.

Statutes of particular relevance to nursing practice include:
- The Human Rights Act 1998.
- The Mental Capacity Act 2005.

Both of these laws uphold the fundamental rights and freedoms of individuals in the UK. They also provide a framework to protect those whose mental and/or physical capacity renders them vulnerable and which might compromise their ability to make decisions for themselves. Other relevant statutes governing the protection of individuals who have a mental health condition are:
- The Mental Health Act 1983.
- The Mental Health Act 2007 (which provided amendments to the original 1983 Act).

Other areas that concern the nursing profession are Acts which relate to confidentiality, such as the Data Protection Act 1998, and various Acts which govern health and safety, the administration of medicines, and aspects of employment law, which delineate the nurse's legal obligation to their employer and vice versa.

All these laws act to guide the power and limits imposed upon the nurse when practising, and thereby act to protect the public by safeguarding their interests. Nurses are legally and professionally obliged to act in accordance with the term and conditions set out within the laws.

Common law
- This is a particularly important area of law. In the UK, this is where decisions around competence and errors in practice are often heard, and where judges preside over cases.
- Litigation in relation to healthcare most often refers to when some form of harm to a person occurs accidentally at the hands of a nurse or other healthcare practitioner. The litigant will normally seek some form of justice, often financial compensation.
- Other examples of common law judgements may include resolution of a dispute between a healthcare practitioner and a patient over treatment decisions. These often revolve around individual rights in respect of treatments being offered.

Negligence

- In relation to medicine and healthcare, the aim of the civil law of negligence is to restore a person who has been harmed to the position in which they would have been, had the harm not occurred. This often involves claims for damages and compensation.
- Often the judgement will focus on the duty of care owed to the person by the healthcare team, whether this duty has been breached, and whether this breach has resulted in harm which was reasonably foreseeable.

Battery

- A claim of battery may be brought if a person believes that non-consensual contact has occurred between themselves and a nurse or other healthcare professional.
- This can include physically examining a patient or moving them against their will, giving an injection, or operating on the person without their consent.
- For this to be considered a criminal act, the person must show that they were competent to agree to the contact, but that the act was conducted against their will or without their consent.
- This type of contact does not necessarily constitute a crime of assault.

Consent

- In legal terms, the need for consent for healthcare interventions is underpinned by respect for autonomy and protection of bodily integrity.
- Consent can also act as a waiver where an act would otherwise wrong an individual or disrupt their legitimate expectations. A person's consent can waive their right or modify their expectations, and so justify an act that would otherwise be unacceptable. Without consent, acts of healthcare may be considered, in law, to be an assault.

The UK Department of Health defines valid consent as that which is:

> '. . . given voluntarily by an appropriately informed person who has the capacity to consent to the intervention in question (this will be the patient or someone with parental responsibility for a patient under the age of 18, someone authorised to do so under a Lasting Power of Attorney (LPA) or someone who has the authority to make treatment decisions as a court appointed deputy). Acquiescence where the person does not know what the intervention entails is not consent'.

In nursing practice, consent given by a person with whom the nurse is working may be verbal or written. So, for example, in order to take a measurement of a person's blood pressure, it would be appropriate to ask their permission to carry out the procedure and for them to give verbal consent. For more invasive procedures, such as surgery, it would be necessary for the consent to be written.

Respect for autonomy, privacy, and confidentiality

Respect for a person's autonomy extends to protection of their privacy and a duty of confidence. The UK Department of Health stipulates that a duty of confidence arises:

> 'When one person discloses information to another (e.g. patient to clinician) in circumstances where it is reasonable to expect that the information will be held in confidence'.

A duty of confidence is a legal obligation that is derived from case law, and it is also a requirement established within professional codes of conduct. A duty of confidence will normally be found within NHS employment contracts as a specific requirement linked to disciplinary procedures. In some circumstances, disclosure of confidential information and acting without consent may be legally and ethically defensible.

If a person does not have sufficient capacity to be able to provide consent, the Mental Capacity Act allows treatment to be given if it is believed that the person will never gain capacity to be able to make such a decision and that their condition is immediately life-threatening.

Breaches of confidentiality may be necessary in the public interest where a failure to disclose information may expose the patient, or others, to risk of death or serious harm. In such circumstances, nurses should disclose information promptly to an appropriate person or authority. Disclosure is also necessary for the prevention or detection of a serious crime. Some statutory instruments may oblige a nurse to reveal information about an individual:

- The Road Traffic Act 1988.
- The Prevention of Terrorism Act 2005.
- The Public Health Acts 1984, 2008.
- The Misuse of Drugs Act 2015.

The other circumstance where it is permissible to disclose confidential information is with a person's consent, if sharing information with members of the multidisciplinary team (MDT) will benefit their clinical treatment. The challenge of maintaining confidentiality for nurses is to achieve a balance between the sharing of information for legitimate purposes and respecting a person's autonomy and privacy.

Clinical governance

Governance is the term used to describe the way in which UK healthcare organizations manage services and information in the health and social care system.

The clinical governance framework charges every UK health provider with a responsibility to work towards delivering safe and high-quality services to the public. It involves identifying risk and managing it appropriately, and extends to ensuring that all healthcare staffs are able to develop their professional skills.

In order to monitor quality standards, clinical audits are regularly conducted against recognized benchmarks, to measure both the clinical and cost-effectiveness of services.

The Care Quality Commission (CQC), National Patient Safety Agency (NPSA), National Institute for Health and Care Excellence (NICE), and NHS Litigation Authority work alongside all parts of the healthcare sector to monitor and advise on issues of clinical governance and care quality standards.

Ethical nursing practice

Ethics can be defined as the moral principles which govern a person's behaviour or the conduct of an activity. It seeks to address questions such as whether we should treat all people the same, and focuses upon our attitudes and behaviour towards, and treatment of, others.

Ethical accountability is defined by societal rules which govern general social conduct. Along with the NMC Code and the UK NHS constitution, ethics help to shape appropriate professional behaviour and provide a framework for ethical nursing practice.

Ethical practice in nursing and healthcare is framed by the World Medical Association (⅋ www.wma.net) Geneva Declaration, which is often used as a pledge made by health professionals at the time of their formal entry into their profession.

'I solemnly pledge myself to consecrate my life to the service of humanity; I will give to my teachers the respect and gratitude which is their due; I will practise my profession with conscience and dignity; The health of those in my care will be my first consideration; I will respect the secrets that are confided in me, even after the patient has died; I will maintain by all the means in my power, the honour and the noble traditions of my profession; My colleagues will be my sisters and brothers; I will not permit considerations of age, disease or disability, creed, ethnic origin, gender, nationality, political affiliation, race, sexual orientation, or social standing to intervene between my duty and my patient; I will maintain the utmost respect for human life from its beginning, even under threat, and I will not use my specialist knowledge contrary to the laws of humanity; I make these promises solemnly, freely, and upon my honour.'

Ethical principles

A number of different philosophical theories are used to describe a moral perspective which guides motivations and conduct. The philosophical positions most often used to understand ethical decision-making in nursing and healthcare are:

- *Utilitarianism* which defines the morality and ethics of an action in terms of its consequences and where the right action is the one which fulfils the greatest good.
- *Duty* where the morality of an action is determined by the reason or motive for the action, not the consequences or utility of the act.
- *Rights* are the justified claims which individuals and groups can make upon other individuals or society. They enable individuals to have the freedom to act without unwanted interference from government. Rights are often the moral position taken when a system is being challenged, and it is important to note that rights are different from needs, wants, or desires.

The philosophical position which many nurses will recognize is *principlism*. This informs the ethical framework most widely used in nursing education, practice, and research and refers to the four bioethical principles of autonomy, beneficence, non-maleficence, and justice.

- *Autonomy* means self-rule, and respect for autonomy means respecting an individual's decisions and values.
- *Beneficence* means doing good by and for others.
- *Non-maleficence* means bringing no harm to another person.
- *Justice* refers to universal fairness and providing due consideration for all.

The four principles framework, alongside the NMC Code, can guide nursing decision-making, to help ensure that nurses always act ethically and in the best interests of patients and the public.

When working with and for people, it is also important to appreciate differences of opinion. Public concepts of health and well-being may differ significantly from those of the nurse or other healthcare professionals.

Ethical nursing practice is underpinned by decision-making which is driven by a rigorous reasoning process and a desire to serve the best interests of people and their families.

Consent in ethical nursing practice

The key principles of ethical nursing practice can be maintained through open and honest communication of information, secure and accurate record-keeping, and respect for persons, through partnership working and securing informed consent for any nursing action to be carried out.

As part of the duty of care to patients and the public, nurses are obliged to ensure that properly informed consent is gained and documented before any invasive action is carried out. People must give their permission for routine procedures and practices, consistent with local policies and protocols.

In order to safeguard the public, and contribute to an ever evolving profession and healthcare system, modern nurses are required to have a range of medico-technical competencies and critical thinking abilities.

Alongside their knowledge and skills, nurses also need to demonstrate caring attributes, humanistic values, professional values, and a due regard for the ethical and legal boundaries of their practice and decision-making.

Useful sources of further information

- For more detailed consideration of negligence and issues relating to duty of care and foreseeable risk, useful resources are Bridgit Dimond's *Legal Aspects of Nursing* and Margaret Brazier and Emma Cave's *Medicine, Patients and the Law*.
- NHS Codes of Practice and legal obligations on confidentiality are available at: ℬ http://systems.hscic.gov.uk/infogov/codes.
- Further information on clinical governance is available at: ℬ www. england.nhs.uk/wp-content/uploads/2014/06/nhs111-coms-stand.pdf.

Values-led nursing research

Nursing research

Nursing research is the mechanism by which the profession develops its theoretical knowledge, advances understanding, and tests ideas related to the practice of nursing. The conduct of nursing research always involves people, so all the nursing values, knowledge, and skills relevant to general nursing practice are also central to nursing research.

There are large numbers of nurses who work with medical or other research teams, often recruiting people into biomedical studies or collecting samples. There are also academic nurses who focus their work on pushing the boundaries of nursing knowledge. General adult nurses may become involved in research when studies are being conducted in their clinical areas, or they may pursue their own research as part of their professional development.

By virtue of the nature of nursing itself, the conduct of nursing research encompasses the full spectrum of scientific and social research methods.

A key feature of nursing research is that it always involves people. This may be at a distance (such as investigations involving physiological samples or collating information from clinical charts) or in a very intimate circumstance (such as interviewing patients and their families about a traumatic health event).

Any research which involves people is bound by the Declaration of Helsinki, a statement of ethical principles governing research which involves human beings and including research conducted on identifiable human material and data (℘ www.wma.net).

People taking part in nursing research studies may also be vulnerable on account of their health condition or their position as a 'patient'. This means that, through participation in nursing research studies, they may be exposed to a degree of risk. This could be a risk of exploitation, psychological harm, or physical harm, or risk of disclosure of information about them or their condition.

Ethical nursing research practice upholds the key ethical principles to ensure that study design, recruitment, data collection, data analysis, and reporting study findings all respect the dignity, rights, safety, well-being, and integrity of participants at all times.

Research governance

In the UK, all health research activity is coordinated through the National Institute for Health Research (NIHR), the purpose of which is (see ℘ www. nihr.ac.uk):

> . . . to maintain a health research system in which the NHS supports outstanding individuals, working in world-class facilities, conducting leading-edge research focused on the needs of patients and public.

Health research practice is also regulated through UK and international laws and regulatory bodies, including:
- The Declaration of Helsinki.
- Professional codes of practice.
- Health and safety legislation.
- Data Protection Act.
- Human Tissue Act.
- EU Clinical Trials Directive.
- Regulations on clinical trials involving medicines.
- Medical Research Council (MRC) guidelines on good research practice.
- Medicine and Healthcare products Regulatory Agency (MHRA).
- National Patient Safety Agency (NPSA).
- UK National Research Ethics Service (NRES).

In the UK NHS, the Research Governance Framework outlines the mandatory principles of ethical research practice and sets explicit standards to assure the scientific quality of health research studies. The national standards for health research practice are described in five key domains.
- Ethics.
- Science.
- Information.
- Health, safety, and employment.
- Finance and intellectual property.

Any proposed nursing, or other health research study, has to be approved by a research ethics committee (NREC), a local Trust research and development (R&D) office, or, in some cases, a University research ethics committee, before it commences.

Approval from NRES is required for all studies in areas covered by legislation and for those involving patients and service users (℘ www.hra.nhs.uk/ research-community/applying-for-approvals/research-ethics-committee/). This includes:
- Clinical trials.
- Studies involving human tissue.
- Studies with adults lacking capacity.
- Studies involving radiation.
- All research involving NHS patients, carers, or service users.
- All research involving adult social care.
- All research involving prisoners or those in the custody of the National Offender Management System (NOMS).

Advice from the regional ethics service should be sought for any studies which propose to use previously collected NHS data, including:

- Identifiable tissue samples.
- Where there are queries about consent.
- Where there is a necessity for new comparative samples.
- Research involving acellular materials (e.g. DNA).
- Research involving previously collected information, particularly where patients or service users could possibly be identified.
- Research involving NHS premises or facilities.

Within the NHS guidelines and arrangements for research ethics committees, local R&D or audit departments are able to give approval to some types of studies:

- Research involving previously collected non-identifiable NHS data or samples.
- Research involving previously collected non-identifiable information.
- Research involving NHS staff.
- Research involving some NHS premises or facilities.
- Clinical audit studies.
- Service evaluation studies.

Ethical approval for nursing research studies

The principal function of research ethics committees is to assess any potential risks to participants and ensure that the study design, procedures and processes, and arrangements for data and information management all uphold ethical principles. Normally, applications for ethical approval are evaluated on the basis of:

- The quality of the science: the study should be well designed and have the potential to add to nursing knowledge or understanding.
- The level of experience of the researchers.
- Whether or not service users or the public are to be involved in any part of the design or management of the research.
- The quality and clarity of study information to be provided to participants.
- The procedures for securing and recording informed consent to participate in the research.
- How any participants and their contributions will be anonymized.
- An explicit risk/benefit analysis which calculates the risks and potential benefits for individuals, society, and the nursing profession.
- The arrangements in place for data management, storage, and archiving.
- Arrangements for the responsible disposal of data (in line with local policies and procedures).
- Procedures for the management of any human tissues or materials (including such things as routine blood samples).
- Clear procedures for dealing with sensitive, embarrassing, or upsetting topics, criminal disclosures, adverse effects, pain, discomfort, distress, inconvenience, or lifestyle changes.

In terms of planning or carrying out a nursing research study, these evaluation criteria mean that any unnecessary duplication of ideas is to be avoided, and study findings should have the potential to enhance existing nursing knowledge or practice in some way.

Duplication can be avoided through a comprehensive review of the existing evidence in the field, including any reported systematic reviews of evidence lodged in the Cochrane database. It is also good practice to seek expert or peer review of proposed nursing research studies, proportional to the scale of the project.

Informed consent in nursing research

The justification for any nursing research project entails rationalizing its potential contribution to knowledge or practice, against the principles of respect for autonomy, beneficence, non-maleficence, and justice.

These four principles are the ethical framework used by the UK NHS research ethics service to make judgements about the potential risks and benefits of any proposed nursing research studies.

Ethical principles can be upheld through careful attention to the way the research study is designed and conducted, and principally the means of providing accurate and honest participant information. The securing of informed consent is essential.

- Acknowledge the right of participants to full disclosure about the study and the nature of their contribution.
- Never engage in covert data collection or deception about the purpose of the study.
- Recognize the need for informed consent and provide accurate and accessible participant information to facilitate decision-making.
- Allow a suitable period of time for prospective study participants to consider their position and, if necessary, discuss their involvement with significant others.
- Respect the right to self-determination and never coerce people into taking part in studies.
- Respect the right to fair and equitable treatment, and do not discriminate if allocating people to different treatment groups or study conditions.
- Provide access to research personnel and psychological or other support to all study participants if required.
- Respect the individual's right to privacy, and minimize intrusion when collecting data.
- Assure anonymity for study participants and that all aspects of the research interaction remain confidential.

(See also ➜ Chapter 1, Professional nursing values and ➜ Chapter 22, Surgery, for consent in nursing practice).

Vulnerable groups

Particular care is needed when seeking to involve people in vulnerable groups in nursing research. They are potentially at greater risk of exploitation or harm through participation in studies.
- Children under 16 years.
- People with mental illness, learning disabilities, dementias, and neurodegenerative diseases.
- People who are unconscious, severely ill, and terminally ill.
- People in clinical emergency situations.
- Prisoners, young offenders.
- People detained in high, medium, or low secure units.
- People who are detained under mental health legislation.
- People in dependent relationships.
- People who do not speak English.

Data management

Research governance arrangements require any data collected during the course of a nursing research study to be securely retained for an appropriate period of time and in such a way that participants' human dignity and confidentiality is maintained.

The NHS research governance arrangements also stipulate a requirement that data are made available to other researchers or auditors, if necessary and appropriate.

This means that close attention needs to be paid to the ways in which data are recorded and stored, ensuring they are treated with respect, equity, and confidentiality.

Data include both 'raw' and processed material which may be in the form of written, recorded, digital, and electronic materials, clinical records, human tissue, cultured samples, transcripts, and spreadsheets.

Trusts and universities will have legally appropriate procedures and processes for archiving research material, and local policies should always be followed.

Evidence-based practice

The concept of evidence-based practice (EBP) first emerged as a means to rationalize an increasing volume of clinical research, with the rapid development of innovative health technologies, and a perceived need to justify an exponentially increasing expenditure on health interventions and treatments.

The origins of the EBP movement are located firmly in the domain of medicine. EBP was conceptualized as a move away from opinion-based clinical decision-making and sought to integrate individual clinical expertise with the best available evidence from robust and systematic research. Sophisticated information and communication technology has enabled international research studies and their findings to be shared and collated for universal access, largely via the Cochrane collaboration ($\wp$ www.uk.cochrane.org/)

As a direct consequence of these conditions, the EBP movement was primarily concerned with medical research, specifically that which could demonstrate the efficacy and effectiveness of treatment interventions and medicines. The EBP movement also developed processes and practices which ordered research into a *hierarchy of evidence*. This hierarchy relates to how useful the different research designs are in determining the *effectiveness* of clinical interventions or treatments.

Alongside the growth of EBP in medicine, the nursing profession also committed to developing an evidence base, and EBP is now a central tenet of nursing education and clinical practice.

The same founding principles apply to EBP in nursing, namely the integration of clinical knowledge and expertise with the findings of robust research, to support nursing decision-making in clinical practice.

EBP demands that nurses are able to recognize good-quality evidence and critically engage with ideas in order to make informed judgements about nursing practice and care. EBP also requires that nurses have the skills and resources to implement and evaluate changes in practice and that practice change is consistent with the needs and desires of service users and the public.

However, the purpose and practice of the research endeavour means that all evidence for practice is inherently 'temporary'. No matter how robust nursing evidence may appear, the nature of nursing will always generate new questions which may challenge the existing evidence base, and perhaps eventually result in a paradigm shift which alters nursing thought, practice, and decision-making.

It should also be noted that within the wider international nursing community, the concept of EBP for nursing holds a contentious position. There is considerable debate about whether the philosophy and principles of EBP are relevant to the essence of nursing or applicable to the type of decisions nurses need to make when working with people. Issues which have been debated include, but are not limited to:

- What constitutes appropriate evidence for the extensive range of nursing practices?
- How is legitimacy conferred on different sources of nursing knowledge?
- How is clinical experience to be used where practice decisions need to be supported by best evidence?
- How are nursing decisions justified in situations where there is no relevant evidence?
- Is there sufficient good-quality nursing research to support practice decisions?
- What influence does the prevailing financial and political climate exert on nursing research, education, and practice?
- What impact does the commitment to EBP have on humanistic nursing values?
- Is the notion of an evidence-based nursing profession masking a depersonalization of core nursing values, resulting in a perceived deficit of care and compassion?

Useful sources of further information

Further information regarding research ethics committees is available from:
- ℘ www.hra.nhs.uk/about-the-hra/our-committees/
  research-ethicscommittees-recs/
- National Institute for Health Research ℘ www.nihr.ac.uk
- National Patient Safety Agency ℘ www.npsa.nhs.uk
- The Cochrane collaboration ℘ www.uk.cochrane.org
- World Medical Association (Declaration of Helsinki) ℘ www.wma.net

Safety in the clinical environment

Patient safety

In addition to upholding professional nursing values and behaviours at all times, nurses also have a duty to ensure that the clinical environment in which they work is safe. This responsibility extends to the safety of patients, the public, colleagues, and any visitors to the clinical area.

The safety of clinical environments is largely regulated by law and managed through strict local policies and operating procedures, but maintaining patient safety is fundamental to all nursing practice. The primary obligation of registered nurses is to always act in a way which safeguards the public (℮ www.nmc.org.uk).

The complexity of modern healthcare carries with it inherent risks to safety. These risks extend beyond the medico-technical aspects of clinical interventions and into the environments in which nurses work.

The clinical decisions which nurses make have a direct impact on the safety and comfort of people in their care, but other decisions relating to the clinical environment and the way nursing work is organized can also impact on the safety of patients, the public, and colleagues.

Environmental risks may result in incidents which affect everyone's safety, and the way individual nurses, other healthcare workers, clinical organizations, and the NHS respond to incidents is an important part of healthcare governance.

In the UK, the Health and Safety Executive (HSE) sets and monitors standards of environmental safety in the workplace. These standards include all aspects of physical geography, emergency procedures, equipment, machinery, and working conditions (℮ www.hse.gov.uk).

The NHS Commissioning Board describes a framework for managing and reporting incidents in clinical environments, to ensure the continued safety of everyone involved in health services (℮ www.england.nhs.uk/patientsafety).

Definition of incidents

- An incident is defined as an event which could have, or did, result in unnecessary damage, loss, or harm to patients, staff, visitors, or members of the public.
- Incidents are also recognized as any circumstance which prevents or compromises an organization's ability to continue to provide healthcare services.
- A serious incident involves unexpected or avoidable injury or death of one or more patient, staff, visitor, or member of the public.
- Incidents which compromise patient safety and are largely preventable are referred to as 'never events' (℮ www.nrls.npsa.nhs.uk/neverevents).

Managing an adverse incident

In the event of an adverse incident of any sort, the quality of written records and the way the incident is reported are of central importance. All healthcare organizations have local policies and internal processes for accident or incident reporting, and these should always be followed.

As far as is possible, a contemporaneous record of the event should be made and reported promptly through the local reporting procedures.

Nurses should always work within their sphere of competence and, in the event of an incident, will need to make decisions about appropriate actions to take:

- Call for help.
- Remain calm and avoid personal danger.
- As far as is possible, minimize danger to patients, visitors, and colleagues.
- Make a clear and accurate report of events and all actions taken.
- Promptly inform the line manager or the person responsible for the shift or sector.
- If the incident involves a patient's care or treatment, ensure the responsible medical team is informed.
- Provide clear and accurate information about the incident to patients and their families.
- Involve other departments, if necessary, such as local safeguarding teams, pharmacy, medical engineering, or security.
- If necessary, refer the incident to relevant outside agencies such as the police, social services, or the coroner.
- A personal reflective account of the incident and the way it was managed may also be useful in a nurse's personal portfolio to facilitate professional learning and development.

Human factors in healthcare

Human factors theories come from a coalition of academic disciplines, including psychology, engineering, and ergonomics, and they seek to understand and describe how behaviour at work is influenced by individual characteristics, the working environment, organizations, and the nature of the job itself.

The potential relevance of human factors for nursing and healthcare is related to patient safety and the reduction of clinical errors. It has been estimated that of all the people admitted to hospital in the UK each year, around 10% will be involved in an adverse event, of which approximately half are preventable ($\wp$ improvement.nhs.uk/improvement-hub/patient-safety/).

It is assumed that widespread attention to human factors could potentially improve patient safety by reducing errors at both individual and organizational levels.

The Clinical Human Factors Group (CHFG) is a collective of healthcare professionals, managers, and service users working with human factors experts to campaign for change in the NHS ($\wp$ www.chfg.org). It is recognized that the risk of errors and incidents increases where the clinical care delivery system is complex. Other known factors include:

- Stress and fatigue.
- Time constraints.
- Poor communication.
- Lack of experience or training.
- Inadequate supervision.

Improving safety through attention to human factors relies on teamwork, open and effective communications between different healthcare professional groups, and, wherever possible, the use of standardized tools to assess clinical and other risks. (See also ➜ Chapter 11, Communication in the procedural administration of care and ➜ Chapter 12, Risk assessment.)

Clinical deterioration

In the hospital and community settings, many patients with clinical disorders may at some point suffer deterioration in their condition. This may be part of the natural progress of a disease or the effect of new treatments or medications. Clinical deterioration may also be the result of neglect or poor healthcare practices or it may indicate the start of the end-of-life phase and a natural process of dying. (See also ➋ Chapter 25, Death and dying.)

It is an important part of nurse decision-making to judge clinical deterioration and to respond appropriately. However, it has been estimated that in the UK, approximately 23,000 hospital inpatients each year suffer a clinical deterioration which is unrecognized or untreated. Unrecognized or untreated deterioration will lead to clinical emergencies, and often to a preventable cardiopulmonary arrest.

The UK NPSA notes that vigilant monitoring of physiological parameters can assist in identifying a deteriorating patient, before a serious clinical event occurs (✍ www.npsa.nhs.uk), and NICE has issued guidelines for effective clinical monitoring (✍ www.nice.org.uk/guidance/cg50).

Summary of NICE guidelines

It is recommended that all adult patients in acute hospital settings should have:
- Physiological observations recorded at the time of admission or initial assessment by health professionals who are trained in the tasks and who understand the clinical relevance of measurements.
- As a minimum, these measurements should include heart rate, respiratory rate, systolic blood pressure, level of consciousness, oxygen saturation, and temperature.
- A clear written monitoring plan, which takes into account the person's diagnosis, co-morbidities, and treatment and specifies which observations should be recorded and how often.
- Observations should be recorded at least 12-hourly, unless a clinical decision to increase or decrease the frequency has been made at a senior level.
- Monitoring frequency should be increased if an abnormality in physiological parameters is detected, and the locally agreed escalation strategy should be initiated in response to any early warning scores (EWS).
- In specific situations, additional measurement of hourly urine output, pain, blood glucose, lactate, and arterial blood gases (ABGs) may also be considered.
- Physiological 'track and trigger' or EWS systems should be used to monitor all adult patients.

Key nursing considerations

Caring for a deteriorating patient is often a stressful and emotional experience for nurses, and it is important that the locally agreed early warning score system and escalation plans are always followed.

Within their sphere of competence, key nursing practices should include:

- Timely and accurate measurement of all physiological measurements, as described in the monitoring plan.
- Timely and accurate recording of all observations of the person's condition.
- Timely and accurate reporting of any changes in observations and condition within the MDT.
- Timely and accurate administration and recording of any prescribed pain relief, symptom relief, and other medications.
- Ensuring intravenous (IV) access is maintained.
- Administering oxygen, if required, to maintain a comfortable respiratory rate and oxygen saturation at >95%.
- Monitoring cumulative fluid intake and urine output.
- Clearly explain all actions and interventions.
- Seek to clearly and honestly allay patient and family anxieties.
- Maintain a safe and calming environment.
- As far as possible, ensure physical comfort.

(For details of specific clinical procedures, see ➔ *Oxford Handbook of Clinical Skills in Adult Nursing*.)

Early warning scores

EWS, or 'track and trigger' systems, monitor and score physiological observations in order to identify any deterioration in a person's condition and stimulate appropriate clinical responses.

Early warning systems have been developed in an effort to predict and prevent clinical deterioration and reduce mortality, and are in widespread use across the UK NHS.

Although there are local variations in early warning procedures and documentation, the key principles have been described by a multidisciplinary working group and published as a national early warning system (NEWS) under the auspice of the Royal College of Physicians (ℛ www.rcplondon.ac.uk).

Principles of early warning score systems

- EWS should be used to improve assessment of acute illness, detect clinical deterioration, and initiate a timely and competent clinical response.
- EWS should not be used in children under 16 or pregnant women whose physiological response to illness can be modified.
- The chronically disturbed physiology of some patients with chronic obstructive pulmonary disease (COPD) can influence the sensitivity of EWS systems.
- EWS can be implemented in pre-hospital, primary, and community care facilities.
- The EWS should be determined from six physiological parameters: respiratory rate, oxygen saturation, temperature, systolic blood pressure, pulse rate, and level of consciousness.
- Each of the physiological observations is scored according to the extent of deviation from the normal range, and where a person is receiving oxygen therapy, an additional score is added.
- Scores on all physiological parameters are aggregated to give a total 'trigger' score.
- A low EWS, normally 1–4, should prompt assessment by a competent registered nurse to decide on the frequency of clinical monitoring or whether care needs to be escalated.
- A medium EWS, between 5 and 6, or a maximum score in just one measure (a RED score) requires urgent review by a suitably qualified clinician.
- A high EWS of >7 necessitates an emergency assessment by the clinical team, and possibly critical care experts.

These are recommendations for a national early warning scoring system, which local services may adapt to their own circumstances. It is therefore essential that nurses are familiar with, and competent in the use of, any local early warning systems.

Standard precautions and infection control

Healthcare-associated infections (HCAIs), also known as nosocomial or 'hospital' infections, are those which are acquired as a result of healthcare. These infections are neither present nor incubating when a person initially comes into contact with a healthcare setting and may also develop after discharge from a hospital or clinical facility.

HCAIs also include occupational infections amongst healthcare workers and are known to be one of the most commonly occurring adverse events in healthcare delivery worldwide. Frequently seen HCAIs include:

- Meticillin-resistant *Staphylococcus aureus* (MRSA).
- Meticillin-sensitive *Staphylococcus aureus* (MSSA).
- *Escherichia coli* (E. coli).
- Surgical site infection (SSI).
- *Klebsiella* bacteraemia.

HCAIs present a significant risk to patients, visitors, and healthcare staff. Their effects can range from mild discomfort to prolonged or permanent disability, and in some cases death.

People most at risk of contracting HCAIs are those who are very old or very young, those undergoing invasive procedures, and those with compromised immune systems.

Prevention of HCAIs is crucial, and the UK Health Protection Agency (% www.gov.uk/government/organisations/health-protection-agency) provides comprehensive guidelines for standard precautions and infection control in healthcare settings.

Standard infection control precautions must be applied by all healthcare workers, and there are five key principles which frame local policy and practice guidelines:

- Hospital environment hygiene.
- Hand hygiene.
- Use of personal protective equipment (PPE).
- Safe use and disposal of sharps.
- Asepsis.

Hospital environment hygiene

The key priority is to make the environment acceptable for patients, visitors, and staff, and specific actions include:

- Removal of dust and dirt so that the environment is visibly clean.
- Regular removal of all non-essential items or equipment.
- Increased cleaning, with the use of disinfectants, in cases of known or suspected infection.
- Decontamination (with recommended manufacturer products) of any shared equipment used in the delivery of patient care.
- All healthcare workers to be aware of their individual responsibilities for cleaning and decontamination in the clinical environment.
- In some cases of known infection, isolation rooms may be used, as determined by local policy. Nurses should be aware of relevant local practice guidelines relating to working with people in isolation rooms.

Hand hygiene

Hand hygiene is a simple, but effective, means of preventing infection and cross-infection. For healthcare staff, it is recommended that when working in clinical environments:

- All wrist and hand jewellery is removed.
- Short-sleeved clothing is worn.
- Fingernails are kept short, clean, and free from nail polish and false nails.
- Skin abrasions and cuts are covered using waterproof dressings.

In many circumstances, hands can be effectively decontaminated using alcohol-based gel hand rub:

- Immediately prior to direct patient contact.
- Clean or aseptic procedures.
- Immediately after direct patient contact.
- Immediately after contact with bodily fluids, mucous membranes, and broken skin.
- Immediately after contact with objects or equipment in a clinical environment that could result in contamination.
- Immediately after the removal of gloves.

In circumstances where hands are visibly dirty, potentially contaminated with bodily fluids, or when working with people with vomiting or diarrhoea, hands should be decontaminated thoroughly using soap and water and an effective handwashing procedure such as the Ayliffe technique.

(For details of the Ayliffe technique, see ➔ *Oxford Handbook of Clinical Skills in Adult Nursing*.)

Personal protective equipment

PPE is used by healthcare workers when risk assessment suggests there is a possibility of transmission of microorganisms or contamination of clothing and skin by blood or other bodily fluids. PPE includes gloves, disposable plastic aprons, full body gowns, surgical face masks, and eye protection.

Gloves

Gloves are worn as single-use items and disposed of immediately after use, in all situations which include:

- Invasive procedures.
- Contact with sterile sites.
- Contact with broken skin or mucous membranes.
- Activities that carry the risk of exposure to blood or bodily fluids.
- Handling sharps.
- Contact with contaminated equipment.

Gloves must be changed between contacts with different patients. Non-powdered, non-sterile latex examination gloves are normally used, except in cases of latex allergy when they are replaced by non-sterile nitrile examination gloves.

Disposable plastic aprons

Disposable plastic aprons should be worn in any situation when there is a risk that clothing may become contaminated by pathogenic microorganisms, blood, or bodily fluids.

If there is a risk of extensive splashing of contaminants or bodily fluids, then a full body fluid-repellent gown should be worn.

Aprons and gowns are single-use only and must be changed between patients and disposed of safely. Surgical masks and eye protection are appropriate when there is a risk of blood or bodily fluids contaminating the face and eyes.

To further prevent the risk of cross- or self-contamination, PPE should be removed in the following order:

- Gloves.
- Apron/gown.
- Eye protection.
- Face mask.

PPE must be disposed of with the clinical waste and in accordance with local policies. Hands must be thoroughly decontaminated (by washing) immediately after removal of PPE.

Safe handling and disposal of sharps

Incidents involving the unintentional inoculation of healthcare workers, with used needles or other sharp materials, are the most common factor in the transmission of blood-borne viruses.

The UK HSE issue guidelines for the safe management of medical devices, needles, and other medical sharps (🕮 www.hse.gov.uk), and they recommend that, wherever possible, unprotected traditional medical sharps should be replaced with safety-engineered devices. Guidelines also suggest that:

- Handling of sharps should be kept to a minimum.
- Sharps should not be passed directly from hand to hand.
- Needles must not be re-sheathed, bent, or disassembled after use.
- Sharps should be discarded at the point of use by the person using the device—another person should never be asked to discard any waste that incorporates sharps.

In addition, the containers for sharps disposal must:

- Be positioned and secured safely, away from public areas and at a height that enables safe disposal by all members of staff.
- Be temporarily closed when not in use.
- Never be filled above the recommended capacity.
- Be disposed of in accordance with the local policy when full.

All healthcare workers have a responsibility to ensure they are familiar with the local policy regarding the action to be taken in the event of a sharps-related injury.

Asepsis

Asepsis refers to the exclusion of harmful bacteria, viruses, and micro-organisms from the body. In clinical environments, the aseptic non-touch technique (ANTT) is used to protect people from the introduction of microorganisms and pathogens during the course of clinical procedures.

The ANTT is a set of mandatory guidelines, which are based on the decontamination of hands and the use of non-sterile gloves, and which may also involve the use of sterile gloves and equipment.

The ANTT should be used for any procedure that breaches the body's natural defences such as:

• Insertion and maintenance of invasive devices.
• Management of IV infusions of fluids or medications.
• Care of wounds and surgical incisions.

(For details of the ANTT procedure, see ➲ *Oxford Handbook of Clinical Skills in Adult Nursing*.)

Safeguarding adults

Registered nurses have a duty to safeguard the well-being of all people in their care. Whilst some people may engage with health services as a direct result of harm from abuse or violence, other vulnerable adults may only be incidentally identified as being unable to protect themselves from harm or neglect.

Vulnerable adults will often require additional safeguarding measures, and appropriate and sensitive care of these people can be extremely challenging.

When concern for patient safety is raised, nurses should initially work in close partnership with the patient, before engaging with family, carers, or partner agencies in the safeguarding team.

An essential element of this partnership working is ensuring that a vulnerable adult has the mental capacity to engage in the decision-making process. Any safeguarding decisions should be made in the person's best interest and in accordance with their values, lifestyles, and beliefs.

Key nursing considerations

If a person presents to the health service with harm from violence or abuse, local protocols for the physical assessment and treatment of any injuries should be carried out first. Where a person is identified as vulnerable, then local safeguarding procedures must be followed:

- Inform the clinical team caring for the person.
- Safeguarding procedures may include completing a risk identification tool, which should only be done with the person's consent.
- People identified as being at high risk should have the opportunity to have their case managed by the local multi-agency risk assessment forum.
- Accurate contemporaneous notes should be made, as they may be required in any future multi-agency risk assessment and safeguarding plans.
- Seek to clearly and honestly allay the person's anxieties.
- Clearly explain all actions and interventions, and give accurate explanations of any other likely events and investigations.
- Maintain a safe and calming environment.
- As far as is possible, ensure physical comfort.
- Provide support and engage family or friends if appropriate.

Management of aggression and violence

Safety in the clinical environment can be seriously compromised by aggression and violence by, or to, patients, the public, or staff. Key facts and nursing considerations in managing aggression and violence can be found in ➲ Chapter 10, Conflict resolution.

Control of substances hazardous to health (COSHH)

There is a legal framework for controlling exposure to substances hazardous to health, and the COSHH legislation requires all employers to ensure that safeguards are in place to protect staff from dangerous substances in all clinical environments (ℰ www.hse.gov.uk).

Substances which are potentially hazardous to health in a clinical environment include chemical preparations, anaesthetic agents, medical gases, disinfectants, solvents and cleaning products, latex, and airborne biological pathogens or those contained in blood or other body fluids.

General principles of COSHH

- Local policies and procedures for the handling of hazardous substances should always be followed.
- Different hazards will require different PPE and procedures.
- Always use appropriate PPE properly.
- Engage in regular training to ensure the knowledge and skills necessary to work safely with hazardous substances.
- Ensure the safety of patients, visitors, and colleagues at all times.
- In the case of people who are cared for in isolation, caregivers and visitors should always wear PPE.
- If exposure to a hazardous substance does occur, local policies and procedures for treatment and notification should be followed.
- Any incidents of exposure to substances hazardous to health should be promptly recorded and reported, according to local procedures.
- Further advice or support about COSHH can be provided by infection control departments, occupational health services, or health and safety teams.

Useful sources of further information

- Department of Health Safeguarding adults policy.℗ www.england.nhs.
  uk/wp-content/uploads/2015/07/safeguard-policy.pdf
- Health and Safety Executive ℗ www.hse.gov.uk
- National Patient Safety Agency ℗ www.npsa.nhs.uk
- National Institute for Health and Care Excellence ℗ www.nice.org.uk
- Royal College of Physicians ℗ www.rcplondon.ac.uk

Medicines management

The safe management of medicines

The administration of medicines, in both hospital and community settings, is a central part of the nursing role. In the UK, all aspects of control, prescription, supply, storage, dispensing, administration, and disposal of medicines are bound by law.

In Europe, medicines are defined as any substance, or combination of substances, presented for treating or preventing disease.

Medicines management refers to the clinically safe use of effective medications, so that any people using prescription medicines gain maximum therapeutic benefit and avoid any harm.

To ensure the continued safety of people taking medicines and that of the nurses administering them, the UK NMC sets standards of practice to which all nurses must adhere when managing medicines and medicinal products.

The NMC recognizes that medicines management is not a routine task but is a nursing action which requires careful thought and professional judgement. The NMC describes standards for the management of medicines, all of which guide safe nursing practice (ℰ www.nmc.org.uk).

The standards clarify that nurses should only supply and administer medicines where there are clear and accurate instructions, which may be in the form of:

• Patient-specific direction (PSD).
• Patient medicines administration chart (inpatient drug chart).
• Patient group direction (PGD).
• Prescription forms.

In addition, nurses also have a professional responsibility to accurately record any medicines given, to be aware of contraindications, and to promptly report any side effects or reactions. It is also incumbent on nurses to record when prescribed medicines have not been given and any reasons for the omission. There are different classes of medicines which nurses administer, which include:

• *Prescription-only medicine* (POM), which are the medicines designed to treat any given condition and where the dosage and route of administration must be prescribed by an authorized prescriber.
• *General sales list* (GSL) drugs are those which are available without prescription such as paracetamol.
• *Controlled drugs* (CDs) are those which are closely regulated, such as powerful opiates, and which are subject to strict local operating procedures. The administration of CDs must be by a registered nurse whose actions are witnessed by another practitioner.
• *Intravenous infusions* (IV) where medicines, such as antibiotics, have been added to a standard solution. The addition of the drug should be carried out by a pharmacist or registered nurse, and the process witnessed. Details of the added drug should be recorded on the solution and in the patient record, in accordance with local policy.

Routes of drug administration

The route of administration of medicines will be determined by several factors. These include the condition of the person and the urgency with which the medicine needs to be given.

The route of administration will influence how quickly a drug will be absorbed and so begin to have an effect. The route of administration will also be determined, to an extent, by the nature of the drug itself and whether it is available as an oral, injectable, or other preparation.

- The *oral* route is for tablets, capsules, linctuses, and other liquids, to be absorbed through the digestive system. A majority of medicines are available in tablet form, and an oral prescription would normally be written as 'O' or 'PO'.
- The *sublingual* route is for tablets or sprays applied under the tongue, which can be absorbed rapidly. The vasodilator glyceryl trinitrate (GTN) is given sublingually in the treatment of angina. A sublingual prescription would normally be written as 'SL'.
- The *inhalation* route is for drugs and preparations which need to be absorbed through the respiratory mucosa and those to directly treat respiratory conditions. Prescriptions for inhaled medications may appear as 'neb' or 'nebulize'.
- The *topical* route refers to drugs to treat a specific local area of the body such as creams for the skin or drops for the eyes and ears.
- Some medicines can also be administered *transdermally* as medicated patches. This route is often used for slow-release pain relief, hormone replacement therapy, and smoking cessation nicotine patches.
- Medicines may also be given by a *rectal* (PR) or *vaginal* route (PV), either for local treatment or a systemic effect by absorption through the mucosa.
- The *subcutaneous* (SC) route is where the drug is administered under the skin for systemic treatment and slower absorption. Insulin, to manage diabetes, and anticoagulant drugs are normally administered SC.
- *Nasogastric* (NG) tubes can be used for medicine administration. If a medication is not available in liquid form, tablets or capsules can be crushed into a suitable liquid medium. Slow-release, long-acting, enteric-coated, or chewable tablets should not be crushed and given through an NG tube.
- *Buccal* administration of drugs allows medications to bypass the digestive system and work more rapidly. Preparations come in the form of tablets, films, or spray and this route of administration is often used for cardiovascular drugs such as glyceryl trinitrate and verapamil. Some opioids (e.g. naloxone, fentanyl) and nausea medicines (prochlorperazine) can also be given this way, as can nicotine replacement therapies.

A large number of medicines are administered by injection, and this may be in response to a clinical emergency situation or where large doses of drugs need to be given over a period of time. Injections may also be used where a person is not able to swallow or cannot tolerate oral preparations.

- *Intravenous (IV)* injections deliver the drug directly into the venous circulation, for rapid absorption and systemic effect.
- *Intramuscular (IM)* injections into muscles in the upper outer quadrant of the buttocks, the anterior lateral aspect of the thigh, or the deltoid muscle of the arm are frequently used for treatment of systemic disorders.
- *Intraosseous (IO)* is the route by which drugs and fluid are injected directly to the bone marrow. It is used when it is not possible to gain venous access or in clinical emergencies. Usual sites for IO access are the upper tibia, the femur, or the head of the humerus, and access is secured through an automatic intraosseous device.
- *Intrathecal injections* are where a medicinal agent is inserted directly into the spinal theca, and they are normally used for anaesthetic purposes.

Vascular access for medicine administration

Peripheral venous access

When people are admitted to Accident and Emergency departments and to some specialist clinical areas, it is routine practice to secure access to the systemic circulation through peripheral veins. Venous access is necessary for taking blood samples, fluid replacement therapy, and medicine administration and can be secured through a range of venous access devices.

- *Peripheral cannulae* are small devices inserted into veins in the hand, arm, or antecubital fossa and secured by taping to the skin. They can also be inserted into the veins of the feet. They are widely used for obtaining blood samples, IV fluid replacement, and administration of some medications such as IV antibiotics.
- *Midline catheters* are inserted through veins near the antecubital fossa and sit in the distal axillary vein in the upper arm. These are normally used when it is necessary to administer medicines which will damage peripheral veins. Midline catheters cannot be used for measurement of central venous pressure (CVP).

Central venous access

Central venous access devices, or central lines, are normally used to monitor CVP in people who are critically ill, or for giving fluids, nutrients, blood products, or medicines over a protracted period of time. They can also be used when peripheral venous access is not possible or for medical procedures and treatments such as plasmapheresis and dialysis.

Different types of central venous catheter will be used, depending on the clinical need. These include multi-lumen catheters (often used in the intensive care unit (ICU)), Hickman lines, tunnelled catheters, and implanted ports. Central lines are normally inserted through the internal jugular vein in the neck, the subclavian or axillary veins of the chest, or the femoral vein in the groin, and once inserted, they sit in the superior vena cava.

Peripherally inserted central catheters (PICC lines) are central lines inserted through the veins in the arm. Common reasons for insertion of a central line for medicine administration include:

- Long-term IV antibiotic therapy.
- Parenteral nutrition.
- Long-term pain control medicines.
- Chemotherapy.
- Administration of caustic drugs such as calcium chloride, potassium chloride, and hypertonic saline.

Supply and disposal of medicines in hospital

The supply and disposal of medicines is regulated by law, and so hospitals and other healthcare organizations will normally have strict procedures in place to monitor medicines management within the organization.

These procedures are important in tracking the movement of medicines, from their distribution by the manufacturers through to their disposal, and the inpatient prescription sheet, or drug chart, is a key part of this audit trail.

Some medicines, such as CDs, need to be transported and stored in locked containers. They may only be administered by registered nurses, and any use has to be properly witnessed.

The registered nurse in charge of a shift or span of duty is the person responsible for safe medicines management in the clinical area, so all local policies and procedures for the safe handling of medicines should always be followed.

- Within hospitals, medicines are normally dispensed and supplied through the pharmacy department, which may be a local or centralized service.
- The role of the pharmacy service is to provide clinical areas with the medicines needed for routine use, and specific medicines required for individual patients.
- In many hospitals, pharmacy staff visit wards and departments on a daily basis to assess the need for stock items, to ensure that stock items are replenished and that prescribed non-stock items are supplied.
- Pharmacy services will normally provide emergency drug supplies from which medicines can be obtained outside of normal pharmacy working hours by designated members of staff. Most hospitals also have a duty pharmacist who can be called out of hours.
- Medicines and medicinal products must always be disposed of in accordance with legislation. Unused, unwanted, or out-of-date stock will normally be disposed of by the pharmacy services.
- Inpatients' own medicines should be returned to any carers or family and taken home. They should only be destroyed or returned to the pharmacy if the person has given their explicit consent.
- If a patient dies in hospital, any medicines which they brought with them should be returned to the family, along with any other personal possessions. With the family's consent, the pharmacy service may dispose of medicines.
- In the community setting, a person may return their medicines to a dispensing pharmacy or their general practitioner (GP) if they are no longer needed, but nurses should not remove any drugs from a person's home unless the person has given their written consent.
- Pharmacists are a very good source of information about medicines and their safe and legal management.

Storage of medicines

In people's own homes, anyone who is taking prescription medicines is themselves responsible for their safe storage. In hospitals, the registered nurse in charge of a clinical area has overall responsibility for the storage and security of medicines.

It is good practice to conduct a weekly stock check of medicines, and CD supplies should normally be checked at least once a day or, depending on local policies, at each shift change.

- Medicines may be stored in locked cupboards, refrigerators, movable medicines trolleys, or individual patient drug lockers.
- Exceptions include emergency drugs in resuscitation equipment and some drugs used in ICUs and operating departments which are in constant use.
- CDs must always be kept in a double-locked drug storage cupboard, and stocks must be checked and verified daily.
- For medicines that require refrigeration, these should be stored at temperatures between 2°C and 8°C, and the temperature monitored daily.
- Medicines treatment charts, prescription pads, and pharmacy requisition forms should also be kept securely.
- Keys for medicine storage cupboards should always be kept securely by the responsible nurse.
- Nurses should be familiar with the local policy on verification and recording of spillages, especially of CDs.
- Medicines brought into hospital by a patient cannot be taken from them without their consent. They may be returned to their family or stored in a locked cupboard until discharge.
- Any loss or apparent theft of medicines, keys, or medicine paraphernalia should be reported promptly, in accordance with local procedures.

Safe practice in the administration of medicines

In the administration of medicines, best practice is focused on patient safety. To minimize medication errors, nurses need to ensure that the correct dose of the prescribed drug is given to the right person at the right time.

This means that nurses need knowledge of the nature and actions of drugs, and always uphold NMC standards for the administration of medicines (℘ www.nmc-org.uk).

Key points of the NMC standards and their implications for nursing practice in drug administration are:

• Nurses must be aware of the therapeutic uses of the medicine to be administered, and its normal dosage, side effects, precautions, and contraindications.

• When administering medicines, nurses must be able to confirm the identity of the patient and ensure that they are not allergic to the prescribed drug and that there are no aspects of the patient's condition which would contraindicate the medicine being given.

• Where there are contraindications, or the patient develops a reaction to the medicines, the prescriber must be informed immediately.

• All prescribed medicines should be given at the time indicated on the prescription.

• Where medication is not given, the reason for not doing so must be recorded.

• Clear and accurate records should be made of all medicines administered, intentionally withheld, or refused by the patient.

• CDs must always be administered by a registered nurse and in line with relevant legislation and local standard operating procedures.

• For the administration of CDs in hospitals, a witness to the process and a second signatory are required.

• In a person's home, where a nurse is administering a CD that has already been prescribed and dispensed to that person, the need for a witness and second signatory should be based on local risk assessment.

• Any medicines administered in substance misuse clinics should be by a registered nurse, and the process witnessed.

• Where student nurses administer medicines, the student's signature must be countersigned by a registered nurse.

• Any medicines to be administered IV should, wherever possible, be checked by two registered nurses.

• Nurses must have successfully undertaken additional training and be competent before administration of complementary and alternative therapies.

Adverse events

• If an error occurs in drug administration, the nurse must take every reasonable action to prevent any potential harm to the patient.

• The error must be documented and reported as soon as possible, in line with local reporting procedures, to the prescriber, the line manager, or employer.

- Information about the medication error must be given to patients and their families, according to local governance arrangements (🖰 www.england.nhs.uk/patientsafety).
- If a person experiences an adverse drug reaction to a medication, nurses must take all reasonable action to remedy harm caused by the reaction.
- Adverse drug reactions must be recorded in the person's medical record.
- The prescriber and the national Yellow Card Scheme (for reporting adverse drug reactions) should be notified immediately. (🖰 www.yellowcard.mhra.gov.uk).

Prescriptions

In primary and community services, the prescription will normally be issued directly to the person, and safe medicines management is their own responsibility.

In some circumstances, community nurses may collect prescriptions for people who would otherwise be unable to have a prescription dispensed (🖰 www.nmc.org.uk).

In hospitals, the prescription is normally prepared and amended online or on a paper record kept with the patient's notes. Prescriptions for inpatient medicines must:

- Be legible and complete and include the patient's full name and hospital number and other required details, in line with local prescribing policy.
- Clearly note any allergies or intolerances.
- Clearly specify the medicine to be given, using the generic or brand name.
- Clearly state the preparation, strength, dose, time, frequency, route of administration, and start and finish dates.
- Be signed and dated by the authorized prescriber.

Abbreviations which are frequently used in prescriptions are noted in Table 4.1.

Table 4.1 Abbreviations used in prescriptions

mg	milligram
g	gram
kg	kilogram
mL	millilitre
L	litre
OD	once daily
BD	twice daily
TDS	three times a day
QDS	four times a day
OM	in the morning
ON	at night
PRN	As required

Key nursing considerations

Nurses who are responsible for administering medicines need to have a sufficient working knowledge of the uses and features of the medicines, so they are able to make appropriate clinical decisions in relation to each person's condition and their treatment.

They also need to be able to address any questions people may have about their medicines. Nurses administering medicines should:

- Check that the prescribed medication and the label on the container are the same, and check the expiry date.
- Check the route and method of administration, the time to be given and the dose.
- Check the patient's identity and administer the medication as prescribed.
- Make a clear, accurate, and immediate record of the medicine administered, and sign.
- Document if the patient refuses or is unable to take the medication, and any actions taken.
- Monitor any effects of the medication and report any abnormal effects or reactions.
- When supervising a student nurse administering medicines, clearly countersign the student's signature.
- Nursing students must never administer or supply medicinal products without direct supervision.
- Some drugs, such as chemotherapeutic agents and vasoactive drugs, should only be administered by nurses who are specifically trained or experienced in the field of practice. Local guidelines and policies should always be followed.

Compliance, adherence, and concordance

The volume of medicines which are prescribed in primary care and hospitals constitutes a large proportion of the total UK health budget. Yet outside of hospital environments, it is estimated that approximately half of the people who are on a prescribed course of medicine do not complete the course or otherwise fail to adhere to the prescribed medicine regime.

This has been a long-term issue for UK health services, resulting in waste, expense, and preventable hospital admissions. NICE guidelines (ℜ www. nice.org.uk) suggest that in order to make best use of medicine treatment regimes and to encourage people to complete treatments, concordance between people, prescribers, and other healthcare professionals is necessary.

Factors which influence compliance with, and adherence to, drug treatment schedules and emphasize the need for concordance are:
• Age.
• Socio-economic status.
• Homelessness.
• Vulnerability.
• Language and fluency.
• Confidence and trust in health professionals.
• Beliefs about health and medicine.
• Perceived benefits of taking the medication.
• Understanding the consequences of not taking medicines.
• Peer, social, or family pressure.
• Complexity of the medication regime.
• Polypharmacy.
• Anticipated side effects.

These factors indicate that nurses have an important role to play in medicine concordance. Nurses need to share their own knowledge of medicines and their actions, and be able to explore people's knowledge, values, and beliefs in relation to medicines, prescriptions, and health.

Non-medical prescribing

The development of non-medical prescribing within the UK health service allows nurses and other health professionals to enhance their roles, skills, and competencies in patient care in a range of settings (℘ www.dhsspsni. gov.uk):

- Management of long-term conditions.
- Medicines management or medication review.
- Emergency, urgent, and unscheduled care.
- Mental health services.
- Services for non-registered patients such as those who are homeless.
- Palliative care.

Registered nurses who wish to prescribe medicines are required to undertake approved training and record this additional competence with the NMC (℘ www.nmc.org.uk).

Independent prescribers

- Independent prescribers are responsible and accountable for the assessment of patients with undiagnosed and diagnosed conditions and for decisions about the clinical management required, including prescribing.
- Independent nurse prescribers are able to prescribe any medicine for any medical condition within their competence, including some CDs.

Supplementary prescribers

- Supplementary prescribing is a voluntary partnership between a medical (or dental) practitioner, a non-medical prescriber, and a patient within the framework of a clinical management plan (CMP).
- Nurses can train and register as supplementary prescribers and may then prescribe any medicine within the patient-specific CMP.
- Supplementary prescribers may only prescribe for patients for whom a clinical management plan exists, and only within the limits of that plan.

Community practitioners

- Community practitioners are able to prescribe independently from a limited formulary comprising some medicines, dressings, and appliances suitable for use in community settings (℘ www.dhsspsni.gov.uk).

Scope of prescribing

Information about the scope of non-medical prescribing is detailed in the *British National Formulary* (*BNF*). All first-level registered nurses may now train to use the extended formulary which includes:

- All medicines in the formulary for community practitioners.
- All licensed pharmacy (P) medicines and all GSL medicines.
- A range of POMs.

These medicines may only be prescribed for use in the specific medical conditions set out in the Drug Tariff and the *BNF*. Nurses cannot prescribe independently outside of these conditions.

Nurse prescribing regulations are regularly reviewed and updated. Once noted on the professional register as an independent or supplementary prescriber, regular updating is necessary. Nurse prescribers are individually and professionally accountable for this aspect of their practice.

Patient group directions

- A PGD is a written instruction for the supply or administration of medicines to a group of patients who may not be individually identified before they present for treatment.
- The protocol is prepared locally by physicians, pharmacists, and other professionals, with advice from relevant professional bodies.
- The protocol must be authorized by a physician (or dentist) and a pharmacist who was involved in writing the group direction.
- PGDs are locally specific. They will normally specify that only certain nurses, working in specified areas of a healthcare organization, can administer the medicines within the patient group.
- PGDs are not a form of prescribing, and there is no specific statutory training that registered nurses must undertake before supplying medicines this way.

Patient-specific directions

- These are written instructions by a doctor, dentist, or nurse prescriber for a medicine to be supplied or administered to a named person. The instruction may be given via a patient's notes or on a drug chart.

Calculating drug doses

Many drug preparations are supplied in a range of doses, which will be dispensed by community or hospital pharmacists. The administration of standard doses of tablets and capsules is straightforward, but when a multiplication of a standard preparation is required, this should always be done with care.

In preparing medicines to be administered IM or IV, it may be necessary to calculate the dose. To do this, it is necessary to know:

- The dose required.
- The volume of the standard preparation.
- The strength of the standard preparation.

For example, a dose of 5mg is prescribed where the strength of the standard preparation is 10mg in a volume of 5mL. The calculation is the dose required × the stock volume divided by the stock strength.

$$5mg \times 5mL/10mg = 2.5mL$$

Infusion flow rates

Many IV infusions are administered through infusion pumps which control the rate of flow, but where mechanical devices are not used, the calculation of flow rate is made through:

- How many drops per millilitre the infusion set delivers.
- The total volume to be infused.
- The period of time over which the infusion is to be delivered.

For example, an infusion of 500mL to be delivered over 4h with an infusion set that has a rate of 20 drops/mL. The calculation is the total volume × the number of drops/mL divided by the number of hours × 60 (minutes).

$$(500 \times 20)/(4 \times 60) = 42 \text{ drops/min}$$

For mechanical infusion pumps, the flow rates are set by dividing the total volume to be infused in millilitres by the period of time.

$$500/4 = 125mL/h$$

(See also ➲ Oxford Handbook of Prescribing for Nurses and Allied Health Professionals.)

Record keeping and social media

Record keeping

Nursing records and documentation are used to communicate details of nursing care provided and to inform other members of the healthcare team of any significant events. Effective nursing documentation is a core nursing responsibility and a means of ensuring continuity of care.

Nursing records are a reflection of the standard of nursing practice. When done well, nursing records can denote the knowledge, skill, and competence of a safe nurse. Good record keeping not only protects patients, but can also support the professional nurse if their practice is ever called into question.

Each practitioner is held legally accountable for what is communicated through written notes and records. Careless or incomplete record keeping typically indicates wider problems with individual practice or how it is managerially organized.

Nursing records can be called as evidence to investigate a complaint: at a local level; at a professional level with the statutory regulatory body; and for criminal or other court proceedings.

In the event of 'never events' or a serious incident or unexpected death, nursing records may need to be closely scrutinized as part of an investigation or reviewed by a coroner's court.

It is therefore crucial that in all clinical environments and healthcare organizations, nursing contributions to care, clinical decision-making, and nursing practice are identified and clearly recorded in appropriate written communication and records.

It is also important to correctly and accurately use any local systems for record keeping. The NMC Code (℘ www.nmc.org.uk) prioritizes the need for nurses to keep clear and accurate records, which includes '*all records* that are relevant to the scope of practice'. In achieving this, the guidelines indicate a need to:

• Complete all records at the time of, or as soon as possible after, an event, recording if the notes are written some time after the event.
• Identify any risks or problems that have arisen and the steps taken to deal with them, so that colleagues who use the records have all the information they need.
• Complete all records accurately and without any falsification, taking immediate and appropriate action if you become aware that someone has not kept to these requirements.
• Attribute any entries you make in any paper or electronic records to yourself, making sure they are clearly written, dated, and timed, and do not include unnecessary abbreviations, jargon, speculation, or subjective statements.
• Take all steps to make sure that all records are kept securely.
• Collect, treat, and store all data and research findings appropriately.

Communication is the cornerstone of effective record keeping and documentation, and promotes continuity of care. In this context, nursing records should provide clear evidence of the way nurses have used their professional values, knowledge, and skills to: assess patient needs; make their clinical and practice decisions; and evaluate the impact of their nursing actions and interventions.

- Good record keeping is a mark of good practice.
- Professional judgement must be used when deciding what to record.
- Entries should be consecutive and follow a continuous sequence.
- Nursing records should be regularly audited.
- Nursing records should reflect safe, competent, and compassionate nursing care.
- Patients have the right of access to records about them.
- The confidentiality of the nursing records must be respected and managed accordingly.

Nursing records

Different local care organizations will have policies, procedures, and requirements for nursing records, which may include:

- Universal risk assessment tools.
- Local risk assessment tools.
- Records of vital signs and observations.
- Fluid balance charts.
- Dietary records.
- Records of accurate and timely drug administration.
- Nursing care plans.
- Nursing notes.
- Records of care pathways for specific conditions.
- Patient diaries.
- Incident reports.
- Root cause analyses.

It is important to ensure an equitable balance between nursing care and record keeping. There is no point in having pristine case notes if the time taken to produce them is detrimental to actual patient care. Nursing records should demonstrate:

- Any assessment made by the nurse on the patient's admission or first contact.
- All risk assessments which have been completed and reviewed.
- Relevant ongoing, and updating of, information regarding the patient.
- Any care planning tools which are used to implement and guide nursing care.
- A record of the patient's priorities for care.
- Entries that demonstrate a diary, or history, of the patient's progress.
- Any relevant observations or instructions used in the care of the patient.
- Evidence that the nursing care has been informed by nursing values, knowledge, and skills.
- That, wherever possible, the person has been involved in the care process.

Accuracy in nursing records

Where a nurse is in the unfortunate position of having their practice questioned or scrutinized, it will normally be the nursing records which are used as 'evidence', often against the nurse.

Effective communication of information in nursing records and documents should always avoid the use of jargon, shorthand, or subjective statements, which are open to misinterpretation.

- Do not use subjective statements such as 'good day' and 'slept well'.
- Always write legibly, including a legible signature.
- Always time and date entries in documentation.
- Always record that local policies and procedures have been followed, particularly on transfer from one clinical environment to the next.
- Always document special needs of patients, such as learning disability, deafness, and blindness, or people who have difficulties feeding themselves.
- Always record conversations and communications between healthcare professionals, including telephone messages.
- Do not follow, or duplicate, what has been written or recorded previously.
- Ensure there is sufficient information on the psychological and mental health aspects of the patient if this impacts on the care process.
- Always complete all areas of an assessment completely.
- Always document any reasons why care was not delivered according to plan.

Social media and professional nursing practice

Terms and context

As a component of globalization, the use of information and communication technology (ICT) has become a feature of modern life. More than 2 billion people around the world now use the Internet.

This exponential growth, in a relatively short space of time, has been accompanied by the popularity of 'social media'—an assortment of Internet groupings and applications which allow creation and exchange of 'user-generated content' (Barry and Hardiker, 2012) where the range of possibilities is classified in terms of six main types (see Table 5.1).

Professional guidelines

The UK NMC *Code* (NMC, 2015, p. 17) clearly states that, as part of promoting professionalism and trust, the nurse needs to 'use all forms of spoken, written and digital communication including *social media* and *networking sites* (emphasis added) responsibly, respecting the right to privacy of others at all times' (⌨ www.nmc.org.uk).

'*Guidance on using social media responsibly*' provides supplementary information which ought to be considered in the context of local policy and employer expectations. It has been estimated that almost half a million nurses, midwives, and health visitors in the UK have Facebook accounts, representing a very small fraction of the 950 million monthly users worldwide.

It is noted that, when used appropriately, social media has the potential to benefit the nursing profession, including:

• Acting as a resource in building and maintaining professional relationships.
• Offering a networking opportunity for nurses in relation to professional support forum.
• Providing an accessible portal to ongoing continuing professional development (CPD).

In the UK, it has been reported that the massive expansion of social media as a communicative tool has value for both nursing staff and service users/patients (Betton and Tomlinson, 2013), pointing out that:

• Social media is changing people's expectations of healthcare services.

Table 5.1 Types of user-generated Internet content

Type	Example
Collaborative projects	Wikipedia
Blogs and microblogs	Twitter
Content communities	You Tube
Social networking sites	Facebook
Virtual game worlds	World of Warcraft
Virtual social worlds	Second Life

Information summarised from Barry J, Hardiker N.R. (2012) Advancing nursing practice through social media: A global perspective. *The Online Journal of Issues in Nursing*, **17** (3) Manuscript 5.

- Universities that offer nurse education programmes around the world are engaging with social media to keep in touch with current students and alumni, to encourage research networking and promote dialogue around international professional issues.
- Social media permits service users with an effective network to share and discuss their experiences of specific conditions and treatment options available.
- In remote, or sparsely populated, parts of the world, social media can increase equity and access to healthcare information and services.
- For a growing number of mental health service users, social media is playing an important role in their recovery by helping them to manage their condition and combat isolation through online support groups.
- Nurses can actively support service users to make use of social media as a way to improve their mental health.
- Nursing staff need to be sufficiently knowledgeable about new technologies to ensure that people they look after can be safeguarded against risk.
- One area of risk, however, for both healthcare staff and service users is the unregulated nature of the Internet, which has prompted calls for health/nursing sites to be quality-appraised.

Conversely, the UK NMC is also emphatic in drawing attention to the ways that reputation can be compromised, and registration revoked, if a nurse acts in a way deemed to be unprofessional or engages in any unlawful activity. Examples given of these concerns include:
- Sharing confidential information inappropriately.
- Posting pictures of patients and people receiving care, without their consent. This also applies to patients who have been discharged.
- Using mobile phones to take photographs in the workplace.
- Posting inappropriate comments about colleagues or patients.
- Bullying, intimidating, or exploiting people.
- Building or pursuing relationships with patients or service users.
- Stealing personal information or using someone else's identity.
- Encouraging violence or self-harm.
- Inciting hatred or discrimination.
- Posting any materials/images that could be considered 'sexually explicit'.

These statements embody the principles of respecting the rights, dignity, and privacy of those people who receive nursing care in a range of settings. As in the clinical/caring context, the need for confidentiality is paramount, and it should be remembered that online discussions or comments can, in a very short space of time, become accessible to a global audience.

The UK NMC notes: 'It is important to realise that even the strictest privacy settings have limitations. This is because, once something is online, it can be copied and redistributed' (NMC, 2015, *Guidance on using social media responsibly*, p. 6).

It is important to remember that, once posted on social media sites, information is in the public domain and can be stored, reproduced, and redistributed. For the professional nurse, *online conduct* and *real-world conduct* are judged by the same standards.

Other users/browsers may post items that are discriminatory or offensive, and maintaining contact, or accepting the link, could be interpreted as an endorsement of those views. In cyber-space, the *past* is ever *present*.

Responsibilities of organizations and employers

Given the widespread use of social media, such as Facebook and Twitter, healthcare employers and institutions that contribute to the training, education, and ongoing professional development of nurses need to engage with these sites in a positive and productive way.

Employing organizations need to produce, and make available to all staff, clear policies relating to the use of social media. This should direct nursing staff and nursing students to appropriate professional guidelines and standards.

A corporate presence on social networking sites, in relation to nursing practice, can enhance credibility and provide a professional and academic platform to promote responsible use.

Managers responsible for implementing policy and making decisions or judgements regarding any perceived professional or legal breaches of protocol should be informed and knowledgeable about the mechanics of social media.

Any complaints made about an online activity should be treated and investigated with the same level of seriousness as real-world behaviours.

Useful sources of further information

- NMC (2015). *The Code* ℘ www.nmc-uk.org
- NMC (2015). *Guidance on using social media responsibly.* ℘ www.nmc. org.uk/globalassets/sitedocuments/nmc-publications/social-media-guidance.pdf
- Barry J, Hardiker NR (2012). Advancing nursing practice through social media: a global perspective. *Online J Issues Nurs*, **17**(3), Manuscript 5. ℘ www.nursingworld.org/MainMenuCategories/ANAMarketplace/ ANAPeriodicals/OJIN/TableofContents/Vol-17-2012/No3-Sept-2012/ Advancing-Nursing-Through-Social-Media.html
- Betton V, Tomlinson V (2013). Benefits of social media for nurses and service users. *Nursing Times*, **109**(24): 20–1

Part 2

Communication and interpersonal skills

Communication in a healthcare context

Communication in a healthcare context

Good communication resides at the core of nursing practice. It is based on theoretical approaches, personal values, and professional qualities, supported by an identifiable set of specific skills.

Together, these represent a key domain of the values, standards, and competencies required by the UK NMC for student nurses to progress through accredited training programmes, and then to practise safely as a nurse and safeguard the interests of people receiving care, their families, and carers.

The Code (℘ www.nmc.org.uk) provides guidelines to achieve effective nursing practice through clear communication, which can be summarized as:

- Using terms that can be easily understood by people in your care, colleagues, and the public.
- Striving to achieve optimum levels of assistance and support to individuals who experience language or communication difficulties.
- Employing a range of verbal and non-verbal communication techniques.
- Consideration of cultural sensitivities to understand and appropriately respond to people's personal and healthcare needs.
- Periodically checking people's understandings to keep mistakes to a minimum.
- An ability to communicate clearly and effectively in English.

Language, power, and empowerment

Language and the construction of the 'other'

Language is central to social life of how we make sense of, and respond to, the everyday world around us. More broadly, the concept of 'communication' refers to the way that human beings exchange information through the spoken and written word or a shared system of signs and signals. In this context, communication is always relational and interactional, involving two or more people in a particular cultural setting, and defined by sets of beliefs, ideas, and values.

In terms of nursing practice, this could include hospital wards, GP clinics, elderly care centres, or people's own homes in the community. In each of these locations, patient needs vary widely, and the physical environment, social–clinical space, and time constraints will impact on the nature of the nurse–patient encounter.

Communication in healthcare is reciprocal and responsive—*talking with*, and *listening to*, people in a way that enhances the quality of care they receive. However, from a social science perspective, language is more than just a system for communicating ideas and information.

The constructionist theory is concerned with exploring how the words that we use in everyday and professional life are part of a set of discourses that perform powerful social actions. Rather than just '*naming* an object', it is argued that language creates, or *constructs*, individuals and identities in particular ways. This can be a positive or damaging experience, depending on the social power differentials between those who apply the *labels* and those who are *labelled*.

Some examples of this, in healthcare practice, are ideologies of 'difference' based on a Eurocentric construction of what constitutes the 'normal'. Typically, these are expressed via dominant white, male, and heterosexist discourses.

The concept of 'cultural competence' in nursing, medicine, and psychiatry, for example, begins from an assumption that individual health problems are somehow inseparable from the cultural history of the 'other' person. Structural inequalities are expressed in terms of social class, gender, ethnicity, sexuality, and age.

In contrast, those who apply this type of model operate from a position of unquestioned cultural neutrality. Women have been more likely, historically, to be diagnosed with 'depression' or some other type of 'neurotic' condition. This, though, says as much about the gendered discourse of psychiatry as it does about the validity of 'objective' scientific assessment.

Health and criminal justice responses toward young black men perceived to be 'mentally ill' or 'dangerous', in terms of diagnosis, disposal, and treatment, are disproportionate and discriminatory, compared to their white counterparts. They are more likely to be sectioned under mental health legislation, detained in secure services, and prescribed anti-psychotic medication, rather than 'talking therapies'.

In this way, some individuals, as part of a larger group, are defined as 'other', marginalized, and socially excluded. To take an extreme historical example of the inherent dangers of unboundaried discrimination, it was a mix of biomedical (psychiatric) science and eugenics that made the Holocaust possible in Nazi Germany. Thousands of mentally ill and physically or intellectually disabled people were murdered as a public hygiene programme, with the complicity of doctors and nurses, with people deemed 'useless eaters' and 'lives not worth living'.

Globally today, it is sadly not unusual to find 'first nation' or aboriginal peoples and displaced populations like Afro-Americans, Latinos, and Mexicans over-represented in prison and forensic psychiatric services. Stark examples of injustice might seem a world away from the daily work of adult general nurses, but inequitable social processes that manufacture exclusion transcend time and space.

In this context, general nurses can take an opportunity to critically reflect on language use in the informal and unmapped territories of care environments. In the 'old days', this type of talk was colloquially referred to as 'tales from the sluice'. It could include comments made after an 'official handover', staff room gossip, or coded messages embellished with 'knowing' gestures and expressions.

Anthropologists might interpret and explore this set of subterranean discourses as the 'story-telling' tradition of a 'tribal group' unified by its own set of totemic beliefs and values. Nowadays, we are more familiar with the corporate-speak of 'ward culture' and 'culture change strategies'.

Empowering the disenfranchised

The concept of 'empowerment' has assumed currency in the vocabulary of the nursing profession, lauded as the panacea of all perceived problems in the care setting, enshrined in 'visions', 'mission statements', and 'care plans'. Rarely, however, is this lofty aspiration explicated in pragmatic terms. It is implied that power is a 'gift' that can be handed to people.

From a theoretical perspective, the issue of empowerment is much more complex, embracing personal, political, and professional issues. To empower an individual, or a social group, requires an understanding of what power *is*, who power *serves*, and how power *operates*. Simply stated, 'power' can be seen in terms of domination, oppression, and repression. Power relations are successful when they are unrecognized and unchallenged—a social world accepted as the way things *are*.

It is important to appreciate that communication in healthcare is part of a 'web of power' that constructs relations between those who deliver and those who receive care. Language is not a neutral category. It conveys individual values, but also acts as a conduit for powerful institutional interests.

Consider the terms, often used interchangeably, to describe recipients of care—'patient', 'client', and 'service user'. Each connotes a different type of relationship and constructs the professional-person roles in different ways. Or think about the colloquial language of the wards and the terms that are used to describe certain individuals as 'good' or 'bad' patients.

There is a danger of professional complacency that such practices are irrevocably behind us, but arguably the nursing profession has a duty to engage with colleagues in trade unions, activist groups, and the academy in combating extremist ideologies that fuel division and hatred. One way of empowering disenfranchised people is to listen to, and learn from, their stories. Often these are untold or unheard. In this sense, we can privilege their narratives as a form of 'evidence' for caring.

In nursing research, the phenomenological approach has become increasingly popular because its philosophical base complements the value base of nursing in attempting to access, through language, the essence or meaning of human experiences.

For the nurse, these debates are central to their practice and professional values, and not remote abstractions that can be consigned to the pages of professional or academic journals.

It is important to remember that what you *say to*, or *write about*, a person can have damaging consequences. People in receipt of care are fundamentally human beings, and not disease entities. They have histories and life experiences that stretch far beyond the diagnosis or condition that brought them into contact with healthcare services.

The risk of seeing and talking about a person only in terms of a 'master status' (e.g. a medical diagnosis or pejorative label) is that it contributes to the process of diminishing their humanity, identity, and personhood.

Interpersonal relations in nursing practice

Effective healthcare communication can be understood in terms of specific skills that can be utilized by the nurse, and the relational contexts that frame their interactions with those receiving care.

It is possible, for example, to learn and deploy a particular skill, but without any meaningful engagement with the other person, this is unlikely to be convincing—and sincerity resides at the core of any relationship based on trust.

Person-centred counselling skills are arguably at the heart of all effective communication and therapeutic relations. The humanist psychologist Carl Rogers identified the core conditions by which people can be supported in their personal growth.

Research studies have consistently shown that the active ingredient in most psychotherapy interventions boils down to the interpersonal qualities of the therapist, and particularly the presence of Rogerian values and skills. Rogers's core conditions for personal growth, which enable any human actor to achieve their full potential, are:

- Empathy.
- Genuineness.
- Unconditional positive regard.

As a part of growing up, each person develops a sense of identity or selfhood, but there can be a disjuncture between how an individual sees her-/himself (the ideal self) and the way other people perceive them (the real self).

This can be in response to illness, disability, social stigma, or external negative forces. Later on, in this section, we look at how 'spoilt identities' characterize many of the people we look after who have been marginalized from mainstream society.

Derived from humanistic psychology, these conceptual conditions put the person at the centre of the enabling interaction. Traditionally, they have been associated with a specific, though influential, school of counselling. This is one where the person/client is encouraged to find solutions or answers to their life concerns through dialogue with a counsellor. It is usually achieved during a course of 'therapy' consisting of a number of scheduled and time-limited sessions.

Humanistic nursing practice

Nursing practice is very different from conventional understandings of therapeutic intervention in that it is not restricted to sessional contact; there is not the time to engage in lengthy, focused interactions, and the working environment is usually marked by competing tasks and duties.

However, the nurse can adopt the generic principles of person-centred working and translate them into their own sphere of practice, and this is the focus of the discussion that follows. First, we explore the core conditions of worth in the context of good nursing practice, noting how these parallel the value base of the profession.

Empathy

- Though they share some similarities, this should not be confused with 'sympathy' which is about an expression of sadness or sorrow. In contrast, empathy describes approaching any humanistic relationship with the desire to understand the feelings and emotions of the other *as they* are experiencing them *at that* time.
- Often, this is explained as trying to 'step into the shoes' of the other person, whilst 'keeping one step back'. The extent to which this can actually be achieved is an existential debate and, for the nurse, should be taken as a message about trying to see and feel 'through the eyes of the other'.
- For example, a young, newly qualified nurse will have little in common with the life experiences of an older person diagnosed with a serious illness. But what they should have is the qualities and skills to be patient, to listen, and to learn.

Genuineness

- In many textbooks and professional papers, this is referred to as 'congruence'. It refers to the way that you, as a nurse, present yourself to the other person as 'real', conveying sincerity and interest in both verbal and non-verbal ways.
- This provides a basis for the other person to trust you and invites them to disclose any concerns or talk about their lives more generally.
- Being genuine has another important attribute in therapeutic communication—it can begin to redress damage done to individuals 'conditions of worth', by valuing them for *who they are*, rather than *what they are*, in the eyes of others.
- This provides a foundation for someone to develop confidence, repair their sense of esteem, and grow emotionally as a person.

Unconditional positive regard

- Again, this is a defining feature of the values that construct nursing practice and the way individual nurses relate to the people they are looking after. It is sometimes described as 'acceptance'.
- In short, it requires that individuals are worthy of our respect and regard, without conditions, regardless of other aspects of the person's life.
- The process of caring and the therapeutic relationship cannot be compromised or contaminated by judgements based on the personal feelings or emotional responses of the care provider.

In many cases, this is a taken-for-granted part of everyday nursing where the suffering, or loss, of the other person engenders compassion and care.

However, for health professionals working with specific groups of people, often described as 'challenging', this requirement is less straightforward. Examples would include individuals whose hospitalization or treatment is the result of antisocial or offending behaviours directed against vulnerable human beings.

Communication skills and behaviours

Having considered how professional nursing practice can be interwoven with a respected set of psychological principles, it remains to look at the skills, verbal and non-verbal, which can be employed to 'bring them to life' in healthcare settings.

The first consideration is with verbal, or spoken, components of communication, though it has been estimated that these actually play a smaller role than non-verbal aspects of communication in person-to-person interactions.

Verbal skills and behaviours

This is often referred to in terms of linguistic (language) and paralinguistic (speech attributes like tone or pitch) components of communication, though each of these should complement the other.

The important thing to remember is that you, as the nurse, are sending a message to another person—information, for instance—and you want it to be received and understood. For this to happen, the UK Royal College of Nursing (RCN) (℞ www.rcn.org.uk) suggests that you need to pay attention to:

- Being courteous and respectful at all times, introducing yourself, and checking that you are addressing, or speaking to, the right person.
- Giving clear, accurate, and culturally appropriate information to the person that you are addressing.
- Speaking at a rate the other person can follow, and allowing time for them to ask questions or clarify their understanding.
- Avoiding technical and clinical language or jargonistic shorthand, and adopting plain English.
- Encouraging the person to talk and expand on issues, so that they are actively involved in conversation. This can be done by employing open-ended, or narrative, questions that invite exploration of issues, rather than the 'yes'/'no' answers generated by closed questions.
- Using paraphrasing, where you abridge the content of the other person's comments, and feed this back to check meaning and interpretation. This also provides evidence that you are actively listening to what is being said.
- Ensuring that your voice does not show indications of needing to complete the task, even if it is a particularly busy time, as this is likely to 'close down' the other person's involvement.
- When we alternate the pitch and tone of our voice, the listener can 'read' *how* we are speaking to them, as well as *what* we are saying to them.

Non-verbal skills and behaviours

These are collectively referred to as 'body language' and comprise the non-verbal signs, cues, and gestures that reinforce the spoken word. They consist of things like:

- *Body posture and proxemics* relate to the posture of the speaker and the physical space between the nurse and the other person. Avoid presenting yourself in a way that connotes dominance, where you are too close (encroaching on 'personal space'), standing over the person, or adopting an authoritarian stance (e.g. folded arms).
- *Eye contact* is really important in signalling interest and attention, but fixed eye contact, like staring, can be perceived as threatening and intimidatory. In some cultures, eye contact is not socially validated and can be interpreted as inappropriate and rude.
- *Facial expressions* have an almost universal code of meaning as a way that we express human emotions, from sadness to pleasure and contentment to rage. As a nurse, it is fairly easy to pick up on these, but self-awareness is about being mindful of how they can manifest and give away our own unspoken thoughts.
- *Therapeutic touch* is a powerful way of conveying, without words, our understanding of emotional distress or upset. A hand placed gently over the hand of another who is suffering pain can be a great comfort or indication that they are not 'alone'.

However, therapeutic touch is one of the more contentious of the non-verbal skills, in that inappropriately used, it can be interpreted as intrusive and invasive. It is also a culturally constructed response and not welcomed by some groups of people. Whenever used, the permission of the other person needs to be gained in advance.

Therapeutic use of *silence* is an important skill to master, but one that can feel quite difficult or embarrassing. In everyday life, we are used to accommodating other people's speech difficulties and experience discomfort with lengthy pauses—often rushing to 'fill the gaps'.

In healthcare settings, silence can be a meaningful and productive part of communication, for both the nurse and the other person. It allows time to reflect, to organize what will be said next, and to act as a way of managing information that is sensitive in the immediate moment of 'here and now'.

The vital connection between verbal and non-verbal communication strategies resides in the concept of *active listening*. This describes the seamless unity of verbal and non-verbal techniques working in a perfect state of balance.

To be effective, the therapeutic focus is intentionally directed at understanding what the person you are listening to is saying. The nurse should take careful note (not on a clipboard) of this talk, so that they are able to repeat it back to the speaker in a form that is acceptable to them.

It does not imply that the nurse necessarily agrees with what is being said, but rather that they comprehend the meaning.

Specialist knowledge and skills

Some nurses have additional training in psychological interventions, and much of the relevant knowledge and skills are useful in the context of therapeutic relationships and effective communication.

From the field of *cognitive behavioural therapy* (CBT), we know that people are more likely to act on assumptions or prejudices, or jump to conclusions, when they are already under stress.

Similarly, they may be more prone to run away with problematic thinking patterns, such as catastrophizing when faced with perhaps manageable difficulties, or being more than usually mistrustful of others' intentions. For all of these reasons, it makes sense to support people to stay as calm as possible in the communication context.

Cognitive psychology also explains how people pay selective attention to what is going on, based upon what they already believe. In essence, we tend to tune into events and information that confirms our own beliefs, and tune out disconfirming evidence without even thinking about it. Again, these thinking errors become more pronounced if our arousal levels are already pronounced, for example if we are very anxious or angry.

Psychologically informed *family interventions* start from a perspective that favours thinking about behaviour in terms of social systems and how people interact together, rather than just focusing on single individuals and presumed psychopathology.

As such, people can then be helped by working with the whole family or network, rather than on their own. Some very simple communication skills have proven to be remarkably helpful in reducing psychosocial stress within families or other groups. These include:

- Expression of positive emotions—appreciating other people by letting them know *they* have done something positive and how this has made *us* feel.
- Making positive requests—being really clear about what we want someone to do and letting them know how it will make us feel if they do it.
- Expression of negative emotions—it is appropriate and honest to inform people if they have done something that has upset us or that we are particularly concerned about. But we need to accomplish this without provocation or escalation of negative emotions. So the behaviour we object to has to be identified clearly, and we need to say, again with clarity, how this has made us feel. Most importantly, we also need to state the alternative behaviour we would prefer to see if the same circumstances arise, reinforcing how we would appreciate the alternative and how it would make us feel.
- Active listening—paying full attention to others and properly hearing and comprehending what they have to tell us. This involves deployment of effective verbal and non-verbal skills to encourage communication.

Useful sources of further information

- Royal College of Nursing. *Person-centred care.* ◈ www.rcn.org.uk
- NHS. *Cognitive behavioural therapy (CBT).* ◈ www.nhs.uk/conditions/cognitive-behavioural-therapy/Pages/Introduction.aspx

Dignity and respect

Promoting dignity and respect

You have the right to be treated with *dignity and respect*, in accordance with your human rights (℅ www.gov.uk/government/organisations/department-of-health).

The concept of 'dignity' resides at the core of nursing practice and nursing philosophy. It is enshrined in the UK NHS Constitution and international and UK legislation around the human rights of those receiving healthcare in all settings. Failure to uphold dignified caring has been central to inquiry reports set up to investigate evidence of poor, or unacceptable, standards of care.

Dignity is a nebulous concept and there have been many attempts to identify its constituent components. Usually it is defined in terms of the moral rights, autonomy, and unconditional worth of each person. Here, though, the emphasis is on pragmatic application of nursing values and skills that can be deployed to provide respectful, empathic, and compassionate care.

Dignity, respect, and rights feature prominently in the NMC Code (℅ www.nmc.org.uk), emphasizing their importance to nursing practice and the prioritization of people receiving care.

Additional guidance is provided to the public regarding older people where research and media reports show little confidence in the dignity and respect accorded to this group of people when they are in hospitals and nursing homes.

In response to claims of a 'compassion deficit' in caring, the UK RCN has prioritized dignity as something that should be 'at the heart of everything' nurses do, centred on three integral dimensions:

• *Respect*: acknowledging the uniqueness of each individual in the care process.
• *Compassion*: not sacrificing the emotional and humanistic components of care to technical and clinical procedures.
• *Sensitivity*: communication and therapeutic use of self, to show genuine concern about the other person.

Dignity can also be compromised by aspects of the physical environment in which care takes place and the way resources are utilized by nursing staff. Often, significant improvements can be made by small changes in the actions and behaviours of the professional. Examples are:

• Ensuring the environment and facilities such as toilets and washrooms are regularly cleaned.
• Properly drawing curtains around the bed when performing intimate or sensitive care where the person could be embarrassed.
• Making sure that cubicle doors are closed when toilets are being used.
• Having single-sex bays on wards where men and women are cared for together.
• Assisting people to put on gowns and tying them securely to avoid unwanted exposure.
• Maintaining privacy whenever the care, or conversation, requires discretion.
• Not talking about an individual, or their health, in a public space such as the ward or bedside where other people can overhear.

- Not assuming that you can use a person's first name without gaining their permission, or an abbreviation of it. For example, Mr Charles Smith should not be referred to as 'Charlie', unless this is how he wishes to be known.
- Avoidance of terminology that can patronize and demean the other person, such as greeting an elderly male patient by saying 'Hiya pops' or 'How are you feeling today sweetie'?
- Avoidance of jargon and acronyms as a 'short-cut' when communicating with a person. This may have meaning for the care team but is unlikely to be understood by non-health professionals and may well be misinterpreted.
- Not allowing a catheterized patient to move around the ward/hospital carrying a full urine bag. These should be frequently and routinely drained and, if the person is able to mobilize, attached to the legs.
- Acknowledging the concept of 'treatment' does not refer only to 'medical treatment' but has much broader meaning in terms of dignity and rights—caring *about* the person as well as *for* them.

The commitment to dignity should also be a central feature of the way nursing staff and other members of the clinical team work together to create, and sustain, a culture that promotes and respects the value and human rights of those in receipt of care—where clinical leaders and ward managers 'role-model' best practice for team members.

NICE (℅ www.nice.org.uk) guidelines suggest how the patient experience in adult UK health services can be constructed around good communication skills:

- Shared decision-making where the person is actively involved in discussions and decisions about their care.
- Use of open-ended questions to invite the person to talk; summarize at the end of discussions to check for understanding; allow time for questions to be asked and addressed, before leaving.
- Giving the person oral and written information to promote active involvement in care and self-management.
- Adopting individualized care that is 'tailored' to each person's health and psychosocial care needs which should be regularly reviewed with the person.
- To allow for feedback on services and care standards, each person should be clearly informed about ways of voicing concerns or making a complaint.
- Encouraging all staff to participate in ongoing CPD and inter-professional learning.
- Developing self-awareness and critical reflection of practice where personal feelings and observations are explored in the context of larger organizational, cultural, and political events.

Nursing identity

The provision of dignified care is inextricably linked to the formation and maintenance of a professional nursing identity. Learning strategies that nurture this should be central to academic programmes leading to nurse registration and professional development, and embedded in the clinical areas in which nurses train and work.

Learning is most powerfully experienced when it is situated within social practices and relationships, and contextual rather than individual. A vital component of positive learning, like communication itself, is authenticity or genuineness where the experience is relevant to the everyday lives of those taking part.

Nurses, for example, who have responsibility to mentor learners in a clinical or community context should ensure that teaching or support is delivered in a way that includes discussion or involvement with all those involved and the opportunity to critically reflect on the outcomes. This means that analysis of the issue(s) should move beyond the micro-dynamics of the interaction and take into account differences in organizational power and status which frame communication.

Social inclusion is pivotal to holistic practice, individualized care, and maintenance of dignity where good communication and interpersonal skills play a key role. The next sections consider the importance of healthcare communication with regard to older people, people who live with dementia, individuals with a learning disability, and those who have mental health issues or experience psychological distress.

Communicating with older people

Globally, there is a growing elderly population. Historically, in a clinical context, those aged over 65 years were collectively described as 'geriatric' or 'psycho-geriatric'. This reflects the dominance of the medical model in defining and constructing the ageing body according to universal sets of diagnoses or typologies. The legacy of this patho-biological perspective persists in the altered status accorded to older people in industrial societies where economic productivity and spending power represent cultural capital; in short, identity and citizenship are constructed by market forces.

With improved standards of living and advances in medical technologies and treatments, many people are living longer lives. Current best practice in health policy and nursing focuses on the care of the 'older person', recognizing that while illness and degenerative conditions can be associated with age, many senior citizens enjoy healthy and fulfilling lives.

A generic set of principles are helpful in communicating with older people, but they do not replace making an individual assessment based on therapeutic relations and observations. As with any communicative interaction, the environment needs to be taken into account. For some older people, there may be a deterioration of vision, hearing, and memory, though it should never be assumed that they are 'blind', 'deaf', or 'demented'. If the ward/room is busy or noisy, this will produce unwanted distractions and impediments. Therefore, try to:

- Minimize the background noise levels, and do not shout.
- Arrange furniture in a way that invites face-to-face talk.
- Speak softly and slowly, using familiar words and short sentences.
- Talk *with* the person, rather than *to* them, and actively listen to what they are saying.
- Reinforce what you are saying with non-verbal signs and gestures.
- Use written information, with a larger font size, if it helps the person to understand what you are saying to them.
- Allow the person time to take in, and reflect on, what you are saying, and do not rush the conversation.
- Avoid complex terminology or nursing/medical jargon.
- Ensure that prescription sensory aids (e.g. spectacles, hearing aids) are available if required by the older person.

On busy hospital wards or in care homes for the elderly, routines and rituals can take precedence over caring *for* and *about* people. Just because someone is staring at the television does not mean they are watching it, or even interested in the programme.

In environments where the radio is permanently playing, talk in general is impeded. In this regard, the concept of 'institutionalization' is of interest. Originally employed by the sociologist Erving Goffman in the 1960s, it described the process by which 'mental patients' became institutional products—a stripping of identity, damaging of selfhood, and ultimately dehumanization of the 'inmate'. There is still much to learn from this work.

Communication with the older person should not always be about clinical care or nursing decision-making. Rather, talk has therapeutic value in, and of, itself.

Older people may have fewer visitors, spending a lot of time on their own. Possibly feeling embarrassed to interrupt younger, and busier, nurses, they can retreat into themselves—passively responding only to requests, rather than actively initiating engagement. Nurses can employ communication skills to help older people maintain a sense of independence and agency, allowing them to retain a degree of control in their lives. General principles could include:

- Acknowledgement of the older person as an individual with unique personal qualities.
- Involvement of the older person through conversation and discussion that is shared and reciprocal.
- Valuing choice by allowing older people to actively participate in decision-making about everyday activities.
- Ensuring that the older person feels they are at the centre of any communicative episode, and using verbal and non-verbal techniques to reinforce this message.

Communicating with people who live with dementia

Another dynamic of people living longer is the increased likelihood of their becoming, at some point, more reliant on health and social care provision. Though the older population is a heterogeneous social group, some will develop disorders in communication as a product of ageing and clinical conditions like Alzheimer's disease and other forms of dementia.

The progressive and degenerative decline of cognitive abilities commensurate with the pathophysiology of the illness means there is a real need to maintain contact with 'reality' through communicative strategies. Over time, there will likely be a significant decline in memory and language use. This will impact on the ability of the individual to organize their thoughts or to rationalize their behaviours.

An unfortunate 'side effect' of the dementia process is that it triggers a parallel social process where the individual is at risk of being marginalized, both within the family and the wider informal support networks.

It is easy for the person with dementia to retreat into an inner, and silent, world—losing touch with, and failing to recognize, friends, loved ones, or the names of professionals who care for them. These people should be treated no differently to other older adults in terms of communication. However, there are some important issues that need to be incorporated into nurse–person interactions:

- Speak clearly and slowly, and keep the content uncomplicated.
- Communication is about more than 'talk' alone. When speech is difficult for the older person, non-verbal factors can assume more importance, so nurses should use gestures and cues accordingly (e.g. accompanying a conversation with a 'friendly smile').
- Remembering the specific impact of dementia on the language use of an individual, nurses will most likely need to take a lead in initiating and prompting talk. Encourage them in this, and do not try to hurry the conversation by finishing sentences or making an assumption about what they are struggling to articulate.
- One way of 'making contact' with an individual who has become withdrawn is to focus on events that have personal meaning. Here, personal histories, memories, photographs, or music can offer productive avenues for talk—but they must also be deployed sensitively to avoid causing distress or recall of painful moments.
- If it feels appropriate, touching the arm or holding the hand of the other person can convey reassurance and a sense of 'being there' for them.
- Because of progressive neural damage within the brain, it is important not to feel emotionally slighted by a sudden change of mood in the other person, but to accept this as a symptom of the disease process.
- Even if you have been working with someone with dementia for a considerable period of time, they may not recognize the longevity of the relationship. Be calm and patient in your approaches, and do not allow yourself to become frustrated.

- 'Active listening' is particularly important when communicating with this group of people, that is using the full range of therapeutic and communicative responses to engage the interest and attention of the other person.
- Of great importance is that nurses do not contradict the person with dementia. Their version of the world may not be factually accurate, but it represents the version of 'reality' in which they are currently living (see also ➔ Chapter 18, Neurological conditions).

Communicating with people with a learning disability

Learning disability is a collective term for a wide spectrum of people, and the degree of impairment will range from very mild to profound.

Some will communicate easily with nursing staff, whilst others will need time, support, and possibly the involvement of a speech and language therapist (ℑ www.rcslt.org.uk). The nursing role is to provide education and promote health, rather than simply manage a clinical episode.

People living with a learning disability experience physical health problems as a result of complex factors unrelated to their individual conditions. This can result from lifestyle, income/economic factors, or lack of access to health screening.

Individuals who are prescribed anti-psychotic medication can experience damaging iatrogenic side effects where the 'problem' is induced as a by-product of treatment. Individuals with a learning disability are at an increased risk of developing heart disease and type 2 diabetes, often made worse by poor diet, lack of exercise, and obesity.

Health needs can be unmet in mainstream primary healthcare services that are poorly equipped or trained to engage with this client group and/or their carers. Life expectancy has increased for people with learning disabilities, but mortality and morbidity rates still remain higher than in the general population.

People with a learning disability have typically grown up and lived with ridicule, bullying, and discrimination. They may be uncomfortable with strangers or uneasy in unfamiliar environments like a clinic or a hospital ward. In circumstances like this, it is important that your approach and presentation of self are welcoming and friendly. This can be reinforced using non-verbal language and cues to reinforce the message of spoken words.

Though adult general nurses use the term 'patient' routinely, people with a learning disability may be more accustomed to 'self-advocate' or 'peer advocate'. This is one way organizations promoting inclusive working resist diagnostic medical discourse in favour of a social model of disability.

National campaigning groups for the learning-disabled community offer generic guidelines. These recommend that you:
- Remember everyone is an *individual* and everyone is *different*.
- Do not make assumptions about a person's ability to understand what you are saying to them.
- Speak clearly and slowly, allowing the person time to process what you are asking or telling them.
- Avoid using jargon or technical language that is more difficult to understand.
- Use open-ended questions that invite the person to communicate with you.
- Always check that what you say has been understood by using polite clarification.
- Observe body language, gestures, and other non-verbal communication of the other person for cues, and also use these to reinforce your message.

For individuals who have greater difficulty in communicating with others, specific techniques have been developed and include:

- Signing systems like Widgit (℘ www.widgit.com) or Makaton (℘ www. makaton.org) which are based on British Sign Language (BSL).
- Commercially produced easy-read pictures and illustrations, or your own quick drawings, to complement spoken and written language.

Communicating with people experiencing mental ill health and psychological distress

From psychiatric illness to mental health movement

For nurses who focus exclusively on caring for individuals diagnosed with a mental illness or personality disorder, communication and therapeutic use of self are the most important attributes of a caring role. But the move from a coercive and controlling system of institutional incarceration to a democratized mental health movement signals the ongoing struggle of service users and survivors, and new ways of engaging with professionals.

From the mid-nineteenth century until around the mid 1960s, psychiatry, located in asylums and mental hospitals, attempted to apply the scientific principles of biomedicine to 'mental diseases'. The power of the medical model has proved remarkably resistant over the years; it continues to dominate the language of healthcare, discourses of aetiology, disease classification, taxonomy, diagnosis, prognosis, and treatment.

The *Diagnostic and Statistical Manual* (DSM), published by the American Psychiatric Association (APA), is an influential source of information for diagnosing mental disorders. It has grown massively in volume since the first edition in 1952. This trend has not been without controversy, given that it proclaims a scientific delineation between 'normal' and 'deviant' human beings.

Historically, the nursing profession responded to diverse care needs in terms of self-contained branches such as *mental illness*, *learning disability*, *adult*, and *child* nursing. This organization of the profession may have utility in relation to specific health and social care needs but masks the universality of ill health, regardless of structural markers such as age, ethnicity, social class, and gender, and promotes a psyche (mind)–body (soma) split.

Regardless of a particular health condition, there is always an affective or psychic component, and general nurses will frequently encounter persons with more serious mental health problems. Nurses should be proficient in effective communication skills to assist in identifying and alleviating psychological components of ill health and supporting those in their care with pre-existing mental health needs.

Those who oppose the institutional apparatus of psychiatry in contemporary society talk about a 'post-psychiatric age'—one which recognizes social and cultural contexts, puts ethics before technology, and works to minimize pharmacological control and coercive interventions.

This brief account of 'psycho-politics' is instrumental in framing the discussion that follows—one premised on the philosophy and principles of *mental health nursing*, rather than *psychiatric nursing*, of *recovery*, not *cure*. It is about working with human needs, not diagnostic descriptors.

The lived experience of mental health

Globally, mental health 'problems' represent a growing public health concern. A corollary of this is measured in suicidal and self-harming behaviours and physical conditions such as ischaemic heart disease. In the UK, it is estimated that one person in four is likely to experience mental health issues and psychological distress. In this chapter, we restrict our discussion to the expressions of mental illness and emotional issues most likely to be encountered by adult general nurses.

It is important to remember that general nurses will be caring for the person in the context of a physical illness. They are not expected to engage therapeutically with any identified mental disorder. As such, the presentation of self, language use, and communication skills will be sufficient to assist in undertaking regular nursing duties.

If someone is admitted who has a previous history or a diagnosis of mental illness, it is important to ensure that any prescribed medications are recorded on the patient prescription sheet and dispensed at the appropriate times.

If someone is behaving in a way that causes concerns about their mental health, this should be reported to the care team, and a referral for specialist assessment requested.

Supporting people living with a thought disorder

In psychiatric literature, certain experiences, which are subjectively experienced, have been explained as evidence of a 'major mental illness' or 'psychotic episode'. This could, if serious and enduring, support a diagnosis of *schizophrenia*. *Bipolar disorder* (previously known as manic depression) shares the same sort of symptomatology, accompanied by extreme mood swings, from elation (mania) to hopeless despair (depression). Features of an enduring psychotic illness include:

- Talking in a way that does not make any sense to other people, and referred to as disorganized thinking.
- Having fixed beliefs about the world that do not match up with the way others see them, referred to as delusions.
- Hearing (auditory) or seeing (visual) things that do not exist, referred to as hallucinations.
- Becoming inward-looking and isolated.
- Being suspicious about the actions of other people.
- A loss of interest in life and the immediate environment.
- Disrupted sleep patterns.
- Lack of attention to personal hygiene, appearance, or dress.

Supporting people who are experiencing a low mood

In the past, depression was sometimes referred to as 'the common cold of psychiatry'. This now sounds dismissive and patronizing to people who live with a depressive disposition, but it remains the case that it is one of the most frequently encountered mental health problems worldwide.

Depression has been variously defined as **aneurotic**, or *minor*, type of mental illness. However, such does not convey the deeply disabling distress and suffering that accompany depressive episodes. Symptoms include:

- Feeling of sadness, remorse, or irritability.
- Losing interest in things that were once enjoyable.
- Diminished levels of energy or motivation.
- Poor levels of concentration.
- Feeling tired for much of the time, accompanied by altered sleep patterns.
- A lack of confidence which can develop into self-loathing and a sense of feeling/being worthless.
- A loss of interest in intimacy, accompanied by sexual self-doubt.
- Having the feeling things are 'so bad' that life is no longer worth living.

Historically, depression was subdivided into *reactive* and *endogenous* types. The former described the onset of depression as a response to something in the life-world of the person (e.g. bereavement), whilst the latter referred to forms of depression that lacked any external reference points, seeming to originate from within the individual themselves.

Presently, such distinctions have been largely abandoned, and psychiatrists tend to make diagnostic decisions in terms of *primary* (internal locus) or *secondary* depression (external locus).

Supporting people who feel anxious

Anxiety is often a component of depressive disorders and, when the manifestations are severe, is equally debilitating. Like low mood, anxiety is a part of everyday life that all people will experience at some point in their lives (e.g. attending for an interview or feeling really nervous before taking an examination).

Where anxiety becomes a recurrent, repetitive, or defining feature of somebody's life—to the extent that treatment in primary care services is required—it is spoken about as 'generalized anxiety disorder'. The physical and psychological features include:

- Increased blood pressure and a rapid heartbeat.
- Feelings of sickness, nausea, and breathlessness.
- Constant state of agitation, without any way to exercise this.
- Disturbed and restless sleep patterns.
- Overwhelming sense of dread.
- Lack of energy and lethargy.
- Inability to think in a logical or rational way.
- Emotional lability and tearfulness.

'Panic disorder', or 'panic attack', is used to describe the condition of people who experience extreme elevations of anxiety. In these situations, physical symptoms such as extreme tachycardia or severe breathlessness are common. These episodes are described in terms of trauma and terror and can rapidly spiral into total loss of control. In parallel, these individuals may feel unable to leave their home, avoiding other people, places, or situations that could trigger another panic attack.

Engaging people who live with 'personality disorder'

The concept of 'personality disorder' is a more recent addition to the diagnostic lexicon of psychiatry. It has not been without its critics, particularly those who express concern about an increasingly medicalized world where diagnosis and treatment can be understood in terms of social control.

As it suggests, a diagnosis of personality disorder constructs the mental health problem in terms of *who a person is*, rather than *what a person has*. The diagnostic criteria focus on persistent ideas, attitudes, beliefs, and behaviours that have a negative impact on how the individual is able to function in everyday social life.

There are a number of sub-categories of personality disorder, including *narcissistic*, *schizotypal*, *paranoid*, and *antisocial*. Diagnosis of the latter is typically associated with actions that cause harm to others and law-breaking behaviours. The attribution of negative characteristics, in what can appear as a judgement of the person's 'self', has witnessed a long history of personal shame and collective stigma to those people described in terms of having a personality disorder. Latterly, though, there is a more enlightened acceptance of this group in terms of real healthcare needs.

In terms of general nursing practice, though, it is more likely you will encounter individuals identified as having a 'borderline personality disorder' (BPD). There is a reminder here of the early origins of the concept of personality disorder, as a way of describing individuals who could be categorized as neither 'psychotic' nor 'neurotic', that is they were situated at the 'borderlines' of psychiatric diagnosis. Typical features of BPD include:

- A weakened sense of self or identity that changes in relation to different people or contexts.
- Acting in an impulsive manner, but feeling bad about this after the event.
- Experiencing emotions intensely, but with regular mood swings.
- An overriding sense of abandonment, and a struggle to maintain attachments and relationships.
- Difficulty in handling frustration, and occasional angry outbursts.
- Brief psychotic episodes.
- Feelings of suicide or self-harm.

Talking with people, and not to disorders

As mentioned previously, the focus of the general nurse in working with people who have mental health problems or experience distress as a product of their clinical treatment is about the *person*, rather than their *diagnosis*.

The best way to engage in a positive and productive way with people is to embrace the core conditions of a humanistic and person-centred approach: empathy, genuineness, and unconditional positive regard (see also ➲ Chapter 6, Communication in a healthcare context). The following suggestions may provide a helpful framework:

- The foundation to any meaningful interaction is based on respect and trust.
- The basis for this is establishing a therapeutic relationship with the other person.
- Some people, because of their mental health needs, are vulnerable to ridicule, abuse, and exploitation.
- As a nurse, you have a duty of care and an advocacy role, to act in their best interests and safeguard their well-being.
- If people are quiet or withdrawn, make an effort to talk to them and keep them involved.
- Where people appear overly worried or suspicious, be sure that you explain everything in an easily understandable way.
- Allow time for the other person to ask questions and address their concerns.
- Always explain what will happen during the day, so that people are informed and prepared.
- If someone becomes anxious or experiences panic, speak clearly, slowly, and calmly.
- Encourage the person to relax and breathe slowly; offer reassurance, and stay with them until the anxiety subsides.
- To the extent that it is possible, try to keep the intrusion of external, environmental stimuli to a minimum.
- Some people may describe events in a way that you do not understand, but accept this as their interpretation, and do not challenge it or attempt to persuade them differently.

Useful sources of further information

- Department of Health. *Personality disorder: no longer a diagnosis of exclusion—policy implementation guidance for the development of services for people with personality disorder.* ℘ http://webarchive. nationalarchives.gov.uk/20120503145059/http://www.dh.gov.uk/en/ Publicationsandstatistics/Publications/PublicationsPolicyAndGuidance/ DH_4009546
- MIND. *Understanding personality disorders.* ℘ www.mind.org.uk/media/ 4792976/understanding-personality-disorders-2016-pdf.pdf
- National Institute for Health and Care Excellence (NICE). Guidelines for borderline personality disorder. ℘ www.nice.org.uk/Guidance/CG78
- Rethink Mental Illness. *Depression: what are the symptoms of depression and how is it diagnosed?* ℘ www.rethink.org/diagnosis-treatment/ conditions/depression/diagnosis

Culturally sensitive communication

Ethnicity, health, and health inequalities

In providing the highest quality of care, a changing global demographic, in terms of ethnic and cultural diversity, is something which contemporary healthcare systems need to address (see Box 8.1). In the UK, the ideal of a pluralist, or multicultural, society has been compromised by significant health inequalities (see Box 8.2). A pattern which, with some degree of variation, is mirrored in developed countries around the world.

Box 8.1 Definitions of race and ethnicity

Race refers to distinctive characteristics shared by a group of people, usually articulated in terms of physical appearance and skin colour, and attributed to genetic or biological differences. How race is socially constructed and enacted in society has dangerous political implications. It can be used as an artificial division between people, based on ideologies of 'superiority' and 'inferiority'. For example, apartheid in South Africa represented a shameful example of legislated prejudice.

Ethnicity refers to shared cultural beliefs, traditions, and practices that set one group of people apart from another. Most commonly, these relate to dress, language, and religious beliefs. Ethnicity describes differences as *socially* learned, rather than *biologically* innate, characteristics.

Box 8.2 Health inequality

Health inequality is defined by the World Health Organization (WHO) as '*differences in health status or in the distribution of health determinants between different population groups . . .* '

Where this is related to external, environmental factors, beyond the control of the individual, they state that:

'. . . *the uneven distribution may be unnecessary and avoidable as well as unjust and unfair, so that the resulting health inequalities also lead to inequity in health*'.

For UK policy makers and international agencies, there is an imperative to address the inequitable morbidity and mortality rates experienced by people from black and minority ethnic (BME) backgrounds.

It is important to recognize that, while culture may play a part, there are other socio-economic factors that contribute to disparities in health and well-being. Material and structural factors characteristic of a 'political economy of health' have long been noted in populations as a product of social class and income.

Ethnicity and economic factors overlap where minority ethnic groups are concentrated in urban areas characterized by high levels of deprivation. Factors that impact on health include:
- Poor housing.
- Poverty.
- High levels of unemployment.
- Low status/high-risk jobs.
- Unskilled/low-income jobs.
- Unhealthy diet.
- Less educational opportunities.
- Increased levels of mortality.
- Inability to access primary care and screening services.
- Living with racism and discrimination.

In the UK, the RCN (℘ www.rcn.org.uk) reported a series of social health determinants that operate outside of individual biology or 'free choice' and cut across cultural, and social, status markers:
- People who live in the poorest parts of England are more likely to die an average of 7 years earlier than those living in the richest areas.
- In England, the average difference in disability-free life expectancy between the most deprived and the wealthiest regions is 17 years.
- Unskilled workers are twice as likely to die from cancer as professionals.
- In Scotland, men from the most deprived areas, on average, will die nearly 11 years earlier than those living in the least deprived areas.
- In Northern Ireland, men living in the poorest areas die an average of 8 years earlier than their counterparts in the richest areas.

In the UK, the *NHS Workforce Race Equality Standard* (WRES) was introduced in 2015 and works strategically alongside the *Race Equality Foundation* to advise NHS Trusts. It has a remit to ensure that all BME employees have equal access to career opportunities and fair treatment in the workplace. The first data to be reported revealed that BME staff reported:
- More experiences of harassment, bullying, and abuse from staff, especially in community provider and ambulance Trusts.
- More experiences of harassment, bullying, or abuse from patients in community provider and mental health and learning disability Trusts.
- More experiences of discrimination at work, from team leaders, managers, or other colleagues.
- Less confidence in the Trust actually providing equal opportunities.

Barriers to communication

No single nurse or team can ever be fully aware of the complete range of cultural factors and individuality to be able to respond on the basis of general knowledge alone. We can attempt to learn as much as possible about different cultures, but there is no substitute for simply asking people about their individual needs, preferences, and beliefs, and how they would like to be cared for.

There can be the additional complication of language barriers, which necessitate the use of interpreting services. Moreover, for certain groups, matters of culture, such as modesty and privacy concerns, can be complicated by consideration of other aspects of diversity such as gender. A number of barriers to communication have been identified:

- *Language barriers*: create obstacles to history-taking and assessment, ascertaining pain levels, arranging transport, explaining medication and side effects, and arranging appointments.
- *Low literacy and anxiety*: this is a problem for some patients, which can lead to loss of independence because of reliance on families to be a bridge to communication, for example supervising ongoing medication.
  - Low literacy can be problematic across cultures, with a particularly negative impact upon confidence and empowerment.
- *Lack of understanding*: most obviously, but not always appreciated by healthcare staff, minority groups can lack understanding of how the NHS or other health systems work.
  - For example, not realizing that a cancelled appointment can lead to a much longer waiting time, or failing to understand medication matters can lead to poor adherence with prescriptions.
- *General attitudes, gender attitudes, and health beliefs*: if an individual's gender preferences are not known in advance, professional encounters can be compromised or cancelled for the lack of a member of staff of the appropriate gender. Aspects of culture interact with health beliefs and perceptions of the nature of a health problem. These can, on occasion, conflict with western medical understandings of specific medical conditions.
- *Retention of information*: complicated by issues of language, people under stress can have diminished capability to comprehend and remember important information. Checking comprehension and retention of information is crucial.

Communicating with traveller communities

Practically and culturally, gypsy, Roma, and traveller people represent 'hard-to-reach' ethnic groups in terms of healthcare access and uptake, and yet collectively, they experience significant health inequalities in comparison to the general population and other minority/ethnic groupings in socially disadvantaged areas within the UK.

This includes the lowest life expectancy and highest infant mortality rates, with high levels of depression, anxiety, and heart disease. Given the nature of travelling cultures, health demographics and healthcare data are, at best, patchy.

Negative attitudes and discriminatory practices witnessed in contemporary societies echo a long history of persecution across Europe. This, in response, generates suspicion and distrust of the non-traveller population generally, and official agencies specifically.

Though some travellers have authorized or semi-permanent dwellings linked to employment, their ethnic identity is self-defined by a nomadic existence. This combination of freedom of movement and cultural separatism has meant that engagement with educational, health, and social care systems has been poorly addressed.

Additionally, minimal attention has been given to gypsy/travellers in policy documents on health inequalities, though there is a statutory requirement in the UK Race Relations (Amendment Act) 2000 to assess the impact of all these policies.

Morbidity embraces both physical and mental ill health, experienced as chronic or enduring health problems. Depression is increased for these groups, though there is often a social sequela, for example racism, harassment, and frequent evictions.

Fear of professional interference or of being given 'bad news' acts as a disincentive to make use of screening services and preventative treatment. Typically, members of these communities will attend accident and emergency departments for immediate attention but fail to avail themselves of ongoing care packages or attend outpatient appointments.

Engaging with travelling people

Communication from the perspective of engaging with travelling communities is about much more than face-to-face interaction or interpersonal skills. Rather, it is about exploring, at systems levels, strategies to work in partnership with representatives of these different groups and break down 'barriers' to healthcare access.

The following points outline some ideas to help achieve this:

- Available literature suggests that initial encounters with healthcare services, usually non-clinical or administrative staff, have been unwelcoming or even hostile. This sort of 'gatekeeper' dismissal needs to be challenged by nurses and medical/healthcare staff.
- Organization of mainstream healthcare services does not have the flexibility to accommodate the cultural needs of travellers experiencing ill health. Within their community, the approach to caring embraces multiple family members.
- The concept of 'carer' is not a feature of traveller culture where looking after a sick person is accepted as a 'family duty'.
- A lack of understanding about traveller culture by health professionals often produces inadequate responses and a feeling of 'being blamed'.
- When travelling people, or those who care for them, do visit a GP, a clinic, or a hospital department, they should be afforded the time and space to talk openly without being made to feel they are 'being judged'.
- Nursing staff need to recognize that the descriptor of 'traveller' represents a diverse, rather than homogenous, social grouping.
- Engagement with these communities has to be genuine, not tokenistic, and involve their long-term collaboration.
- Cross-agency planning and working, alongside partnerships with local traveller communities, should underpin all health policy and practice initiatives regarding the health needs of these people.

Reaching out to refugees and asylum seekers

Box 8.3 UK definitions of asylum seeker and refugee

Asylum seeker

Is a person who has asked for protection, but (a) has not received a decision regarding their application to become a refugee, or (b) is waiting for the outcome of an appeal.

Refugee status

Relates to someone who has been recognized as a refugee within the meaning of the 1951 Refugee Convention. Initially, the person is granted permission to stay in the UK for up to 5 years, pending review. The outcome often results in the individual being granted an 'indefinite permit' to stay.

Cultural competence

The world, in contemporary speak, is often described as a 'global village'—a convergence of political, economic, and ideological interests. Central to the phenomenon of 'globalization' are advancements in technology and mass communications that shrink 'space' and 'time'.

The dominance of 'new' or 'neo'-liberalism which prioritizes the free market and the pursuit of profit is characteristic of a coalition of wealthy nations, typically referred to as the developed world. The availability of healthcare as a fundamental human right is hostage to the drivers of competition, corporatism, commodification, and capitalism—manifested in health inequalities, both nationally and internationally.

Powerful brokers in world trade happily move money and fiscal resources around the planet but are much less willing to afford the same value or freedoms to people. In this context, the mass movement of refugee and migrant populations, often fleeing poverty, war, and persecution, presents a new set of challenges for nursing and healthcare staff.

Indeed, the tragic lives and unparalleled suffering experienced by countless men, women, and children are now considered to constitute a specialist field of healthcare practice. The trauma associated with these kind of 'diasporas', such as the European colonial trade in African slaves or forced mass movement of people, are now described in terms of post-traumatic stress disorder (PTSD). Typical symptoms or manifestations of this are:

- Depression, anxiety, grief, and general distress.
- Memory loss, inability to concentrate, and a sense of helplessness and hopelessness.
- Anger, hostility, and distrust.
- Sleep disturbances, nightmares, and terrifying 'flashbacks' of prior events.
- Confusion, feelings of shame, self-blame, suicidal thoughts, and self-harming behaviours.

At the same time, research evidence suggests 'cultural competence' in nurses is poorly understood and that knowledge and skill requirements are much more specific than those developed through working with established ethnic and cultural communities.

Cultural competence as a way of working with ethnic diversity and improving the health outcomes of minority populations is generally described in terms of three interdependent concepts:

- *Awareness*: is about self-awareness and self-reflection of questioning personal and 'taken-for-granted' ideas and assumptions about the world. This entails critically thinking about how our own prejudices, or lack of awareness, can be detrimental to the care that we deliver.
  - It has been suggested that positive emotional and professional growth is often the product of a 'disorienting dilemma' where an uncomfortable realization prompts alternative ways of seeing a particular situation.
- *Knowledge*: is focused on education and understanding of different cultures; also knowing about the epidemiology, prevalence, and treatment of sickness and disease associated with migratory trends.
- *Skills*: is about being able to incorporate culture into assessment and care planning, with the help of skilled interpreters.

Healthcare entitlements for migrants entering the UK are complex, but victims of torture and human rights abuses do not face any monetary costs under current regulations. This includes:

- GP and nurse consultations.
- Emergency treatment at accident and emergency departments or 'walk-in centres'.
- Services dedicated to the diagnosis and treatment of communicable diseases.
- Services dedicated to the diagnosis and treatment of sexually transmitted diseases (STDs).
- Family planning services.
- Specialist services that focus on the support needed to manage the physical and psychological effects of torture, sexual violence, and female genital mutilation (FGM).

Like all health professionals, nurses need to ensure that they deliver equivalent care of the highest possible standard. In likelihood, many of the healthcare needs associated with migration will be managed by professionals with specific expertise, supported by an interpreter.

In terms of basic care needs, though, therapeutic communication skills—based on the core conditions of worth—will enable the nurse to combine a *humanitarian* philosophy with *humanistic* practice.

Advocacy

As part of an advocacy role, however, there are more general issues where nurses can play a key role in developing sensitive services:

- Given their personal histories, many refugees (see Box 8.3) are frightened and distrustful of all forms of 'authority'. Healthcare is typically based on hierarchical and status-laden power structures—enacted in forms of address, role delineation, and uniform or dress codes which are incomprehensible to people newly arrived from other parts of the world.
- The nurse is well placed to act as a 'friendly face' and 'go-between' in making movement through the system easier and more understandable.
- Levels of racism and xenophobic bigotry are still a real problem in many Western societies where people from different cultural and ethnic backgrounds are the target of discrimination, harassment, and hate crime (see also ➜ Chapter 9, Communicating concerns in healthcare). This is sadly still the case for those people born in the host country—where nationality is defined by birth, not skin colour, language, or religious belief.
- Asylum seekers (see Box 8.3) face even more direct attacks on their personhood and personal well-being. As a profession rooted in the dignity, humanity, and unconditional worth of every individual, the nursing profession can champion fairness and equity. One way of demonstrating this is to participate in collective actions against discrimination, challenging ignorance, intolerance, and stereotyping.
- Championing fairness and equality can also be achieved through recognition and celebration of the contributions made within the UK healthcare system by professional and ancillary staff from overseas.
- And if it occurs, acknowledging and confronting the overt and insidious impact of institutionalized racism on the ethos of the nursing profession, provision of unconditional care, and inclusive teamworking.

Interpreter and translation services in healthcare

Professional interpreters provide a vital service at the interface of health, social care, and the law. They guarantee accurate information and respect for confidentiality. In planning to talk to a person, with the assistance of an interpreter, it is recommended that the following issues are given consideration:

- Prior to the meeting, ascertain whether the person/patient has a preference in terms of the gender of the interpreter and also the dialect with which they are familiar.
- Allow extra time for the appointment, as information will need to be spoken, translated, and then related back.
- Make the meeting room as comfortable and 'inviting' as possible.
- Speak slowly and clearly, avoiding jargon, with regular breaks in speech so that the interpreter is able to provide as accurate a translation as possible.
- Remember that the focus should be on the person, using eye contact and active listening skills, rather than 'talking to' the interpreter.
- Ensure that everything said to the interpreter is translated for the other person. Even casual social exchanges, if they are not accounted for, can generate suspicion and mistrust.
- If possible, try to have a short debrief with the interpreter when the planned interaction is completed.

Occasionally, the person may decline a professional interpreter in favour of asking a family member or friend. This might be an issue of trust where the information is not only personal, but also highly sensitive. If this happens, the following points need to be taken into account:

- Each hospital or Trust will have its own set of policies and procedures which should be adhered to.
- If a non-professional is used to translate, this should be recorded in the patient records and a disclaimer obtained.
- If a family member undertakes the job of interpreting, it can compromise the integrity of the information that is shared. Women, for example, are less likely to talk about things like rape or sexual violence with someone who belongs to their kinship network.
- Children should never be allowed to undertake this role.

Useful sources of further information

- Freedom from Torture. ℘ www.freedomfromtorture.org
- NHS Equality and Diversity Council. *NHS Workforce Race Equality Standard Report 2015: data analysis report for NHS Trusts.* ℘ www.england.nhs.uk/wp-content/uploads/2014/10/WRES-Data-Analysis-Report.pdf
- patient.info. *Ethnicity and health.* ℘ www.patient.info/doctor/ethnicity-and-health
- Public Health England. *Migrant health guide.* ℘ www.gov.uk/topic/health-protection/migrant-health-guide
- Race Equality Foundation. *Interpreting and translation services in the UK.* ℘ www.raceequalityfoundation.org.uk
- Royal College of Nursing. *Health inequalities and the social determinants of health.* ℘ https://my.rcn.org.uk/__data/assets/pdf_file/0007/438838/01.12_Health_inequalities_and_the_social_determinants_of_health.pdf
- Suurrmond J et al. (2010). Cultural competence among nurse practitioners working with asylum seekers. *Nurse Educ Today*, **30**(8), 821–6
- Race Equality Foundation. *The health of gypsies and travellers in the UK: better health briefing 12.* ℘ www.better-health.org.uk/sites/default/files/briefings/downloads/health-brief12.pdf
- Wagner KS et al. (2014). Migrant health and infectious diseases in the UK: findings from the last 10 years of surveillance. *J Public Health (Oxf)*, **36**(1), 28–35
- World Health Organization. *Health impact assessment—Glossary of terms used.* ℘ www.who.int/hia/about/glos/en/index1.html

Communicating concerns in healthcare

Communicating concerns in healthcare

Whilst each practitioner is individually accountable, singular incidents often reflect larger cultural problems or systemic factors. In a safeguarding context, when nurses adopt an advocacy role, they may have to raise concerns over patient care issues via the appropriate organizational channels.

On rare occasions, when managers or services do not adequately attend to deficiencies in care or the abuse of patients, there will be an obligation to escalate concerns. Usually, employers would be expected to have a policy for raising and escalating concerns over patient welfare.

For nurses acting to express concerns in this way, it is vitally important that they follow established procedures to protect themselves from any adverse consequences, which may include the employer taking disciplinary action against them if their actions are viewed as frivolous or vexatious.

For these reasons, whistle-blowing—taking one's concerns outside of the organization or making them public—should be seen as a very last resort (see also ➜ Chapter 30, Nursing collectivism).

Recognizing and reporting hate crime

All of the groups discussed in ➔ Chapters 7, Dignity and respect and ➔ Chapters 8, Culturally sensitive communication (older people, people living with dementia, people with a learning disability, people with mental ill health and psychological distress, traveller communities, refugees, and asylum seekers) can all be described as vulnerable and at risk for discriminatory behaviours and antisocial or criminal acts.

Often they are casualties of stigma, discredited and rejected from society, where the negative reactions of others profoundly damage their sense of who they are (identity) and social worth (esteem), accompanied by fears for personal safety. It is usually associated with stereotyping of visible physical characteristics such as skin colour, ethnic dress, weight, size, or disability. As a nurse, it is important to be aware of the negative impact this has on the physical and mental health of people.

In the UK, the Police Service, Crown Prosecution Service, and Prison Service, along with other agencies that comprise the Criminal Justice System, have produced a commonly agreed definition of hate crime, with five centrally monitored strands.

Hate crime is defined as any criminal offence perceived by the victim or another person to be motivated by hostility or prejudice towards an individual, based on a visible personal characteristic. The five strands are race, religion or faith, sexual orientation, disability, and gender identity. Examples of hate crime include:

- Name-calling.
- Verbal abuse.
- Bullying and harassment.
- Befriending, or 'mate crime', where vulnerable people are exploited by predatory individuals who typically steal money and valuables, move into their home, take control of finances, and socially isolate them from neighbours and local communities.
- Obscene or offensive phone calls, texts, and e-mails.
- Graffiti, property damage, and arson.
- Physical violence and assault.

It is very possible that general nurses will encounter victims of hate crime in an emergency or acute hospital setting, or in the community where the police might already be involved.

As an advocate of the person/patient, nurses have a responsibility to ensure that a crime is reported and that sensitive and compassionate communication is employed to engage with the individual. If it is suspected that someone has been the victim of a hate crime, you need to:

- Find out what happened and remember that some people may not understand that what they experienced constitutes a hate crime.
- Appreciate that the person is likely to be traumatized, so when speaking to them, proceed slowly and use clear language to ask questions.
- Try and engage a suitable interpreter/translator where English is not the first language of the person.
- Ensure that, once there is sufficient information to justify concerns, the appropriate personnel in the organization (e.g. the individual with a responsibility for hate crime) are contacted.

If this level of support is not available, it will be necessary to contact the social services adult protection team or a third-party reporting centre such as Victim Support or Crimestoppers. In serious cases, the police will need to be involved.

Most importantly, nurses need to act quickly to protect and support the individual in terms of healthcare needs and human rights.

Recognizing and reporting elder abuse

Sadly, any old person can become the victim of abuse and negative attitudes and behaviours, and these often constitute a criminal offence. Broad categories of elder abuse include: financial exploitation (or defrauding), sexual abuse, physical violence, psychological damage, and general neglect. Action on Elder Abuse (⌘ www.elderabuse.org.uk) offer examples of actions or behaviours that are classed as 'abuse':

- Stealing from an older person or forcing them to hand over money or other valuables.
- Making decisions, but not consulting with the person involved.
- Treating someone in a way that makes them feel embarrassed, threatened, or unimportant.
- Touching another person in a way that they do not want to be touched.
- Harming someone in a way that causes physical harm and pain.

Nursing staff increasingly work with older people in a range of healthcare settings, privately run care facilities, as well as the person's own home, and the potential for abuse crosses all of these.

In the case of 'family abuse', it is often more difficult for the person to raise or voice concerns because of the inter-familial relations and context. Regardless of the setting, the person perpetrating the abuse is usually well known to the individual at risk, and in this case elder abuse is also:

- A betrayal of trust by someone with a close relationship—be that a paid carer or a family member.
- Deliberate emotional or financial exploitation.
- Not always intentional—and might result from a lack of resources and skills to cope with an ageing, or dependent, member of the family. This, though, does not lessen the impact of abuse on the older person.

Elder abuse is defined by an imbalance of power and control between the perpetrators of abuse and the people experiencing it. It might be a spontaneous act of opportunism or a longer-term and calculated set of behaviours, compounded and made worse when older people become socially isolated and cut off from peer support networks.

Alongside their advocacy role, nurses have a safeguarding duty and it is important that they promote self-protection, are aware of the signs and indications of abuse or neglect, and understand the appropriate actions to take.

Action on Elder Abuse provide a concise account of indicative signs of elder abuse in its various manifestations, and these are drawn on here in relation to physical, psychological, and sexual abuse, and factors that are suggestive of neglect.

Signs of physical abuse of the older person

These can often be disguised by abusers or by the person themselves, but given the range of caring duties, from bathing and toileting to everyday interactions and conversations, nurses in hospitals and the community are ideally placed to recognize untoward indicators such as:

- Cuts, bruises, black eyes, and open wounds.
- Bone fractures, skull fractures, and burns.
- Poor skin condition/hygiene and discoloration.
- Weight loss.
- Soiled clothing or bed linen.
- Broken spectacles (glasses) or spectacle frames.
- Evidence of the person having been restrained or having restricted mobility.
- Mismanagement of medications—either under- or over-usage.
- The older person reporting that they have been hit, slapped, or otherwise mistreated.

Signs of psychological abuse of the older person

This, it is suggested, is the most common form of elder abuse. Often it takes the form of 'emotional blackmail' where there is a threat that things of value will be withheld or denied if the person refuses to comply with demands.

This could be, for example, access to grandchildren or visits from relatives. Psychological abuse typically makes itself known through changes in mental state, mood, or behaviour. Examples of such include:

- Uncharacteristic behaviours such as rocking, rubbing the hands together, or retreating from the company of others.
- Implausible stories to explain away the concerns of other people or health professionals.
- Sudden angry outbursts for which there is no apparent reason.
- Reluctance to talk openly or in public spaces.
- Appearing frightened and nervous without any obvious reason.
- An older person telling you that they are being verbally or emotionally mistreated.

Signs of sexual abuse of the older person

Though difficult for many people to comprehend, sexual abuse of older people is an unpleasant reality and a serious criminal offence.

This partly explains why it can go unrecognized and unreported to authorities. Alongside this, older people are socially constructed as asexual or non-sexual beings, redundant in terms of reproduction and child-rearing which are status markers in industrial societies. Physical signs of sexual abuse include:

- Bruising of the breasts or genital area.
- Unexplained STDs or recurrent urinary tract infections (UTIs).
- Unexplained vaginal/anal bleeding.
- Difficulty in walking or standing upright.
- Ripped or bloodstained underclothing or nightwear.
- An older person telling you that they have been raped or sexually assaulted.

Signs of neglect in the care of an older person

This does not always represent deliberate actions of one individual or systematic institutional abuse, and might arise because of financial difficulties or a carer who themselves is elderly or unwell.

Whatever the cause though, the effect on the person experiencing neglect can be extremely damaging in terms of their well-being and sense of identity/esteem. Here, a distinction is made between 'intentional' and 'passive' abuse. Signs of neglect that nurses should look out for include:

• An unclean and dirty living environment and the smell of faeces/urine.
• Skin rashes, sores, and body lice.
• Evidence of an older person being malnourished or dehydrated, where it is possible they are not being given assistance in eating and drinking.
• Poor personal hygiene and unkempt or unwashed attire.

If a nurse is concerned that an older person in their care might be the victim of one or multiple types of abuse, they have a professional and legal responsibility to take appropriate actions and raise these concerns:

• Nurses should maintain the safety, dignity, and respect of the person deemed to be at risk, ascertaining if they are in immediate danger.
• Before reporting suspected abuse, nurses should first speak with the older person and gain their permission to do so. If the person is deemed to lack mental capacity, an informed decision will need to be made regarding between raising a safeguarding issue and the best interests of the individual.
• Any legal offence, such as assault and fraud, should be reported to the police—and subject to criminal investigation. In the UK, this is done through liaison with the safeguarding representative of the Local Authority.
• In hospital settings, it is the manager or chief nurse who should be made aware of concerns.
• In care homes, the Local Authority should be made aware of concerns about abuse and neglect.

Specialist social workers in social services deal specifically with neglect or risk of abuse. In the first instance, contact should be made through the adult protection or safeguarding coordinator.

Useful sources of further information

- Action on Elder Abuse. ✍ www.elderabuse.org.uk
- Age UK. ✍ www.ageuk.org.uk
- Crimestoppers. ✍ www.crimestoppers-uk.org
- Stop Hate UK. ✍ www.stophateuk.org
- Victim Support. ✍ www.victimsupport.org.uk

Conflict resolution

Conflict resolution

A certain amount of conflict in relationships is quite normal and healthy. Healthcare can be replete with powerful emotions, differences in power, and contradictory opinions of what to do for the best. This can be complicated by possibilities for people to act irrationally or find themselves in confused, anxious, or paranoid states. The latter can result from altered physiologies or be associated with mental health fluctuations.

Taken together, there is always a potential for conflict between caregivers and care recipients, so nurses need to be alert to such possibilities and adept at dealing with conflict, should it arise. Not all conflict is between patients, families, and staff.

People can disagree with their relatives, and staff within care teams can disagree with each other. In a context of employment relations, staff can be in conflict with managers and employers over terms and conditions.

General attempts to equalize relationships, facilitate shared decision-making, and respond with empathy to patients' concerns can go a long way to preventing conflict from arising. Attention to signs that people are 'on edge' or losing their temper can point to the need to commence de-escalation strategies that can prevent anger or the escalation of aggression.

Respectful listening to people's views, concerns, and complaints can allow for venting of frustration without this escalating into aggression or violence. Even if we personally disagree with people's perspective, we can agree that raising concerns is legitimate and attempt to understand what is driving any upset or powerful emotions. Skilled nurses can model how to respond in conflict situations:

- Look at the person with a healthy, but not intrusive, amount of eye contact.
- Stay calm and speak calmly.
- Keep communication simple, and articulate your message clearly.
- Offer open body posture.
- Maintain a safe distance (at least arm's length) with unobstructed passage to exit routes.
- If possible, attempt to have everyone involved sit down and relax.
- Actively listen to what is being said, avoid interrupting, and confirm what you have heard.
- Respond honestly, even if you disagree, and emphasize your commitment to finding a constructive solution.
- Make your favoured solution absolutely clear.

In circumstances of ongoing difference of opinion between people and/or their families and care teams, solutions can be sought through negotiation or mediation. As such, these interventions and some of the above conflict resolution tactics can be seen to share principles and skills drawn from family therapy practice.

Being appreciative of the skills, talents, and positive contributions of others can assist in minimizing conflict. Independent advocates or service managers can be useful participants if mediation is required.

Management of violence and aggression

It is an unfortunate fact of life in healthcare settings that nurses and other members of the clinical team commonly experience patient aggression and occupational violence. Such episodes have a negative impact on professional relations, the treatment environment, and the safety of patients and staff.

Longer-term effects of these incidents for staff include stress, 'burn-out' and low morale, reduced job satisfaction, and increased absenteeism. The RCN promotes dynamic risk assessment as part of an organizational culture predicated on the well-being of nurses and the people they care for (℘ www.rcn.org.uk).

The HSE (℘ www.hse.gov.uk) defines work-related violence as 'any incident in which a person is abused, threatened or assaulted in circumstances related to their work'. This ranges from direct threats or acts of violence to harassment and psychological abuse expressed in sexist or racist language. In practical terms, this can include:

- A nurse who is bitten by a person with a learning disability during their normal care of that person.
- An angry visitor who shouts at a staff nurse in the belief that their relative is not being looked after properly.
- A nurse who is verbally abused and threatened because a patient is unwilling to accept their medication.
- A care assistant providing refreshments to elderly people who has tea thrown at her by a confused resident.

Triggers to violence and aggression

The antecedents of antisocial or abusive actions are complex and multiple, but some healthcare employees, who work in specific contexts or with specific client groups, might experience enhanced levels of risk. Such include:

- Working with people under the influence of alcohol, substance misuse, or the effects of withdrawal.
- Working in the community or travelling alone as part of a clinical role.
- Working with people diagnosed as having a mental illness or personality disorder.
- Clinical factors such as pain, side effects of prescribed medications, confusional states, or behaviours resulting from a fluid and electrolyte imbalance.
- Environmental factors such as busy accident and emergency departments or overcrowded clinics.
- Anxiety and frustration expressed by people who have experienced delays in treatment and lack of information.
- Negative attitudes and behaviours of nurses or healthcare staff.
- Poor communication skills.
- Avoiding or ignoring an escalating problem.

Employing organizations need to communicate information that clearly states an overall position on violence in healthcare settings and procedures for dealing with it. For example:

- Notifying the public that aggressive and abusive behaviours toward health workers will not be tolerated.
- Compiling information about individuals with a history of antisocial behaviour as a way of alerting staff to potential risks.
- Identifying specific areas where risk of violence is elevated. Typically, this includes emergency departments, though thought needs to be given to individuals who work alone in community settings.
- Making available technological alarm and security systems to nurses who are more likely to be exposed to hostile incidents.

Good communication and interpersonal skills are an essential part of the de-escalation process. At the outset, however, it has to be emphasized that 'heroism' in healthcare should be confined to the quality of care that is administered to sick individuals, and not translate into combative interactions.

If a nurse is faced with a threatening situation which could become potentially life-threatening, hospital security staff and the police will need to be notified and the safety of other people and patients in the vicinity prioritized. Important steps that nurses can take to maintain personal safety and de-escalate potentially violent situations whilst acting in an appropriate and professional manner include:

- Keeping individuals regularly informed about their treatment and care plan, and involving them in discussion about any changes that might need to be introduced.
- Using effective communication skills to communicate frequently with the people being cared for.
- Ensuring active listening to the things people and patients are saying.
- Always treating people in a polite, respectful, and dignified manner.
- Taking time to make individuals feel safe and valued.
- Where possible, provide space or a quiet environment.
- Check for any previously recorded episodes of violence or aggression.
- Within healthcare teams, make efforts to understand, or learn from, violent or aggressive events if they do occur.

Helpful suggestions to manage physically and emotionally challenging situations, and to learn from them, include strategies to reduce the level of perceived threat, accurately report the incident, and post-incident support for the staff involved.

De-escalation

Establishing a therapeutic relationship means that nurses are more likely to notice any mood changes or signs of agitation, and be able to explore these at the earliest opportunity.

One member of the clinical team should take a lead responsibility for communicating with the individual who is agitated or disturbed, *responding* rather than *reacting*.

This nominated individual should attempt to ascertain the reason for the aggressive behaviour in a non-confrontational way that cannot be interpreted by the other person as a counter threat.

- Nurses should attempt to remain as calm as possible under the circumstances, be conscious of their body posture, non-verbal signals (e.g. eye contact or staring), language used, and tone of voice.
- Avoid overly close proximity whilst talking to an angry individual, and do not invade their personal space.
- Do not fold arms across your chest, as this can be interpreted as a defensive and authoritarian posture.
- Keep your hands low and unclenched, and avoid pointing at the other person.
- If possible, try to encourage the agitated individual to talk in a more private setting such as an interview room, but nurses should not allow themselves to become isolated which could increase the level of personal risk.
- Be prepared to stand-off and not intervene to stop destruction of property.
- Reserve physical interventions for risk of harm to self or others.

Any situation where a nurse is dealing with an aggressive individual should be continually monitored to assess whether the individual is becoming calmer or if the level of anger is escalating. In the latter case, and if the situation is deemed dangerous, support or help may be required from more specialist practitioners/agencies such as:

- A mental health or learning disability liaison team member.
- A member of the alcohol/addiction liaison team.
- A doctor/psychiatrist if the person is acutely unwell or in need of pharmacological management or emergency sedation.
- An emergency response team.
- The police.

Debriefing and post-incident support

Where an incident is described as 'serious' or 'severe', it is recommended that clinical managers have a responsibility to ensure that:

- All those involved are reassured and receive appropriate medical attention, and treatment if needed.
- The nurse(s) involved should be removed from the vicinity of the incident, be allowed to take a break, spend time in a quiet area, or undertake different duties.
- The incident is documented via the appropriate reporting systems, including personal notes from the staff involved.
- The incident, if considered sufficiently serious, is reported to the police.
- An optional debriefing exercise is offered to all staff involved. This should proceed on the basis of a learning culture. A no-blame standpoint can assist with free exchange of views and feelings appropriate to better future planning.
- If deemed appropriate, an incident review should be undertaken where levels of future risk can be assessed and communicated to all staff.
- The behaviour of the aggressor is explored in relation to clinical symptomatology where this might contribute to care planning.

Useful sources of further information

- Royal College of Nursing. ℘ www.rcn.org.uk
- *Oxford Handbook of Mental Health Nursing* (2nd edition)
- UK Health and Safety Executive. ℘ www.hse.gov.uk
- UK NHS Security Management Agency. ℘ www.nhsbsa.nhs.uk

Chapter 11

Breaking 'bad news'

Breaking 'bad news'

It is a fairly common occurrence for nurses to find themselves in the position of having to impart information to patients, families, or friends that is difficult to take on board. In situations where the information relates to a potentially life-changing or life-limiting diagnosis, this is often referred to as 'breaking bad news'.

It is important to remember though that what constitutes bad news will be shaped by the social context and the individuals concerned. The most obvious of these are circumstances of death or dying, including progression of terminal illness or suicide, but can also include moments of diagnosis or coming to terms with disability or loss of function. Dealing with parents of sick children can be particularly emotion-laden work.

In everyday nursing practice, what constitutes bad news is also shaped by context and circumstance. For example, where an inpatient is expecting to be discharged home and has to be told they are unable to because some blood results have not been returned from the clinical laboratory, or where a person has been prepared for surgery which is then cancelled at short notice.

The terminology of breaking bad news is itself quite loaded, and not ideal, but it is the language used in most formal guidance.

• The extent to which news is 'bad' will ultimately be in the impact for the recipient of the news, so nurses need to be vigilant at all times when information exchange deals with significant matters likely to cause upset.
• It is equally important that nurses deal with patients and families with equanimity and humanity, communicate honestly and compassionately, attend empathically to their concerns and needs for further information or elaboration, and respect the fact that people will respond differently.
• It will not always be absolutely clear that people are ready, or even wish, to hear bad news, so nurses need to ascertain their preparedness to receive difficult information before beginning the process.

Models for breaking bad news do exist, expressed as sequential stages, for example the *SPIKES* strategy based on the work of Robert Buckman: *Setting* up the interview; assessing the patient's *Perspective*; obtaining the patient's *Invitation*; giving the patient *Knowledge* and information; managing the patient's *Emotions* with empathic responses; and strategy and *Summary*.

Originally, interventions like this were developed for physicians where the nursing role was to bear witness and offer support to the patient. Latterly, with the development of specialized roles, particularly in the community, nurses play a much more significant part in the process of delivering bad news. This has been explored and developed in the context of nursing practice under the following headings.

Preparation

This is about setting the scene in environmental and emotional terms. For example:

- Making sure there is a 'safe' space to guarantee privacy and minimal interruption.
- Deciding who needs to be present.
- Making sure individuals involved understand the interaction is about a specific issue, rather than a routine meeting (sometimes referred to as 'firing a warning shot').
- Being well informed and taking time to consider how the encounter will be organized.

Information giving

This is about ensuring the message is delivered with clarity, in a way that can be understood.

- Ambiguous language and euphemisms, which can be interpreted in different ways, should be avoided, for example using the word 'cancer' rather than 'growth', or 'died' rather than 'no longer with us'.
- Give the information in manageable 'chunks', allowing time for the person to think about what has been said and to ask questions.
- Constantly check for understanding and reassure those involved that you or a colleague will be available, should further concerns arise.

Responding to reactions

This is about anticipating some type of emotive response from the person receiving the news. If this happens:

- Allow the person to ventilate their feelings.
- Validate the response by acknowledging their distress or anger.
- Do not close down the interaction, and allow for questioning and further discussion.

Planning the next step

Breaking bad news is normally a process, rather than a single event. As part of the healthcare team, nurses will need to develop a plan for future working together and ideally, the patient, relatives, and carers should be involved in this. If appropriate, written information should be provided.

Debriefing

This stage is focused on the emotional labour of breaking bad news and the effect it has on nursing staff. Within nursing or healthcare teams, there are often mechanisms in place to address the impact of stressful experiences.

It is a responsibility of senior managers to provide both time and opportunity for reflection and professional guidance—particularly for students or more junior members of staff.

In everyday nursing practice, it may not always be necessary for nurses to debrief after breaking bad news.

Breaking bad news in everyday practice

Bad news in everyday healthcare situations is not necessarily going to be of the magnitude of life-changing information, but nonetheless it is important that nurses address this in a sensitive and compassionate manner.

Whilst the *SPIKE* framework is useful for structuring a 'bad news' interaction, from a person-centred approach, it needs to be acknowledged that the terminology is clumsy and limiting.

An empathic understanding of the potential impact particular information may have on a person is important, particularly in relation to issues that may seem of little consequence to nurses or the healthcare organization. Nurses should never assume, or predict, the emotional impact of a piece of news without talking to those who are personally involved.

For example, a single old person who has come into hospital for minor elective surgery may have spent a great deal of time organizing security for their home, care of their pet, transport to and from the hospital, and support once they return home. So the cancellation of surgery at short notice could be devastating to them.

The principles of preparation, giving information, responding to reactions, and planning the next step are all important in breaking bad news in everyday situations, and in some situations debriefing may also be useful.

In everyday 'bad news' situations, the way nurses give information, respond to emotional reactions, and plan the next steps will be central to maintaining a dignified and respectful interaction.

Useful sources of further information

- Buckman R (2005). Breaking bad news: the S-P-I-K-E-S strategy. *Community Oncology*, **2**(2), 138–42
- National Institute for Health and Care Excellence. ℅ www.nice.org.uk
- Warnock C (2014). Breaking bad news: issues relating to nursing practice. *Nurs Stand*, **28**(45), 51–8

Part 3

Nursing practice and decision-making

Risk assessment

Safety and risk assessment

General adult nurses work with people in hospitals, hospices, community care services, and people's homes. Irrespective of location, there will be many routine procedures which are an important part of reducing risk to people and organizing subsequent nursing work. It is recognized that all organizations will have different risk assessment tools and recording procedures, but there are generic principles of safety which underpin all these tools.

Understanding and managing risk and maintaining patient safety are fundamental to all nursing practice and decision-making, and the primary obligation of registered nurses is to always act in a way which safeguards the public (www.nmc.org.uk). The complexity of modern healthcare carries with it inherent risks to safety, not only through clinical decisions and practices, but also through risk associated with healthcare technology and environments.

In the UK, standards of environmental safety in healthcare workplaces are set and monitored by the HSE (www.hse.gov.uk). These standards and reporting procedures inform the safe use of such things as medical equipment, medical gases, or hazardous substances (see also Chapter 3, Safety in the clinical environment).

Nursing decisions and practices will normally have a more immediate impact on safety, not only patient safety, but also that of colleagues and members of the wider public. An important part of safeguarding people is to make informed decisions and organize nursing work in such a way that any events which could result in unnecessary damage, loss, or harm to patients, staff, visitors, or members of the public are avoided.

The UK NPSA describes incidents which compromise patient safety and are largely preventable as 'never events', and these have to be reported. All healthcare organizations will have accident or incident reporting procedures which must always be followed (www.nrls.npsa.nhs.uk/neverevents).

Events which result in unexpected or avoidable injury or death of patients, staff, visitors, or members of the public are known as serious incidents and are always investigated.

Whilst the likelihood of 'never events' and serious incidents may be small, the possibility of them occurring emphasizes the importance of keeping timely and accurate nursing records, which clearly demonstrate informed decision-making and appropriate nursing practices and interventions.

Whilst it is impossible to eliminate all risk in healthcare, it is also important that risks to people are identified and recorded, along with the steps taken to reduce them.

There are a range of clinical risk assessment tools that have been developed for assessing and monitoring commonly occurring risks, and some of these tools also include recommended risk management strategies and expected outcomes.

The choice of risk assessment tools will normally be determined by local policy and preferences, but wherever these are in place, they should always be completed and followed up as instructed.

ABCDE(F) assessment

The ABCDE(F) assessment is fundamental to nursing practice in any community or clinical environment. The acronym should be used when making an assessment of a person's general condition, for example on admission to hospital, and always in clinical emergency situations.

The ABCDE system allows nurses to make a global judgement about a person in their care, and we also add an 'F' for Family. When a person is unwell, whether in hospital or outside, it may well be that the nurse is the person who assumes, or is given, the task of informing or comforting family or significant others.

- *A – Airway*: assess airway patency, which should be established prior to moving on to the next part of the assessment. In people who have suffered a trauma, it is important to be aware of the risk of a potential injury to the cervical spine with some airway manoeuvres.
- *B – Breathing*: assess the efficacy of breathing. Any life-threatening conditions, such as asthma, tension pneumothorax, or pulmonary oedema, should be treated immediately.
- *C – Circulation*: assess circulation and, if impaired, treat the cause. Ensure that IV access has been established, in case emergency drug administration or fluid replacement is needed.
- *D – Disability*: assess the level of consciousness (LOC) through noting alertness, voice, pain, and unresponsiveness (AVPU). Aim to establish the cause of any loss of consciousness, as this may require reassessment and urgent treatment of ABC.
- *E – Exposure*: assess the patient's overall condition and any injury by exposing the body for inspection, whilst maintaining the patient's dignity at all times.
- *F – Family*: candour and effective communication with the family and significant others are an important nursing responsibility, particularly when dealing with people in clinical emergency situations.

The outcome of the ABCDE(F) assessment will provide a baseline for risk assessment and monitoring, and determine the next steps to be taken.

ABCDE(F) assessment in clinical emergencies

All healthcare organizations will have their own policies and procedures for responding to clinical emergencies, and these should always be followed.

Most local protocols and procedures will incorporate the UK Resuscitation Council's recommended approach and the guidelines for basic and advanced life support (ℬ www.resus.org.uk/resuscitation-guidelines/abcde-approach/).

The principles of the ABCDE approach to the critically unwell or injured person allow for systematic assessment of both the person and the situation. Each element is assessed, and any life-threatening problem corrected, prior to moving on to the next step in the assessment.

The ABCDE approach facilitates early recognition of the need for help, promotes a team approach to emergency interventions and care, and supports ongoing reassessment and evaluation of the person and the situation.

In the community or outside a clinical environment, it may not be possible to correct all the immediate clinical problems, but nonetheless the ABCDE(F) approach should be used to guide assessment and facilitate an accurate 'handover' to the emergency services.

(➔ See also Chapter 15, Cardiovascular conditions and ➔ Chapter 26, Clinical emergencies.)

Pressure ulcer risk assessment

A pressure ulcer is an area of skin and its underlying tissues which are damaged as a result of direct pressure and impaired blood supply. Pressure ulcers are localized wounds which are often, though not always, associated with bony prominences. The known risks of developing a pressure ulcer include:

- Significantly limited mobility.
- Significant loss of sensation.
- Significantly restricted movement.
- A previous or current pressure ulcer.
- Nutritional deficiency.
- Significant cognitive impairment.
- Serious illness.
- Neurological conditions.
- Fragile or damaged skin.
- Old age.

All people are potentially at risk of developing a pressure ulcer, but those who have more than one of the known risk factors will normally be considered to be at high risk.

UK health policy requires that pressure ulcer risk assessment is carried out and documented, using a validated risk assessment tool, for all people who are receiving care in primary and community care settings or emergency departments, and all people who are admitted to secondary care facilities or care homes.

A pressure ulcer risk assessment needs to be completed within 6 hours of the initial admission or episode of care. The risk must be reassessed if there is any change in the person's condition, and the frequency of routine reassessments will depend on individual circumstances and local policies and guidelines.

In some healthcare organizations, pressure ulcer risk assessment will be a requirement for all people, irrespective of whether they have any of the known risk factors.

There are a number of tools which have been developed for pressure ulcer risk assessment such as the Norton risk assessment scale, the Braden scale, and the Waterlow score. ($\wp$ www.mayflower-medical.co.uk/downloads.html).All assessment tools will assess some or all of the known risk factors such as aspects of mobility, continence, skin integrity, and general health status. In specialist clinical areas, there may also be additional known risks, which apply specifically to the clinical specialty.

It is important to acknowledge that whether specialist or generic, all pressure ulcer risk assessment tools should only be used to framing assessment and monitoring of risk, and should not replace nursing judgement.

If a pressure ulcer does develop despite all preventative interventions, then the European Pressure Ulcer Advisory Panel ($\wp$ www.epuap.org) publishes universal classifications of pressure ulcer grades, along with guidelines for treatment. (See also ➲ Chapter 20, Musculoskeletal conditions.)

Skin assessment

People who have been identified as being at high risk of developing a pressure ulcer will normally be offered a skin assessment by a tissue viability nurse or other specialist healthcare professional.

Skin inspection and assessment examines the skin integrity in areas of pressure and notes any colour changes or discoloration and whether any erythema or discoloration is blanchable. The examination will also note any variations in heat, moisture, and firmness of the skin, and identify any evidence of moisture-associated skin damage.

For people at high risk of developing a pressure ulcer, preventative measures may include some, or all, of the following interventions:
• Continence assessment and management.
• Regular skin assessment and inspection.
• Regular recording of a pressure ulcer risk assessment.
• Regular repositioning of people who are immobile.
• Pressure redistributing devices (alternating airwave mattresses, or high-specification foam mattresses or cushions according to local policy).
• Nutritional assessment and/or dietetic referral.
• Maintaining and monitoring hydration.
• Pain management.

Effective preventative skin care is also likely to include:
• Helping people with personal hygiene.
• Cleansing the skin with a pH-balanced foam cleanser.
• Using moisturizers to restore epidermal function.
• Applying topical barrier creams.
• *Skin massage or rubbing should never be used to prevent the development of pressure ulcers.*

Malnutrition screening

Malnutrition is a growing health concern which can affect people in any age group. Isolated older people, homeless people, drug users, and those young children and families who live below the poverty line are particularly vulnerable. It has been estimated that approximately one in three people admitted to primary or secondary care are either undernourished or at risk of becoming clinically malnourished (℞ www.nhs.uk).

Malnutrition and dehydration are both causes and consequences of illness and have significant impacts on health outcomes. The UK NHS recommends nutritional screening for people at risk of malnutrition, and some healthcare organizations will carry out routine nutritional assessments for all people using their services.

A widely used nutritional assessment tool is the Malnutrition Universal Screening Tool (MUST) devised by the British Association for Parenteral and Enteral Nutrition (℞ www.bapen.org.uk).

The MUST assessment is a five-step process which can use either objective measurements to obtain a score and a risk category, or subjective judgement to estimate a risk category but not a score. The risk assessment process is illustrated in ➲ Appendix 2.

It is recommended that malnutrition risk assessment is routinely carried out for:

- All people who are hospital inpatients—on admission and each week thereafter, or when there is a clinical concern.
- All people who are hospital outpatients—at the first appointment and when there is clinical concern.
- All residents of care homes—on admission and repeated each month.
- At initial registration in GP surgeries and annually for people aged over 75 years, where there is clinical concern, and at other opportunities such as health checks or vaccinations.

Falls risk assessment

Falls and fall-related injuries are a widespread and potentially serious health problem, particularly in the older population. People aged 65 and over have the highest risk of falling, with estimates that around 30% of people over 65 and 50% of people over 80 will fall at least once a year (www.nice. org.uk).

Falls can cause injuries such as fractures or wounds which necessitate surgery, and they may also have a profound impact on quality of life. Even when a fall does not result in serious injury, they can cause strains, sprains and bruising, pain, distress, loss of confidence, reduced function or mobility, and loss of independence. In older people, falls can also have a considerable impact on family members and carers.

Older people who are inpatients in hospital are at particular risk of falling and injuring themselves due to their underlying illness, general frailty, confusion, and the clinical environment itself. There are also significant risks to older people in the community, particularly those in care homes and nursing homes, and those suffering from dementia.

Identifying people at risk is the first stage of falls prevention, and a multifactorial falls risk assessment should always be carried out for people admitted to primary or secondary care, or engaging with other healthcare services.

Multi-factorial assessment should involve discussions with the person at risk and any relevant family members or carers. Falls risk assessments are likely to include an evaluation of any existing long-term conditions that affect mobility or balance such as arthritis, diabetes, stroke, Parkinson's disease, and dementia. Falls risk assessments may also consider:

- Gait.
- Balance.
- Osteoporosis.
- Known mobility problems.
- Neurological conditions.
- Cardiovascular conditions.
- Urinary incontinence.
- Medicines review.
- Impaired functional ability.
- Visual impairment.
- Cognitive disorders.
- Fear of falling.
- Home hazards.

Polypharmacy and the use of particular drugs can increase the risk of falls, particularly in older people. Many older people have prescribed antihypertensive medicines, which can cause postural hypotension and so increase the risk of falling, as can psychoactive drugs such as benzodiazepines and antidepressants.

Where people are identified as being at risk of falling, other members of the multidisciplinary healthcare team, such as GPs, physiotherapists, occupational therapists, podiatrists, or psychologists, may be involved in developing an individualized falls prevention plan or risk reduction strategy.

Individualized risk reduction will need to address any identified risk areas wherever possible. This may include changes to prescribed medications, exploring new treatments or interventions for identified risk factors, or making changes to the environment.

If a person in hospital is identified as at high risk of falls, then pressure pads and sensor alarms which alert staff when a patient moves from their chair or bed can be used. However, any nursing decisions to use these devices as safety tools must be balanced against the dignity, privacy, and the rights of the person.

Safe use of bed rails

Bed rails are widely used to reduce the risk of falls in hospitals, and although they are not suitable for all people, they can be very effective when used correctly.

In some instances, particularly where a person may be disorientated, be confused, or have some cognitive disorder, then the use of bed rails can increase the risk of harm through falls or other serious incidents. Risks to people when bed rails are used include:

• Entrapment in the rails.
• Climbing over the rail.
• Climbing over the footboard.
• Violently dislodging the rail.
• Injury through violent contact with bed rail parts.

Bed rails can also be perceived as a form of restraint if they are used in a manner which prevents someone from leaving their bed, and in making a decision to use bed rails, specific consideration must be given to people who lack capacity.

Local policy and guidance should always be considered when making decisions about the safe use of bed rails, and a risk assessment of the equipment and the person should be carried out by a competent professional.

Safe moving and handling

The moving and handling of people is a regular undertaking in all aspects of healthcare but, if not done safely, can cause serious injury to patients and staff. All healthcare employers are legally obliged to provide a safe working environment for their staff and also have a statutory obligation to minimize risk associated with moving and handling. The HSE (% www.hse.gov.uk) also requires healthcare employers to:

• Assess the risk of back injury at work.
• Reduce the risk to the lowest level reasonably practicable.
• Provide training for staff on safe practice.
• Supervise staff to ensure compliance with the regulations.

All healthcare organizations will have local policy and guidelines on safe moving and handling, and will require nurses to attend regular training. This is normally done as part of an induction programme when commencing work for an organization, followed by mandatory training every year.

To ensure the safety of both nurses and patients, any moving and handling task will need an individual risk assessment to consider the specific moving and handling case, whether assistance or equipment is required, and how many people are needed to complete the task. The acronym TILE is used to frame a risk assessment for moving and handling:

• *T – the Task*: does the activity involve twisting, stooping, bending, excessive distance, pushing, pulling or precise positioning of the load, sudden movement, or team handling?
• *I – the Individual*: does the individual require unusual strength or height for the activity? Are they pregnant, disabled, or suffering from a health problem? Is specialist knowledge or training required?
• *L – the Load*: is the load heavy, unwieldy, difficult to grasp, sharp, hot, cold, or difficult to grip? Are any contents likely to move or shift?
• *E – the Environment*: are there space constraints, uneven, slippery or unstable floors, variations in floor levels, extremely hot, cold or humid conditions, poor lighting, poor ventilation, or clothing or PPE that restrict movement?

Any moving and handling risk assessment undertaken as part of nursing decision-making should be accurately documented according to local policy. Healthcare organizations will also provide equipment to help moving and handling people, and these should always be used correctly and in line with local policy.

Venous thromboembolism

Venous thromboembolism (VTE) is recognized as an important cause of death in hospitalized people, and in the UK NHS, a comprehensive VTE prevention programme has evolved to encompass risk assessment, mandatory reporting of risk rates, and standardized guidance on VTE prevention.

Although all healthcare organizations will have their own policy guidelines for VTE risk assessment and prevention, these will have been informed by the NICE excellence quality standards (🖰 www.nice.org.uk).

VTE and bleeding risk assessment

- All people, on admission, should receive an assessment of VTE and bleeding risk using the clinical risk assessment criteria described in the national tool (see ➔ Appendix 3).

Verbal and written information on VTE prevention

- Patients and/or carers are offered verbal and written information on VTE prevention as part of the admission process.

Anti-embolism stockings

- People who are provided with anti-embolism stockings have them fitted correctly and monitored.

Reassessment

- Patients are reassessed within 24 hours of admission for risk of VTE and bleeding.

VTE prophylaxis

- Patients assessed to be at risk of VTE are offered prophylaxis in accordance with local guidelines.

Information for patients and carers

- Patients and carers should be offered verbal and written information on VTE prevention as part of the discharge process.

Extended VTE prophylaxis

- Patients are offered extended (post-hospital) VTE prophylaxis in accordance with local guidelines.

(See also ➔ Chapter 20, Musculoskeletal conditions.)

Healthcare-associated infections

HCAIs are those which develop as a direct result of healthcare interventions or treatment. People can also develop HCAIs from being in contact with a healthcare setting.

The term HCAI covers a wide range of infections, but the most common ones are meticillin-resistant *Staphylococcus aureus* (MRSA) and *Clostridium difficile* (*C. difficile*).

People who are unwell in hospital are particularly vulnerable to HCAIs, and they can cause significant morbidity to people infected. HCAIs also pose a risk to healthcare staff and visitors.

The prevention and control of HCAIs is therefore a key priority for the UK NHS, and NICE (⚲ www.nice.org.uk) publishes and updates guidelines for the necessary precautions to reduce the risk of HCAIs. These include environmental hygiene, hand hygiene, the use of PPE, and the safe use and disposal of sharps and other equipment.

All healthcare organizations will have local policies and procedures for the prevention of HCAIs and may also routinely screen for pathogens such as MRSA. All local policies should always be followed.

(See also ➲ Chapter 3, Safety in the clinical environment.)

Useful sources of further information

- Falls ⚲ www.nice.org.uk
- Healthcare risk assessment ⚲ www.npsa.nhs.uk
- Infection control guidelines ⚲ www.nice.org.uk
- MUST tool ⚲ www.bapen.org.uk/screening-and-must/must-calculator
- Safe moving and handling ⚲ www.hse.gov.uk
- VTE ⚲ www.nice.org.uk

Physiological measurements

Physiological measurements

An important part of nursing decision-making, in both hospital and community settings, is interpreting the results of physiological measurements. These may be used to assist in making a diagnosis, monitoring the effects of treatments, or assessing changes to a person's health condition. Physiological values are always interpreted within the context of what is known about the person and their health state, and can guide nursing practices and interventions.

Physiological measurements can provide important indicators of organ function, disease processes, electrolyte balance, and the effectiveness of medicines. Clinical laboratories offer a wide range of tests for blood and other biosamples which are used to assist in clinical diagnosis of physiological and biochemical states and to support decisions regarding treatment and care.

In different clinical specialties, there will be physiological measurements which are routinely used, and it is important that nurses are familiar with those which apply to their own area of work.

Reference values for the different physiological measurements are dependent on many factors, including a person's age and gender, sample populations, and the testing methods used by clinical laboratories.

Differences in test methods and measurements mean that results will vary in different laboratories, and reference ranges will be relevant to the local healthcare setting. Most clinical laboratories present results in a way which highlights any values which are outside the reference ranges. In this context, all local policy and procedures for collecting samples and interpreting physiological results should always be followed.

Full blood count

The full blood count (FBC) is a broad screening test to assess general health, as well as screen for specific conditions such as anaemia or infection. The number of red blood cells, white blood cells, and platelets are measured in a blood sample.

Many health conditions will result in an increase or decrease of these cell populations, some of which may require treatment and some which will resolve spontaneously.

See Table 13.1 for reference ranges.

Table 13.1 FBC reference ranges

White cell count (WCC)	3.6–11.0mcL (microlitre)
Neutrophils	1.8–7.5mcL
Eosinophils	0.1–0.4 mcL
Lymphocytes	1.0–4.0mcL
Monocytes	0.2–0.8mcL
Basophils	0.02–0.1mcL
Platelets	140–400KmcL
Haemoglobin (Hb)	Men = 130–180g/L Women = 115–165g/L
Reticulocytes	0.2–2.0%
MCV (mean corpuscular volume)	80–100fL
MCH (mean corpuscular haemoglobin)	27–32pg
HCT (haematocrit)	Men = 45–52% Women = 37–48%

Renal profile (U&E)

Urea, electrolytes, and creatinine levels (U&E) in the blood are collectively referred to as U&Es and are a measure of kidney function. Abnormalities of these biochemical measurements indicate that the kidneys are not filtering blood effectively.

However, inefficiencies in renal function may be related to a primary renal condition or secondary to a disorder in another body system such as sepsis, dehydration, or hypovolaemia. Blood biochemistry levels outside the normal range can also give rise to symptoms such as muscle pain or dysfunction and cardiac arrhythmias.

Unusual results in blood biochemistry normally indicate that further clinical investigations are needed to identify and treat the underlying cause.

See Table 13.2 for reference ranges.

Table 13.2 U&E reference ranges

Urea	2.5–6.7mmol//L
Creatinine	60–110mmol/L (men)
	49–90mmol/L (women)
Sodium (Na^+)	135–145mmol/L
Potassium (K^+)	3.5–5.3mmol/L
Calcium (Ca^{2+})	2.05–2.6mmol/L
Magnesium (Mg^{2+})	0.75–1.05mmol/L
CK (creatinine kinase)	24–195U/L
LDH (lactate dehydrogenase)	10–250U/L
Amylase	60–180U/L
Lactate	0.6–1.8mmol/L

Liver profile

Liver function tests (LFTs) are used to detect liver damage or disease and focus on functionality, cellular integrity, and some disorders of the biliary tract. LFTs are often used as part of general health screening and may be required when a person has symptoms which could be indicative of a liver condition such as:

- Jaundice.
- Dark urine and light-coloured stools.
- Nausea.
- Diarrhoea and vomiting.
- Swelling or pain in the abdomen.
- Blood in stools.

See Table 13.3 for reference ranges.

Table 13.3 LFT reference ranges

Bilirubin	<21mmol/L
Alanine aminotransferase (ALT)	<40IU/L
Alpha fetoprotein (AFP)	35–129IU/L
Total protein	60–80g/L
Albumin	35–50g/L
Gamma glutamyl transferase (gamma GT)	7–51IU/L

Coagulation screen

Coagulation, or clotting, screening is a group of blood tests, normally used preoperatively to assess a person's risk of bleeding during or after surgery. It is also used to monitor people with diagnosed bleeding and clotting conditions, and the effects of some drug treatment regimes, including:

- Liver failure.
- Disseminated intravascular coagulation (DIC).
- Haemophilia.
- Vitamin K deficiency.
- von Willebrand disease.
- People taking warfarin.
- People using heparin.

See Table 13.4 for reference ranges.

Table 13.4 Coagulation time reference ranges	
Prothrombin time (PT)	11–14s
Activated partial thromboplastin time (APTT)	24–37s
Fibrinogen	1.50–4.50s
International normalized ratio (INR)	0.9–1.3s

Arterial blood gases

An arterial blood gas (ABG) test measures the amounts of oxygen and carbon dioxide dissolved in arterial blood, which are expressed as partial pressures. The test provides information relating to a person's level of oxygenation and the adequacy of ventilation, and is also used to monitor the acid–base balance of the body.

Alterations to ABG measurements and pH may be associated with several health conditions, and some people, such as those living with COPD, usually manage for some time with ABG measurements outside the normal range.

Serious and uncompensated disturbance to the acid–base balance causes a systemic respiratory or metabolic acidosis or alkalosis, which normally requires urgent treatment. ABG analysis typically measures:

- pH (a measure of acidity or alkalinity of the blood).
- PO_2 (partial pressure of oxygen).
- PCO_2 (partial pressure of carbon dioxide).
- Base excess (the buffer base).
- HCO_3 or bicarbonate (derived).
- Lactate (lactic acid).

See Table 13.5 for reference ranges.

Table 13.5 ABG reference ranges

pH	7.35–7.45
PO_2	10–14kPa
PCO_2	4.5–6kPa
Base excess	−2 to 2.0mmol/L
HCO_3	22–26mmol/L
Lactate	0.5–2.0mmol/L

Cardiac enzymes

Cardiac enzyme tests measure the levels of proteins and enzymes that are linked to damage to the heart muscle and are used in the diagnosis of acute coronary syndrome (ACS) and myocardial infarction (MI).

The enzymes are also present in skeletal muscle, so raised enzyme levels would be significant where myocardial damage was suspected and a person had no other obvious cause of muscle damage. Measures of cardiac enzymes need to be made within defined time frames, so to ensure accuracy, and local policy and procedures should always be followed.

See Table 13.6 for reference ranges.

Table 13.6 Cardiac enzyme reference ranges

Troponin T	<50ng/L
CK-MB (creatine phosphokinase isoenzymes)	0–5.0 micrograms/L
Myoglobin	1.0–5.3nmol/L
Brain natriuretic peptide (BNP)	<400ng/L

C-reactive protein

Measures of C-reactive protein (CRP) in the blood are generally used as a non-specific marker of infection and inflammation. Serum CRP is also used for monitoring arthritis, autoimmune diseases, and sometimes after surgery or other invasive procedures.

Repeat CRP measures are useful in the management of chronic inflammatory conditions, such as rheumatoid arthritis and systemic lupus erythematosus (SLE), and can help determine whether treatment has been effective.

Serum CRP levels tend to rise with ageing, and CRP concentrations can be higher in the later stages of pregnancy and in women who use oral contraceptives or hormone replacement therapy (HRT).

The normal reference range for CRP is 5–10mg/L.

Cholesterol

Cholesterol levels in the blood are a combination of high-density lipoprotein (HDL), low-density lipoprotein (LDL), and triglycerides. HDL has protective properties, but high levels of LDL are known to be a contributory factor in the development of atherosclerosis.

High cholesterol is one of the many risk factors associated with the development of cardiovascular disease, and total cholesterol is an important predictor of cardiovascular events. Blood lipids are normally routinely monitored in people over the age of 40.

See Table 13.7 for reference ranges.

Table 13.7 Blood lipid reference ranges	
LDL	<3.0mmol/L
HDL	>1.50mmol/L
Triglycerides	0.45–1.69mmol/L
Total cholesterol	<5.5

Blood glucose

Blood glucose testing measures the amount of glucose in the blood, and it is a key clinical investigation in the diagnosis, monitoring, and treatment of diabetes (see also ➜ Chapter 19, Diabetes). Stress response to injury or infection may also cause blood glucose levels to rise, and this is particularly common in those people who are critically ill. Raised blood glucose can also delay healing and recovery in various health conditions.

Blood glucose is normally tested through a random sample, but for diagnostic or monitoring purposes, a fasting blood glucose or HbA1c test may be used. HbA1c refers to glycated Hb levels and can indicate the average level of blood glucose over a period of around 8–12 weeks.

See Table 13.8 for reference ranges.

Table 13.8 Blood glucose reference ranges	
Random glucose	4.0–11.1mmol/L
Fasting glucose	4.0–6.1mmol/L
HbA1c	<42mmol/mol (6.0%)

Thyroid function tests

Thyroid function tests (TFTs) is a collective term for blood tests used to check the function of the thyroid gland and is necessary for diagnosis and monitoring a hyper- or hypothyroid condition. The test is also used to monitor the effectiveness of thyroid medications and HRTs.

TFTs typically include measurement of thyroid hormones and levels of thyroxine and triiodothyronine, but specific measures used will depend on local policy.

See Table 13.9 for reference ranges.

Table 13.9 TFT reference ranges

Thyroid-stimulating hormone (TSH)	0.2–4.0mIU/L
FT4 (active thyroxine)	10–20pmol/L
FT3 (active triiodothyronine)	0.9–2.5nmol/L

Tumour markers

Tumour markers are proteins made by normal cells, which, in the presence of a cancerous tumour, appear at elevated levels in blood or other biosamples. Tumour markers can also be identified in the urine, stools, or biopsied tumour tissue.

Normally tumour markers are used to support a diagnosis of suspected malignant disease but can also be used to assess responses to treatment for a range of cancers.

(See ➔ *Oxford Handbook of Cancer Nursing*.)

Microbiology screening

Blood, cerebrospinal fluid (CSF), wound swabs, urine, stools, sputum, aspirate, vomit, pus, or any other bodily fluid or tissue can be used as a sample for microbiological culture and sensitivity (C&S) testing.

C&S is the procedure whereby a biosample is used to grow and identify a pathogen, and isolate its sensitivity to particular antibiotics or other treatments.

As with physiological measurements, microbiological test methods will vary in different clinical laboratories, and test results and treatment recommendations will be relevant to the local healthcare setting. In this context, all local policy and procedures for collecting microbiology samples and responding to results should always be followed.

Procedures and practices for infection control are the remit of specialist advisors and practitioners, and most healthcare organizations now have access to infection control specialist nurses. These specialist teams can advise on specific pathways and procedures for treating resistant strains of bacteria and HCAIs, and preventing the spread of each of the different pathogens (see also ➔ Chapter 3, Safety in the clinical environment).

(Details of procedures for safely taking blood or other biological samples can be found in ➔ *Oxford Handbook of Clinical Skills in Adult Nursing*.)

Useful sources of further information

- UK pathology, biochemistry and microbiology services ℘ www.nhs.uk/ NHSEngland/AboutNHSservices/pathology
- Blood tests ℘ www.nhs.uk/conditions/blood-tests
- Human Tissue Authority ℘ www.hta.gov.uk/
- Diabetes UK ℘ www.diabetes.org.uk
- British Heart Foundation ℘ www.bhf.org.uk
- National Kidney Federation ℘ www.kidney.org.uk
- British Association for the Study of the Liver ℘ www.basl.org.uk
- British Thyroid Foundation ℘ www.btf-thyroid.org

Respiratory conditions

Respiratory disease

Respiratory conditions can be an acute health problem, or a long-term and debilitating health condition. They are common in the adult population, and many aspects of respiratory care are carried out by advanced practitioners and specialist nurses. General adult nurses are likely to encounter people with respiratory disease across all care settings.

Respiratory disease refers to pathological conditions affecting the lungs. The function of the lungs is to provide vital oxygen (O_2) supply to the cells, and to remove the carbon dioxide (CO_2) that is a by-product of cellular metabolism. Respiratory disease occurs when lung function is compromised.

Respiratory disease encompasses all conditions affecting the upper respiratory tract, trachea, bronchi, bronchioles, alveoli, pleura, and pleural cavity.

It can be acute, acute-on-chronic, or chronic, and people who have chronic respiratory disease will normally have an illness which follows a typical disease trajectory: declining respiratory function, intermittent acute exacerbations of their condition, a gradual worsening of symptoms, and involvement of other body systems.

Living with respiratory disease is socially limiting and many people also suffer from severe anxiety and depression.

Acute respiratory conditions

Respiratory failure

Acute respiratory failure describes any condition where the body is unable to maintain adequate gas exchange in the lungs, and therefore O_2 saturations in the blood. In healthy adults, with a normal respiratory rate of between 12 and 20 breaths per minute, blood oxygenation levels, measured with an O_2 saturation probe, should be 97%, or higher, on room air.

Acute respiratory failure is categorized according to abnormal blood gas measurements, and there are two types of failure.

Type I
- Type I is the most common type of acute respiratory failure.
- It is when the partial pressure of arterial oxygen (PaO_2) is <8kPa, and arterial saturation (SaO_2) is <92%.
- It may occur in people with severe acute asthma, pneumonia, pulmonary embolus (PE), emphysema, fibrosing alveolitis, and acute respiratory distress syndrome (ARDS).

Type II
- Type II respiratory failure is also known as hypercapnic respiratory failure.
- It is recognized by a low PaO_2 (<8kPa), a high partial pressure of carbon dioxide ($PaCO_2$; >6.5kPa), and a blood pH that is normal or acidotic.
- It normally occurs in people with acute exacerbations of COPD or in neuromuscular disorders such as Guillain–Barré syndrome, polio, and myasthenia gravis, or in drug overdose of opiates or barbiturates.

People with acute respiratory failure will often have dyspnoea or show changes in their normal respiratory rate or pattern. They are also likely to be extremely anxious or otherwise distressed, and may appear confused, have a reduced LOC, and appear critically ill. Treatment modalities for respiratory failure include invasive and non-invasive ventilation (see ➔ the subsection on Treatment approaches in this chapter, p. 178).

Pneumothorax

- Pneumothorax refers to the condition in which air is abnormally accumulated within the pleural space, causing the lung to collapse.
- Pneumothoraces are diagnosed by clinical examination and chest X-ray (CXR), and people are treated with O_2 therapy and either a needle aspiration or a chest drain.
- Spontaneous pneumothorax occurs when there is no chest trauma and often in previously fit young people. It may be due to damaged lung surface in patients with COPD or in people with an underlying lung disease such as asthma.
- Traumatic pneumothorax occurs when chest trauma or surgery allows air in through the chest wall.
- Tension pneumothorax occurs when a large amount of air builds up within the pleural space during inspiration but does not exit during expiration. This causes pressure to build up in the chest which can compress the heart and decrease cardiac output. Tension pneumothorax is a medical emergency.

Haemothorax

- Haemothorax refers to the presence of blood in the thoracic cavity and can occur following blunt chest trauma or a penetrating injury.
- A simple haemothorax is where blood loss into the thoracic cavity is <1500mL.
- A massive haemothorax is where blood loss is >1500mL, and normally these people will be critically ill.
- CXR can identify fluid in the thoracic cavity, but an aspiration is needed to identify the presence of blood.
- Haemothorax is treated by chest drainage, and if the amount of blood evacuated is >1500–2000mL, an open thoracotomy may be performed.

Pleural effusion

- A pleural effusion describes a collection of fluid in the pleural cavity which compresses the lung, making breathing difficult.
- Transudate effusions are low in protein and commonly caused by heart, liver, or renal failure.
- Exudate effusions are high in protein and can be caused by a chest infection, trauma, lung cancer, and commonly mesothelioma (primary cancer of the pleura).
- A pleural effusion causes the chest area to sound 'dull' on examination and CXR is used to confirm diagnosis.
- Fluid withdrawn from the pleural cavity through a needle aspiration should be sent for laboratory analysis to determine the cause, and a chest drain may be used to drain the effusion fluid.

Pulmonary embolism

- A pulmonary embolism (PE) is a collection of particulate matters (gaseous substances, liquids, or solids) that become lodged in the pulmonary vascular system.
- A blood clot is the most common form and usually arises from venous thrombosis in the pelvis or legs.
- Large emboli obstruct the pulmonary arterial system, causing a severe decrease in O_2, hypoxia, and potentially death.
- Symptoms vary from mild breathlessness to severe pleuritic chest pain, haemoptysis, dyspnoea, tachycardia, and hypotension.
- The person may be pale and clammy, with dizziness and confusion.
- A CT scan of the pulmonary circulation may be needed to confirm a diagnosis of PE, which is treated with anticoagulant therapy.

Chronic respiratory conditions

Chronic obstructive pulmonary disease (COPD)

- COPD is the term used for a group of respiratory conditions which include chronic bronchitis and emphysema. It is an irreversible and progressive multisystem disorder that is characterized by airway obstruction.
- In COPD, destructive changes take place in the alveoli which compromise gas exchange. People often experience difficulty in expiration, which is sometimes evident through 'purse-lipped' breathing and the use of accessory muscles of respiration in the shoulders and abdomen.
- COPD is treated by bronchodilators, inhaled steroids, and antibiotics. If necessary, weight loss, diet, exercise, and smoking cessation are recommended, as are influenza and pneumonia vaccines.
- Individuals who smoke but have not yet developed COPD can prevent the disease by quitting, and those who smoke and have already developed COPD can slow the progression of the disease by stopping smoking.
- People with COPD are normally treated and monitored in the community by an MDT or by specialist respiratory care nurses.
- People with COPD are often re-admitted to hospital with an acute exacerbation of their condition which may be a result of clinical deterioration or social factors such as an actual or perceived inability to cope at home.
- These people may often have profound anxiety, severe breathlessness, cyanosis, severe peripheral oedema, impaired consciousness, and poor physical function.
- People with COPD often suffer acute exacerbations of their condition, which can be due to infective or non-infective causes. An acute exacerbation is manifest as a worsening of respiratory symptoms such as breathlessness and cough.
- Persistent coughing can be extremely tiring for people with COPD and they may need treatment with bronchodilator and corticosteroid medication, or temporary ventilator support.

Asthma

- Asthma is a chronic inflammatory airway disorder resulting from hyperactivity in the airways, caused by a variety of non-specific stimuli, leading to variable degrees of airway obstruction. Over many years, asthma may become irreversible and chronic.
- An acute asthma attack is characterized by expiratory wheeze, and mounting anxiety as breathing becomes more difficult.
- Peak flow tests are used to monitor the disease, and asthma is normally managed through avoidance of known triggers and the use of bronchodilator and steroid inhalers.
- The British Thoracic Society (BTS) has a standard plan for asthma management known as the 'asthma stepladder' (⊕ www.brit-thoracic. org.uk).

Sleep apnoea

- Sleep apnoea is defined as breathing disruption during sleep that occurs at least five times per hour and lasts at least 10 seconds.
- The most common cause of sleep apnoea is upper airway obstruction.
- A change in sleeping position or weight loss may resolve sleep apnoea.
- Some people may use continuous positive airway pressure (CPAP) machines to treat sleep apnoea, or devices to prevent obstruction of the tongue and neck structures. In severe cases, surgical intervention may be offered.

Cystic fibrosis

- Cystic fibrosis (CF) is one of the most common serious inherited diseases among children and young people. Although CF is life-limiting, many people survive into adulthood.
- It is a multisystem disease characterized by recurrent infections of the lower respiratory tract, as well as inadequate functioning of the pancreas, high salt content of sweat, and male infertility.
- Abnormal viscid mucus is formed in the lungs, pancreas, and bowel, and in the lungs, this mucus allows bacteria to multiply, causing recurrent infections.
- People with CF may have shortness of breath, dyspnoea, fatigue, cough, and wheezing.
- Recurrent chest infections are treated with IV antibiotics, indwelling IV lines, and nebulized antibiotics, which are often administered at home. In advanced stages of CF, people may need continuous O_2 therapy. Intensive chest physiotherapy is often needed to help clear mucus secretions.
- Some people with CF will eventually need lung transplant surgery.

Cor pulmonale

- Cor pulmonale is right-sided heart failure caused by primary pulmonary disease, with 90% of cases resulting from COPD.
- Chronic airflow limitation increases the workload on the right side of the heart. Blood vessels narrow as the disease progresses, leading to enlarged and thickened heart chambers.
- People with cor pulmonale may have dyspnoea, peripheral oedema, fatigue, syncope, tachycardia, cyanosis, and raised jugular venous pressure.
- Treatment of cor pulmonale includes O_2 and diuretic therapies, and pain management.

Pulmonary fibrosis

- Pulmonary fibrosis is known to be caused by inhalation of particles such as metal dust, asbestos, and wood fibres. Pulmonary fibrosis may also be an adverse effect of drugs commonly used to treat connective tissue diseases.
- Dyspnoea and dry cough, cyanosis, and heart failure can develop as a result of fibrosis, and the condition is diagnosed by CXR, CT scan, and lung biopsy. Treatment is with steroids and O_2 therapy.

Sarcoidosis

- Sarcoidosis is a multisystem granulomatous disorder of unknown cause that normally affects adults aged 20–40 years. The lungs (as well as other organs) become scarred, leading to difficulty in breathing.
- Symptoms of sarcoidosis include coughing, dyspnoea, and general chest discomfort. The condition is diagnosed by CXR, CT scan, lung function tests, and bronchoscopy. Treatment is by prescribed steroids.

Occupational pulmonary disease

This is caused by occupational or environmental irritants such as dust, gases, or bacterial or fungal antigens, and exposure can result in a variety of respiratory disorders.

- *Pneumoconiosis*: pneumoconiosis affects miners and is caused by inhaled coal dust lodging in the lungs. Symptoms are related to the amount and frequency of exposure to coal dust. Initial symptoms are similar to bronchitis. Pneumoconiosis can progress to emphysema and COPD.
- *Asbestosis*: asbestosis is a condition of diffuse fibrosis of the lungs, caused by inhaling asbestos fibres, and may affect people who have worked in the production of paints, plastics, brake, and clutch linings, and with insulation in buildings. People can be exposed over many years (20–40) before symptoms appear, and these include breathlessness and cough. There is an increased risk of bronchial adenocarcinoma with asbestosis.
- *Silicosis*: silicosis is a condition of chronic fibrosing of the lungs caused by inhalation of free crystalline silica dust such as dust from potteries. Symptoms depend upon the length of exposure to the dust and range from mild breathing difficulties to significant dyspnoea and extensive fibrosis that can be seen on CXR and CT scan. Hypoxia, anorexia, and weight loss may also occur.

Lung cancer

- Lung cancer is one of the leading causes of cancer-related deaths in the UK. Primary lung cancers, which arise from the bronchial epithelium, are called bronchogenic carcinomas.
- The main types of lung cancer are small cell carcinomas which occur in one in ten people with lung cancer, and non-small cell carcinomas which occur in nine out of ten people diagnosed.
- The most common non-small cell carcinomas are adenocarcinoma and squamous cell carcinoma.
- In the early stages of lung cancer, most people are asymptomatic and finding the disease may be incidental.
- Symptoms of lung cancer can include mild breathlessness, persistent cough, pain, poor appetite or unexplained weight loss, fatigue, night sweats, stridor, and bloodstained sputum.

- Clinical investigations include tissue specimens for biopsy obtained by bronchoscopy, CT-guided biopsy, or endoscopic bronchial ultrasound (EBUS).
- Chemotherapy and immunotherapy treatments can be used to treat lung cancer, but because of the organs at risk in the thorax, radiotherapy can be difficult.
- Surgery is often only offered to around 20% of people, normally those who have early-stage lung cancer and are functionally fit for surgery.

(See ⮕ *Oxford Handbook of Cancer Nursing*.)

Respiratory infections

Influenza

Influenza is a viral infection that can be fatal in the very young and elderly people and in those with COPD or autoimmune diseases.

People who are otherwise immunocompromised, such as those receiving cytotoxic therapy, people who have had bone marrow transplantation, or people with human immunodeficiency virus (HIV), are at particularly high risk for fatalities from viral respiratory infection.

Pneumonia

Pneumonia is an acute lower respiratory tract infection that is usually associated with fever, malaise, laboured breathing, and hypoxia. Treatment of pneumonia includes antibiotic therapy and analgesia. Pneumonia that is inadequately treated may progress to lung abscess or empyema.

Empyema

Empyema is a collection of pus that forms in the pleural space. This must be drained with a chest drain and treated with antibiotic therapy. Surgical intervention may be required.

Tuberculosis (TB)

TB is a highly contagious infection caused by *Mycobacterium tuberculosis*. Cough and sputum are common symptoms of TB. Other features include night fever and sweats, anorexia and weight loss, and general malaise.

TB may be active or non-active, and treatment is normally by isolation and specific anti-TB medication.

Lung abscess

Lung abscess can be caused by bacteria that reach the lung through aspiration or through the blood. Infected material lodges in the small bronchi and produces inflammation, which results in retention of secretions beyond the obstruction.

Eventually, lung tissue will become necrotic. Lung abscess is treated with antibiotics and may require surgical drainage.

Clinical investigations

Various non-invasive methods are available for investigating the lungs and lung function, most of which involve measuring a person's breathing and lung capacity. Prior to any clinical test, people should be provided with a full explanation as to why the investigation is being carried out, what is going to happen, and what is expected of them.

Peak flow measurement

- Peak expiratory flow is the maximum rate of breathing out, after having taken a full breath in.
- The peak flow meter used for this test is a small tube with a mouthpiece and a gauge. People are instructed to take a full breath in, place their lips securely around the mouthpiece, and give a hard, fast breath out.
- The flow rate is measured in litres per minute and varies according to age, sex, height, and ethnicity. Peak expiratory flow is useful in the diagnosis and monitoring of asthma.

Spirometry

- This test is performed in a lung function laboratory. Spirometry measures the rate of expiration and lung capacity at the same time. Taken together, these two measurements help distinguish between obstructive and restrictive lung disease.
- People having a spirometry test are asked to take a full breath in, place their lips tightly around the mouthpiece, and then breathe out hard and in a controlled way until they have breathed out all the air (maximum expiration).
- Two measurements will be taken. The first is the volume of air expired in the first second, known as forced expiratory volume or FEV1. The second measurement is the amount of air breathed out in total, known as the vital capacity or VC.
- The ratio of one measurement to the other helps define the type of lung disease. A ratio of FEV1/VC of less than approximately 80% indicates an obstructive respiratory condition.

Carbon monoxide transfer

- This test is also performed in the lung function laboratory and measures the functional surface area of the lung and the amount of gas exchange.

Laboratory tests

- Serum U&Es.
- FBC and clotting.
- Serum allergen-specific antibodies.
- ABGs to assess acid–base status.
- Blood cultures.
- Sputum samples may also be tested in the laboratory for culture and sensitivity if an infection is suspected.

Medical imaging
- CXR.
- CT.
- Magnetic resonance imaging (MRI).
- Positron emission tomography (PET).

Specialist investigations
- Pleural biopsy.
- Bronchoscopy.
- Lung biopsy.
- EBUS.
- CT-guided biopsy.

Treatment approaches in respiratory conditions

The treatment of respiratory disease aims to maintain an adequate level of blood oxygen saturation, and in addition to any prescribed medicines, there are a range of physical interventions which can be used to help maintain a clear airway and enhance gas exchange in the lungs.

People with respiratory disease often have excessive secretions in their respiratory tract, and interventions which can be used to aid sputum clearance and improve respiratory function include:

• Physiotherapy and postural drainage.
• Positioning.
• Hydration.
• Nebulized medications.
• Suction.

The frequency of interventions will depend on the viscosity and volume of the sputum, and the clinical stability and physical comfort of the patient.

People who have severe respiratory difficulties may need some form of non-invasive or invasive ventilator support.

Continuous positive airway pressure (CPAP)

• CPAP devices maintain a single level of positive airway pressure throughout the respiratory cycle to keep the airways open and improve gas exchange in the lungs.
• CPAP is only suitable for people who are able to breathe spontaneously and initiate all their own breaths.
• CPAP machines can be used in hospitals, community services, and people's homes using air or oxygen. Some CPAP machines also feature humidifiers.
• CPAP is normally delivered through a face mask, but oral and nasal–oral masks can also be used.
• CPAP is widely used in the treatment of sleep apnoea, and high-flow CPAP systems are often used in critical care units to treat acute pulmonary oedema.

Bi-level positive airway pressure (BiPAP)

• BiPAP is another form of non-invasive mechanical ventilation, which maintains two different levels of positive airway pressure.
• BiPAP is operated on either a time cycle or a flow cycle.
• BiPAP generates positive airway pressure on both inspiration (IPAP) and expiration (EPAP), to complement the person's own respiratory cycle.
• This mechanical support helps reduce the effort of breathing and increase the efficiency of the lungs, so it is useful in treating COPD.

Invasive mechanical ventilation

This is a specialist intervention for critically ill people and is normally delivered in a critical care or intensive care unit. Invasive mechanical ventilation requires endotracheal intubation or tracheostomy.

People with respiratory disease who need invasive assisted ventilation will be normally critically ill and, in the event of recovery, will be particularly vulnerable during weaning from long-term mechanical ventilation.

(See also ➔ Oxford Handbook of Critical Care Nursing.)

Tracheostomy

A tracheostomy is an opening in the anterior wall of the trachea, which may be temporary or permanent. Tracheostomy may be an emergency treatment for an acute airway obstruction, part of the strategy for living with a long-term neurological disorder, or for people needing long-term mechanical ventilation.

In respiratory failure, a tracheostomy can be used for people who require assisted ventilation over a protracted period or need regular removal of bronchial secretions.

In the hospital environment, people who have a tracheostomy will often be a patient in a high-dependency or intensive therapy unit (ITU) area, and if they are receiving mechanical ventilator support, it is important that any inspired gases are humidified and that accidental extubation is avoided.

(See also ➔ Chapter 21, Conditions of the eyes, ears, nose, and throat.)

Suction

Suction is the procedure performed when people are unable to clear their own secretions from their airway.

- People who are breathing spontaneously may need suction to their mouth and oropharynx, which can be carried out using a clean technique and a hard suction catheter. Care must be taken to avoid damage to the mouth and teeth.
- People who are intubated or have a tracheostomy tube in place will require endotracheal suction. The procedure should always be performed with care, by a suitably experienced person, to avoid distressing the patient or causing damage to the upper airways.
- Oxygen should be given before endotracheal suction is carried out, and sterile suction catheters and gloves should always be used to minimize the risk of infection.

(See ➔ Oxford Handbook of Clinical Skills in Adult Nursing for details of the suctioning procedure.)

Inhalers

Inhalers are widely used for delivering respiratory and other drugs, and there are different types of inhalers which can be used.

Metered-dose inhalers (MDIs)

- MDIs deliver drugs directly into the lung, and the device is activated on inspiration.
- Side effects of medicines are reduced, as only a small amount of the drug enters the general circulation.
- Spacer devices can also be added to an MDI, and these are useful for people who find it difficult to simultaneously press the device whilst inhaling. Spacers may also be helpful for people who find the propellant causes irritation.

Breath-actuated inhalers (BAIs)
- BAIs are similar to MDIs, but a slow inspiration triggers the device to release the drug. People often find them simpler to use than an MDI.

Dry powder inhalers (DPIs)
- DPIs are activated by a deep breath and are designed as another alternative to MDIs.

Humidifiers

- Humidifiers are used to prevent drying of the mucous membranes and secretions in people who are having continuous oxygen therapy.
- Humidified circuits can either be 'cold' or 'warm' and as such, their delivery circuits and heating systems differ.
- The humidifier is filled with sterile water and connected to the oxygen flow meter. When the oxygen is turned on, it produces a fine mist which is inhaled.
- Water often collects in the tubing, which should be emptied regularly.

Nebulizers

- A nebulizer is a device for turning a drug solution into a mist of fine particles that can then be inhaled directly into the lungs. It is driven either by an electronic compressor or from a flow meter at 8L/min of oxygen or air.
- People experiencing acute exacerbations of asthma or COPD are likely to be prescribed nebulized drug therapies.
- For people with COPD, nebulized medicine must be driven by medical air, until their risk of type II respiratory failure has been assessed by a clinician.
- The medication is added to the nebulizer container, and drugs such as bronchodilators can be administered.

Pulse oximetry

- Pulse oximetry is a widely used measure of oxygen saturation levels, and a normal measurement is between 97% and 100%.
- A sensor is placed on a finger, toe, or earlobe, and saturation is measured by a beam of infrared light.
- Pulse oximetry can detect desaturation before any clinical signs are apparent.
- Measurements can be affected by hypothermia, decreased peripheral circulation, oedema, and nail varnish.
- All breathless people and those with acute respiratory failure should have continuous pulse oximetry monitoring.

Oxygen therapy

Oxygen therapy is extensively used in both acute and chronic respiratory conditions. As a medical gas, oxygen therapy needs to be prescribed.

The only clinical indication for oxygen therapy is hypoxaemia, which may be physically manifest as dyspnoea, tachypnoea, and cyanosis.

Pulse oximetry is the method normally used to measure oxygen saturation levels and determine the need for oxygen therapy. However, ABG analysis is a more accurate measurement of oxygen saturation.

Oxygen delivery devices

Various devices are available to deliver oxygen therapy (see Table 14.1), and the type of system used is dependent on several factors:
- Oxygen concentration required.
- Accuracy and control of the oxygen concentration.
- Patient comfort.
- Need for humidity.
- Mobility.

Variable performance devices

Variable performance devices enable people to inhale some ambient air in conjunction with oxygen therapy, and the amount of oxygen delivered depends upon the patient's breathing pattern. Methods of administration include:
- *Nasal cannulae*: nasal cannulae are often used for people with chronic lung disease and for those who require long-term oxygen therapy. However, the percentage of oxygen delivered by nasal cannulae is not controlled, as it depends on the minute volume of the patient. Nasal cannulae are also used for low-concentration oxygen delivery in the acute setting, as well as weaning from oxygen therapy which has previously been delivered at higher concentrations by simple face masks.
- *Simple face masks*: simple face masks are used to deliver oxygen concentrations of 40–60% for short-term therapy or for weaning from more complex forms of respiratory support.

Table 14.1 Oxygen delivery devices

Device	Flow of oxygen delivered
Nasal cannulae	24% at 1L/min
	28% at 2L/min
	32% at 3L/min
	40% at 4L/min
Simple face mask	40% at 5L/min
	45–50% at 6L/min
	55–60% at 8L/min
Reservoir mask	Estimated >80%
Venturi™ masks	24–60% at 4–10L/min

- *Reservoir masks*: in cases where patients require a high concentration of oxygen (up to 100%), reservoir masks are used. Reservoir masks are for short-term emergency use when the SpO_2 is <85%, ($\wp$ www.brit-thoracic.org.uk). The reservoir bag must be fully inflated before application and the oxygen delivered at 15L/min to avoid CO_2 retention. Urgent medical review and assistance will be needed.

Fixed-performance devices

Fixed-performance devices include the Venturi™ systems which are colour-coded and specify the flow of oxygen required to deliver 24%, 28%, 31%, 35%, 40%, or 60% oxygen.

These systems provide a flow rate that is adequate to meet total inspiratory effort and are used for acutely ill people, when it is particularly important to know the precise concentration of oxygen being delivered.

In people with COPD, there is a danger of CO_2 retention with oxygen therapy. Acute hypercapnia (high CO_2) is a medical emergency and may lead to death. A person with hypercapnia would have a flushed facial appearance, bounding pulse, increasing drowsiness or confusion, and increased heart rate and blood pressure. In maintaining environmental safety, nurses should always be aware of the fire risks associated with oxygen use.

Key nursing considerations

All people admitted to hospital with an acute or chronic respiratory condition are likely to be in a state of heightened distress and anxiety.

Nurses working with people with respiratory conditions have to deal with an urgent or life-limiting clinical condition, and also with all the psychological, socio-cultural, and emotional implications of the respiratory disorder.

A lot of nursing practice in respiratory care is now the domain of specialist and advanced nurse practitioners, physiotherapists, and occupational therapists, and many people manage their respiratory conditions at home with support from community practitioners

When working with people with respiratory conditions, nursing decision-making and practice are focused on technical knowledge, skills, and competence, teamwork, and also on the effective communication skills necessary for building trust with the person and their family.

Initial assessment and examination of people with respiratory problems

People with respiratory conditions presenting to health services are likely to have considerable anxiety related to their inability to breathe properly.

Before any clinical investigations are carried out, it is possible for nurses to make a rapid assessment of a person's respiratory condition and collate a wealth of important clinical information, by looking, listening, and feeling (see Box 14.1), and by interpreting their observations within the framework of professional nursing knowledge and values.

> ### Box 14.1 Chest examination
> - *Inspection*: observe the patient's chest, comparing one side with the other.
> - *Palpation*: touch the chest and observe movement, abnormalities, and vibrations.
> - *Percussion*: tap the chest wall for sounds of density.
> - *Auscultation*: listen for breath sounds.

Look
- Evaluate the degree of dyspnoea.
- Assess the use of accessory muscles.
- Nasal flaring and/or purse-lipped breathing.
- Cyanosis (peripheral and/or central).
- Respiratory rate (normal range = 12–20 breaths/min).
- Pattern of chest wall movement.
- Oxygen saturation (normal SpO_2 >95%).
- Evidence of clubbing or oedema.
- Sputum and type, amount, colour, and consistency.
- Any deformities, discoloration, scars, lesions, or chest wall masses.

Listen
- Pattern of speech.
- Respiratory sounds such as stridor or wheeze.
- Cough (whether productive, dry, or hacking).
- Breath sounds.

Feel
- Position of the trachea.
- Chest wall symmetry.
- Crepitations in the chest.

Experienced respiratory nurses may also auscultate chest sounds, assess the use of accessory muscles of breathing, examine the lymph nodes, and perform percussion of the chest and listen or feel for vibrations (fremitus).

(For details of specific clinical procedures, see ➡ *Oxford Handbook of Clinical Skills in Adult Nursing*.)

Clinical history

It may not be possible to explore a person's clinical history until any immediate respiratory symptoms have been treated, but when it is possible, listening to the person's story can provide important information to guide the MDT's treatment plan.

Subsequent care and treatment would be determined by the nature of the clinical diagnosis, the needs of the person and their families, and the decisions of the healthcare team.
- Assess smoking history and identify any allergies.
- Review employment history and possible environmental factors related to the respiratory condition.
- Review social and living conditions, recent surgery, or travel abroad.
- Identify any particular risk factors relating to the condition.
- Assess any previous use of non-invasive ventilation.
- Evaluate any confusion, agitation, anxiety, or distress.

Nursing actions and interventions

Nursing care for people with respiratory conditions aims to support the breathless person, whether in hospital or home, and help them to manage their condition, so they can achieve a level of function and quality of life that is acceptable to them.

Depending on the nature of the clinical environment, other members of the respiratory care team, and local policies and procedures, nursing responsibilities are likely to involve:
- Preventing and managing respiratory failure.
- Managing oxygen therapy and non-invasive ventilation.
- Symptom control and management.
- Supporting lifestyle modifications such as smoking cessation, nutrition, and exercise.
- Providing complex psychological support.
- Contributing to pulmonary rehabilitation.
- Palliative and end-of-life care.

Early symptoms of respiratory disease may often be ignored by members of the general public. Individuals and families should be encouraged to seek proper medical attention if they have symptoms such as persistent cough, difficulty in breathing, production of discolored sputum, shortness of breath, and nose and throat problems that do not subside.

Nursing actions in acute respiratory care

- Accurately measure and record vital signs, particularly breathing rate, pattern, and PO_2 (pulse oximetry).
- Timely and accurate administration and recording of any prescribed pain relief, symptom relief, and other medications.
- Safe and accurate administration of any prescribed IV fluids, and accurately record fluid balance (which may be restricted).
- Secure IV access and obtain relevant blood samples (U&Es, FBC and clotting time, serum allergen-specific antibodies, ABGs, blood cultures if sepsis is suspected).
- Administer oxygen, as required, to maintain a comfortable respiratory rate and oxygen saturation at >95% (only use oxygen therapy with medical advice if the person is known to have COPD).
- According to BTS guidelines, the target oxygen saturation in the acutely unwell adult patient, without a risk of type II respiratory failure, is 94–98%. Oxygen saturations of <94% are often acceptable in stable patients over the age of 70.
- Administer nebulized bronchodilators and oxygen, as prescribed, to maintain the required level of oxygen saturation.
- Calculate EWS and adjust care in accordance with local track-and-trigger escalation plans.
- Promptly and accurately report any changes in the patient's condition within the MDT.
- Continually assess the effects of medicines and clinical treatments.
- Assist with coughing and note the condition of any sputum.
- Provide suction, if necessary, to clear upper airways.
- Encourage postural drainage of secretions.
- Clearly explain all actions and interventions to the person and any family or carers present.
- Give accurate explanations of likely events and investigations such as spirometry.
- Maintain a safe and calming environment for recovery.
- Seek to clearly and honestly allay patient and family anxieties.
- As far as possible, ensure physical comfort.

Smoking cessation

Smoking is a major risk factor in most health conditions, and is a particular irritant in respiratory disease. Smoking cessation should always be encouraged and supported.

Specialist services are available to help people stop smoking, through pharmacies, walk-in centres and support groups, alongside the availability of a wide range of nicotine replacement therapies.

Nicotine replacement therapy (NRT) reduces short and medium-term nicotine withdrawal symptoms. NRT is available as slow release patches, chewing gum, micro-tablets, lozenges and sprays. NRT is available on prescription and on general sale in pharmacies.

Surgical interventions

In some circumstances, people with respiratory conditions may need emergency or elective surgery. Local procedures and policies for preoperative preparation should always be followed.

Post-operatively people who have had thoracic surgery may have a chest drain for a period of time. (See also ➲ Chapter 22, Surgery.)

Thoracotomy (open excision)

- Thoracotomy is a surgical opening into the thoracic cavity to locate and remove tumours, perform biopsies, or identify sites of bleeding or injury.
- A thoracotomy may also be performed to remove the lung (pneumonectomy) or a portion of the lung (lobectomy).

Lobectomy

- Lobectomy is resection of a single lobe of a lung and is normally performed when there is a tumour confined to one lobe. After lobectomy, the remaining lung tissue usually expands to fill the space within the rib cage.

Pneumonectomy

- Pneumonectomy is removal of the entire lung and is normally performed for large, centrally located bronchogenic tumours. It is a major surgical procedure which may have some involvement of a main stem bronchus or the main pulmonary artery.
- Post-operatively, care must be taken to ensure that the patient is not positioned on the affected side, as doing so can place pressure on the bronchial stump incision line and decrease lung expansion.
- Following pneumonectomy, it is common for patients to have a chest drain inserted with a clamped drainage tube, which is released each hour to assess for bleeding.

Video-assisted thoracic surgery (VATS)

- VATS is keyhole surgery, which can be used for lobectomy, biopsy, excision of a mass, or drainage of a pleural effusion. VATS normally accesses the surgical site using between one and three entry points.

Chest drains

Following thoracotomy and VATS procedures, patients will often have a closed chest drain system in place to drain any air and bleeding in the surgical site. Different types of chest drains can be used:

- Underwater seal drains.
- Mechanical drains.
- Ambulatory bag drains.

Whichever type of device is used, careful monitoring of the drain is essential. Function and type of drainage are normally monitored every hour, and the acronym *CHATS* identifies the key features of chest drains which need to be observed (see Box 14.2).

Box 14.2 CHATS

Colour of drainage
Hourly volume drained
Air leak
Total drainage
Suction amount

- The collection bottle for underwater seal chest drains should always be kept below the level of the patient's chest to prevent siphoning.
- Some drains are attached to suction devices, but the majority which are inserted outside of surgical wards do not use suction.
- Chest drain tubing should be regularly inspected for any obstruction, and the insertion site should also be checked for local bleeding, leakage, or signs of infection.
- The fluid in the drain should be observed for bubbling. Intermittent bubbling indicates a small air leak, and continuous bubbling indicates a large air leak.
- If the fluid in the chest drain is swinging, this indicates pneumothorax. Swinging reduces as the pneumothorax diminishes, but if it stops abruptly, this normally indicates an obstruction.
- Drainage tubes should only be clamped on medical instruction or if the drainage bottle needs changing.
- The position of drainage tubes can be checked by X-ray, and care must be taken to ensure that tubing is not damaged in any way.
- For people with an ambulatory chest drain system, it is important to clearly and accurately explain the function of the drain, to encourage them to mobilize and carry out regular deep breathing and coughing to promote pleural drainage.
- In some circumstances, people who need longer-term chest drainage can be discharged home with an ambulatory chest drain and monitored remotely by specialist respiratory services.

(See also ➲ Oxford Handbook of Clinical Skills in Adult Nursing.)

Pulmonary rehabilitation and long-term care

The progressive nature of chronic respiratory disease means that the overall aim of treatment is not curative but to support people living at home with a long-term health condition.

Home health services are normally managed by an MDT, with a focus on helping people and their carers manage symptoms, maintain the best quality of life, and avoid recurrent hospital admissions.

Community services for people with respiratory diseases are normally delivered by GPs, respiratory physicians, specialist physiotherapists, occupational therapists, and community nurses and specialist respiratory nurses.

Within the limitations of the person's respiratory condition, long-term healthcare interventions aim to work with people and their families and carers to maximize quality of life. Through concordance and multidisciplinary teamwork, strategies can be developed to:

- Reduce dyspnoea.
- Increase exercise tolerance.
- Increase peripheral and respiratory muscle stamina.
- Improve peripheral and respiratory muscle strength.
- Improve functional performance of everyday activities.
- Reduce use of steroid drugs and oxygen therapy.
- Increase knowledge of their respiratory condition.
- Promote self-management and functional independence.
- Manage anxiety.
- Manage lifestyle factors, smoking cessation, exercise, and diet.

Useful sources of further information

- Asthma UK ✆ www.asthma.org.uk
- British Lung Foundation ✆ www.blf.org.uk
- COPD Foundation ✆ www.copdfoundation.org
- British Thoracic Society ✆ www.brit-thoracic.org.uk
- National Institute for Health and Care Excellence ✆ www.nice.org.uk
- NHS Choices ✆ www.nhs.uk/conditions

Drugs frequently prescribed for respiratory conditions

Common drugs used for respiratory disorders are listed in Table 14.2. *All drug doses listed in this table are adult doses.* This table is only to be used as a guide, and the current *BNF* should be consulted for further advice. Nurses should involve themselves only in the administration of medications which fall within their sphere of competence.

Table 14.2 Drugs frequently prescribed for respiratory conditions

Cough suppressants	Dose	Common side effects
Codeine linctus BP (15mg in 5mL)	5–10mL 3–4 times daily	Constipation; possible sputum retention; in high doses may cause dependence and respiratory depression; others noted with high dose include excitement, convulsions, drowsiness, and confusion
Pholcodine linctus BP (5mg in 5mL)	5–10mL 3–4 times daily	As above
Expectorants	**Dose**	**Common side effects**
Simple linctus	5mL 3–4 times daily	
Beta-2 agonists (NB. All inhalers below refer to aerosol MDIs, not DPIs)		
Salbutamol	Inhaled: 100–200 micrograms, up to 4 times daily Nebulized: 2.5–5mg up to 4 times daily	Fine tremor (particularly hands), nervous tension, headache, muscle cramps, palpitations, tachycardia, arrhythmias, peripheral vasodilatation
Salmeterol	Asthma dose: aerosol inhaler 50–100 micrograms twice daily COPD: inhaler 50 micrograms twice daily	As above, but with potential for paradoxical bronchospasm (calling for discontinuation and alternative therapy)
Terbutaline	DPI 500 micrograms up to 4 times daily	As for salbutamol
Antimuscarinic bronchodilators	**Dose**	**Common side effects**
Ipratropium bromide	Inhaler 20–40 micrograms 3–4 times daily	Dry mouth, nausea, constipation, and headache; tachycardia and atrial fibrillation also reported
Tiotropium	COPD: inhalation powder, 18 micrograms once daily; inhalation solution, 5 micrograms once daily	Dry mouth, nausea, constipation, and headache; tachycardia and atrial fibrillation, taste disturbance, oropharyngeal candidiasis

(Continued)

Table 14.2 (*Contd.*)

Xanthines	Dose	Common side effects
Theophylline	Dose depends on the product used. It is important that the product used achieves a plasma concentration of 10–20mg/L (55–110 micromoles/L) since there is a narrow margin between therapeutic and toxic dose. Due to different bioavailability of different products, the patient must maintain the same brand	Tachycardia, palpitations, nausea, and other gastrointestinal (GI) disturbances, headache, central nervous system (CNS) stimulation, insomnia, arrhythmias, convulsions
Aminophylline	As for theophylline, but dose in obese patients should be calculated on the basis of ideal weight for height	As for theophylline

Corticosteroids	Dose	Common side effects
All the corticosteroids are described individually; however, many exist as compound preparations with other inhaled medicines. For further information on combinations available, doses, and indications, see *BNF*.		
Beclometasone	Inhaler—various doses used according to product selected and patient condition (see *BNF* for details) NB. Preparation must be used regularly	Hoarseness and candidiasis of the mouth and throat; high doses and long-term use have the potential to induce adrenal suppression, reduce bone mineral density, and increase risk for glaucoma; potential for paradoxical bronchospasm (calling for discontinuation and alternative therapy)
Budesonide	As above	As above
Fluticasone	Asthma: Inhaler 100–500 micrograms twice daily, up to a maximum of 1mg twice daily	As above

(Continued)

Table 14.2 (*Contd.*)

Antihistamines	Dose	Common side effects
Chlorphenamine	4mg every 4–6 hours (orally). Maximum 24mg daily	Drowsiness, headache, psychomotor impairment and antimuscarinic effects such as urinary retention, dry mouth, blurred vision, and GI disturbances
Cetirizine	10mg daily	As above, but incidence of sedation and antimuscarinic effects low
Loratadine	10mg daily	As above, but incidence of sedation and antimuscarinic effects low
Drugs used in CF	Dose	Common side effects
Pancreatin (various preparations)	Dosage adjusted according to size, number, and consistency of stools	Nausea, vomiting, and abdominal discomfort; can cause irritation of perioral skin, buccal mucosa, and perianal skin
Dornase alfa	By jet nebulizer— 2500U (2.5mg) once daily (patients >21 years may benefit from twice-daily dosage)	Pharyngitis, voice changes, chest pain

Drugs for PE: common drugs used for cardiovascular disorders (see ➲ Chapter 15, Cardiovascular conditions, Anticoagulants)

Drugs used for pleural effusion and pneumothorax: see local hospital guidelines

Cardiovascular conditions

Cardiovascular disease

Cardiovascular disease (CVD) is a growing, and significant, health condition. It is often associated with other long-term health disorders, and affects a large proportion of the adult population. CVD includes all the disorders of the heart and circulation such as hypertension, angina, myocardial infarction (MI), and heart failure. CVD is characterized by atherosclerosis, which is a generalized, progressive disease process. This process involves complex changes in the artery walls, an accumulation of fats (lipids), blood products, and fibrous tissue, which forms into a fibrous plaque in the blood vessels that eventually obstructs blood flow in the circulatory system. Sudden occlusion can also occur where the plaque ruptures, causing bleeding and thrombus (clot) formation.

The incidence of CVD is increasing globally, and in an ageing population, it is often found alongside other pathologies or long-term health conditions. However, there are also many people who will first become aware of CVD when they suffer an acute coronary episode, which may be life-threatening.

Risk factors for CVD are multi-factorial and include:
- Male >45 years.
- Female >55 years.
- Cigarette smoking.
- Raised serum low-density lipoprotein-cholesterol (LDL-C) and/or reduced high-density lipoprotein-cholesterol (HDL-C).
- Hypertension.
- Diabetes.
- Metabolic syndrome.
- Family history of CVD.
- Clotting abnormalities.
- Lack of exercise/physical inactivity.
- Diet high in saturated fat.
- Obesity.

All general adult nurses, whether hospital- or community-based, are likely to encounter patients with some degree of CVD.

Acute cardiac conditions

Acute coronary syndrome (ACS)

ACS is an umbrella term for a range of manifestations of coronary heart disease. The term covers angina, unstable angina (UA), non-ST elevation myocardial infarction (NSTEMI), and ST elevation myocardial infarction (STEMI).

- ACS is usually a response to the rupture of an atherosclerotic plaque in the coronary arteries.
- The rupture triggers a chain of events (platelet activation, adhesion, and aggregation) that may lead to thrombus formation in the damaged vessel.
- In UA and NSTEMI, the thrombus partially occludes blood flow in a coronary artery, starving the heart muscle of oxygen and nutrients.
- This physiological process can result in symptoms, with or without electrocardiogram (ECG) changes, and cardiac enzyme release (troponin T, troponin I, creatinine kinase).
- If the thrombus totally occludes the blood vessel, a section of the myocardium will become starved of oxygen and die.

Stable angina

Angina is chest pain or discomfort (e.g. pressure, heaviness, tightness, or squeezing) that can occur in people with coronary heart disease. The discomfort or pain results from a transient, reversible episode of inadequate coronary circulation.

- The reduced blood supply to the myocardium normally results from arterial narrowing due to atherosclerosis.
- An episode of angina typically lasts 2–5 minutes.
- With stable angina, the symptoms have a regular pattern, are relatively constant, and are usually associated with exertion.
- Diagnosis is normally confirmed by ECG, exercise tolerance test, and cardiac catheterization.
- Treatment of stable angina involves health and lifestyle modification, regular monitoring, and medication including nitrates such as GTN, β-blockers, calcium channel blockers, statins, and antiplatelet drugs (aspirin, clopidogrel, ticagrelor).

Unstable angina

In UA, there is an unstable atheromatous plaque within a coronary artery. People experience increasing episodes of angina symptoms, not necessarily associated with any particular activity and which may begin to occur whilst they are at rest. The symptoms are not relieved by usual amounts of GTN.

- People with UA are at risk of MI if the artery blocks off completely.
- People with UA should be promptly assessed, either in a GP surgery or an acute hospital.
- Distinguishing between UA and MI in the acute setting is normally dependent on observed ECG changes and changes in cardiac enzyme levels.

- Treatment is focused on the restoration of adequate blood flow to the myocardium (revascularization), which may involve angioplasty, insertion of arterial stents, or coronary artery bypass graft (CABG) surgery.
- Treatment will also include symptom relief through analgesia and anti-anginal medication.

Myocardial infarction (MI)

The term myocardial infarction (often also referred to as heart attack or coronary thrombosis) refers to necrosis of a portion of the myocardium. It is usually the result of a blood clot (thrombus) that blocks all or part of a coronary artery.

Management and treatment options for MI are now divided into two categories—NSTEMI and STEMI, based on whether ST elevation is visible on the ECG tracing.

Non-ST elevation MI (NSTEMI)

- Clinical presentation and cardiac enzyme testing are positive, which indicates myocardial damage; no ST changes are seen on the 12-lead ECG.

ST elevation MI (STEMI)

- Evidence of ST segment changes on the 12-lead ECG and positive cardiac enzyme testing confirm total blockage of a coronary artery resulting in muscle damage to the myocardium.
- Restoring blood flow to the damaged myocardium (reperfusion) is an important part of treatment and must be initiated as soon as possible for it to be effective.
- Preferred reperfusion therapy is cardiac angiography performed within 90 minutes of the initial onset of pain. IV drug therapy (thrombolysis), which dissolves the blood clot to restore blood flow, can also be used.
- Care and management of people with either category of MI should be undertaken in a specialized cardiac or coronary care unit where patients can be closely monitored and life-threatening complications, such as cardiac arrhythmias, can be treated immediately. Clinical care of people who have suffered an MI includes:
  - 12-lead ECG recording.
  - Continuous cardiac monitoring.
  - Regular observation and recording of vital signs.
  - Reduction in myocardial oxygen demand through bed rest.
  - Medications for pain and symptom relief.
  - Alteration of early physiological changes using angiotensin-converting enzyme (ACE) inhibitors.
  - Secondary prevention of further damage involving an antiplatelet and a statin.
  - Psychological support.
  - Supporting lifestyle moderation.
  - Referral to a cardiac rehabilitation programme.

Cardiac arrhythmias

The ECG is a simple, non-invasive technique to identify cardiac damage and conduction disorders. Normal cardiac rhythm is described as sinus rhythm, which means the heartbeat originates in the sinoatrial (SA) node. It is represented graphically as the PQRST cycle, which is illustrated in Figure 15.1.

- P wave is associated with atrial electrical activation in the SA node.
- PR interval is measured from the beginning of the P wave to the beginning of the QRS complex. This interval represents the spread of electrical conduction (depolarization) from the SA node, through the atrial muscle and the atrioventricular (AV) node (normally 0.12–0.2s, represented by 3–5 small squares on the ECG trace).
- QRS complex represents electrical activity of the ventricles (normally <0.12s = 3 small squares).
- ST segment represents the end of ventricular activity and the beginning of ventricular recovery or repolarization.
- T wave represents ventricular recovery/repolarization.
- QT interval represents ventricular depolarization and repolarization.
- U wave represents the recovery period of the Purkinje fibres (rarely seen).

This normal cycle would be seen on an ECG trace as sinus rhythm (see Figure 15.2).

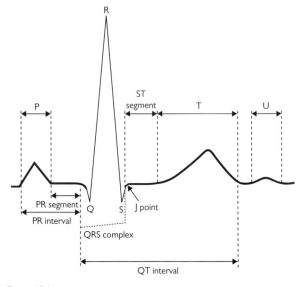

Figure 15.1 The phases of the cardiac cycle.

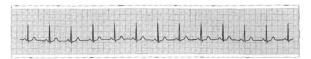

Figure 15.2 Sinus rhythm.
Reproduced with the kind permission of the Resuscitation Council (UK).

An arrhythmia is a disorder of the heart's electrical conduction system. It may be caused by the electrical impulse starting somewhere other than the sinus node of the right atrium or by the electrical impulse following an abnormal route through the heart muscle as a result of myocardial damage or necrosis.

- Blood biochemistry with measures outside the normal ranges of potassium, magnesium, calcium, and thyroid levels can also cause arrhythmias.
- Arrhythmia can be life-threatening, particularly in the period immediately after an acute MI.
- Cardiac arrhythmia can also lead to significant alterations to cardiac output or a thrombus.
- A person with a cardiac arrhythmia may experience a range of symptoms, including chest pain, shortness of breath, light-headedness, collapse, reduced exercise tolerance, and palpitations.
- A diagnosis of arrhythmia is made from the clinical history, physical symptoms and examination, and ECG.

Sinus tachycardia
Heart rate is >100bpm (see Figure 15.3). This rate occurs with exercise, infection, pain, and blood loss. The urgency of treatment depends on the symptoms and any other underlying conditions.

Sinus bradycardia
- Heart rate is <60bpm (see Figure 15.4). A rate of <60bpm can be normal for athletes and those on β-blocker therapy. If the individual has no symptoms, treatment is not indicated.
- A resting sinus bradycardia of 55–60bpm, achieved through β-blocker drugs, is recommended for people with left ventricular systolic dysfunction heart failure (% www.nice.org.uk).

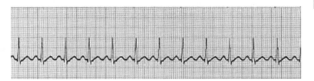

Figure 15.3 Sinus tachycardia.

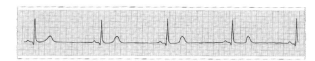

Figure 15.4 Sinus bradycardia.
Reproduced with the kind permission of the Resuscitation Council (UK).

Atrial flutter

- Rapid, but usually regular, atrial contraction >200 bpm, seen on ECG with a characteristic 'saw-tooth' pattern (see Figure 15.5). This is a stable rhythm that can progress to atrial fibrillation. It should be reverted back to normal sinus rhythm by drug therapy or electrical cardioversion.

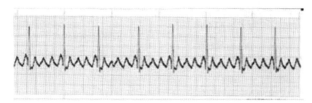

Figure 15.5 Atrial flutter.

Atrial fibrillation

- An irregular, often rapid, heart rate. There are no P waves on the ECG (see Figure 15.6). This is the most common arrhythmia encountered in clinical practice, and many people live with chronic atrial fibrillation. Treatment depends on the ventricular rate, haemodynamic state, and the risk of clot formation.

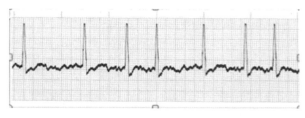

Figure 15.6 Atrial fibrillation.

Ventricular tachycardia

- Characterized by widened QRS complexes on ECG, due to an accelerated heart rate of between 120 and 250bpm (see Figure 15.7). P waves and T waves cannot be identified. Ventricular tachycardia is a serious arrhythmia which can produce shock and cardiac arrest, and can progress to ventricular fibrillation. Normally requires urgent treatment.

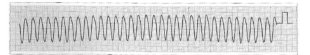

Figure 15.7 Ventricular tachycardia.
Reproduced with the kind permission of the Resuscitation Council (UK).

Ventricular fibrillation

- On ECG, ventricular fibrillation displays as a chaotic waveform, with no P waves, QRS complexes, or T waves, and with a rate between 150 and 500bpm (see Figure 15.8). In this rhythm, the heart is an ineffective pump and the patient will have no cardiac output. Immediate lifesaving treatment is essential.

(For details of the principles of cardiopulmonary resuscitation in the treatment of life-threatening cardiac arrhythmias, see ➲ Chapter 26, Clinical emergencies.)

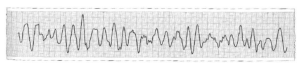

Figure 15.8 Ventricular fibrillation.
Reproduced with the kind permission of the Resuscitation Council (UK).

Heart block

Conduction disturbances of the normal electrical impulse are referred to as heart blocks and may be classified as first-degree, second-degree, or complete heart block.

First-degree atrioventricular (AV) block

- Is present when the PR interval on ECG is >0.20s (see Figure 15.9). It represents a delay in conduction through the AV junction (the AV node and immediately adjacent myocardium). First-degree AV block rarely causes any symptoms and, as an isolated finding, rarely requires treatment.

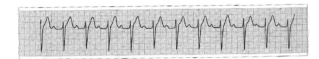

Figure 15.9 First-degree AV block.
Reproduced with the kind permission of the Resuscitation Council (UK).

Second-degree AV block
- Is when some, but not all, P waves are conducted to the ventricles. On ECG, there is a resulting absence of a QRS complex after some P waves. There are two types of second-degree block—Mobitz type I (also called Wenckebach) and Mobitz type II.

Mobitz type I
- On ECG, the PR interval shows progressive prolongation after each successive P wave, until a P wave occurs without a resulting QRS complex. This cycle repeats (see Figure 15.10).

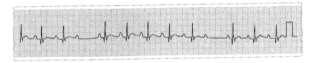

Figure 15.10 Mobitz type I (Wenckebach) block.
Reproduced with the kind permission of the Resuscitation Council (UK).

Mobitz type II
- There is a constant PR interval in the conducted beats, but some of the P waves are not followed by QRS complexes. This may occur randomly, without any consistent pattern (see Figure 15.11).

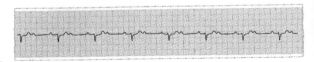

Figure 15.11 Mobitz type II block.
Reproduced with the kind permission of the Resuscitation Council (UK).

2:1 AV block

- Alternate P waves are followed by a QRS complex (see Figure 15.12). A 2:1 AV block may be due to Mobitz type I or Mobitz type II, and it may be difficult to distinguish.

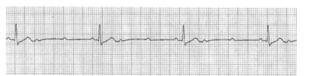

Figure 15.12 2:1 AV block.

Complete heart block (3:1 AV block)

- Here the P wave has no relation to the QRS complex (see Figure 15.13), and electrical impulses to maintain cardiac output are generated from below the AV node. The patient may suffer ventricular standstill, resulting in syncope if the block is self-terminating or sudden cardiac death if prolonged.

Treatment for all heart blocks is aimed at restoring normal rhythm and will usually be delivered on a specialist cardiac unit. Compete heart block requires pacemaker insertion to increase ventricular rate and improve cardiac output.

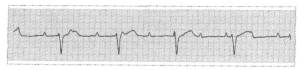

Figure 15.13 Complete heart block.
Reproduced with the kind permission of the Resuscitation Council (UK).

Treatment of cardiac arrhythmias

Cardioversion
- Atrial flutter and atrial fibrillation can be medically or electrically converted back to a normal sinus rhythm.
- For electrical cardioversion, a predetermined dose of electrical current is delivered through a defibrillator.
- The electrical current stimulates the repolarization of cardiac cells, allowing an opportunity for the sinus node to resume its role as the pacemaker.
- People who are conscious should be lightly anaesthetized or sedated for this procedure.
- This procedure can be performed as an outpatient intervention or in an emergency situation. It is usually carried out in the cardiac catheter lab or on the coronary care unit.
- Cardioversion is not always successful nor permanent.

Temporary pacemaker
- Temporary pacemakers are used to treat symptomatic bradyarrhythmias in emergencies or if symptom management is needed for a short time.
- The insertion of a temporary pacemaker is an invasive procedure requiring specialist intervention.
- Under X-ray guidance, small wires are inserted into the myocardium, and electricity is then delivered to the heart at a given rate, using an external mains-operated pacemaker unit.

Permanent pacemakers
- These are used when long-term control of the heart rhythm is necessary and are implanted in an operating theatre, normally by a cardiologist.
- With X-ray guidance, electrical wires are passed through a vein into a chamber of the heart.
- The wires are connected to a pacemaker unit which is then placed in a 'pocket' made between the skin and muscle under the left collar bone.
- Impulses from the pacemaker stimulate the atrium, the ventricles, or both. They operate at a set rate or at a rate that corresponds to the person's own heart rhythm (i.e. on demand).
- Permanent pacemakers may require day-case surgery in order for the batteries to be changed; however, expected battery life is around 10 years.
- The ECG rhythm of a person with a pacemaker (temporary or permanent) will show a pacing 'spike' which corresponds to the external electrical stimulus delivered by the device (see Figure 15.14).

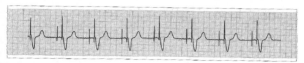

Figure 15.14 Paced rhythm.

Reproduced with the kind permission of the Resuscitation Council (UK).

Internal cardioverter–defibrillator (ICD)

- ICDs are used for people who have survived, or who are at risk of, a life-threatening arrhythmic event.
- ICDs monitor heart rate, initiate pacing, and deliver cardioversion and/or defibrillation if needed.
- The procedure for ICD insertion is similar to that of a permanent pacemaker, but this battery-operated device is implanted in the subcutaneous cavity of the chest.
- If a person with an ICD is reaching the end of their life, it is important that the device is deactivated to prevent the delivery of inappropriate shocks.
- People offered this treatment require considerable and ongoing monitoring and lifestyle and psychological support.

Catheter ablation therapy

- Radiofrequency energy (similar to microwave heat) targets and destroys the tissue in the heart that is causing arrhythmias.
- The procedure takes between 2 and 4 hours and is performed under local anaesthesia, with X-ray guidance.
- People may experience palpitations during ablation therapy, which nonetheless is normally carried out as a day-case intervention.
- Catheter ablation therapy is useful when medicines are not effective in controlling cardiac arrhythmias or the person is suffering from side effects of drug therapy.

Drug therapy

- Cardiac drugs which are designed to restore and maintain normal sinus rhythm and/or maximum cardiac output may also be prescribed to treat cardiac arrhythmias.
- Prescription medicines may be used alone or as an adjunct to other treatments (see ➲ p. 226 for frequently prescribed cardiac medicines).

Clinical investigations in acute cardiac conditions

Blood tests

Blood tests that are useful in cardiac assessment include:
- Serum U&Es.
- Liver function tests (LFTs).
- FBC.
- Troponin T in suspected ACS.
- Plasma lipid profile.
- Plasma glucose.
- D-dimer test to rule out PE or deep vein thrombosis (DVT).
- BNP or NT-proBNP in chronic heart failure.
- Blood gas analysis (ABGs).

Chest X-ray

CXRs are normally ordered to help the clinical team assess heart shape and size, any lung vessel changes, and any degree of pulmonary oedema.

Electrocardiogram

- A 12-lead ECG displays the pathway of electricity through the heart and is able to show areas of myocardial damage, rhythm, rate, any conduction disorders, and arrhythmias.
- It is the most common and useful diagnostic tool used in cardiac care.
- The printed reading which is produced by an EGC machine gives 12 electrical 'views' of the heart which are labelled I, II, III, avR, avL, avF, V1, V2, V3, V4, V5, and V6. Each of these readings gives an indication as to where any myocardial damage has occurred. These are summarized in Figure 15.15.

I Lateral wall	avR (cavity)	V1 Septum	V4 Anterior wall
II Inferior wall	avL Lateral wall	V2 Septum	V5 Lateral wall
III Inferior wall	avF Inferior wall	V3 Anterior wall	V6 Lateral wall

Figure 15.15 Areas of myocardial damage represented by abnormalities in 12 lead ECG readings.

Shaded = Damage to the lateral surface of the myocardium

Diagonal lines = Damage to the inferior surface of the myocardium

Cross-hatched = Damage to the septum

Horizontal lines = Damage to the anterior surface of the myocardium

Continuous cardiac monitoring

- Continuous cardiac monitoring also shows electrical activity in the heart and is normally carried out in pre-hospital settings, emergency departments, and high dependency, critical care, or coronary care units.
- Hospital inpatients can also be monitored remotely through telemetry.
- Three or five disposable electrodes are fixed to the patient's chest, and the wires are connected to a cardiac monitor. Electrodes attached to the patient's chest should be changed every 48 hours to maintain efficacy.
- Continuous monitoring of cardiac rate and rhythm allows changes to be identified promptly, and the effects of therapy to be monitored.
- Telemetry allows patients more freedom of movement and is useful for patients who are able to mobilize.

Central venous pressure monitoring (CVP)

- A CVP recording is a direct measure of venous pressure and gives a guide to right heart function.
- In patients who are haemodynamically unstable, it may be necessary to monitor this aspect of cardiac activity with invasive devices.
- The normal range of measurement is 4–10cmH$_2$O or 0–8mmHg.
- The CVP rises in fluid overload and falls in decreased circulatory volume. Measurement is useful to estimate the patient's fluid status and acts as a guide to fluid replacement and other treatment.
- Blood samples can be obtained from a CVP line and are very useful in patients with difficult or no IV access.

Echocardiography (Echo)

- Echocardiography is a multi-dimensional (2- to 4-dimensional) ultrasound picture of the heart, which is used to diagnose and monitor cardiac conditions.
- Echocardiograms are normally performed in specialist cardiorespiratory departments but may also be performed in an emergency situation. Portable echocardiogram equipment can also be used to perform the procedure in the community or people's homes.
- Echocardiograms are particularly useful when a person with heart failure or MI is showing signs of rapid clinical deterioration. It is also useful for detecting valve disease or defects in the septum.
- A hand-held transducer is placed on the patient's chest, which picks up sound waves reflected from various parts of the heart.
- A recording device is connected to the transducer, so that the reflected sound waves are converted into images and displayed on a screen.

Transoesophageal echocardiography (TOE)

- This imaging procedure uses a 2-dimensional transducer on the end of a flexible endoscope, which is introduced into the oesophagus, to obtain more detailed images of the aorta, heart, and atria.
- The procedure is normally performed in a specialist cardiorespiratory unit, with or without sedation.

Stress testing—exercise tolerance tests (ETTs)

- Stress testing is used to assess the heart's response to increased demand. It is used to confirm suspected coronary artery disease, determine functional capacity, and assess prognosis.
- The heart is monitored under increasing aerobic stress that is induced either pharmacologically or with graduated exercise (ETT).
- During ETT, aerobic stress is induced by stair climbing, a treadmill, or a bicycle.
- The person's ECG, blood pressure, and heart rate are compared before and after the graduated exercise or pharmacological interventions.

Ambulatory ECG monitoring

- Continuous ECG monitoring is used to record arrhythmias and conduction defects that may not be picked up by a standard ECG.
- The person wears an ECG recorder, whilst carrying out usual activities, for a period of 24 hours.
- They also keep a diary and record any symptoms which are later matched with the ECG trace.

Implantable loop recorder (ILR)

- An ILR is a small recording playback device which is used to monitor and record heart rhythm irregularities over a prolonged period.
- An ILR is introduced under the skin at the left side of the chest wall under local anaesthesia, and can provide cardiac surveillance on a loop recording for up to 1 year or longer.
- A patient with a prolonged history of unexplained dizziness or collapse may be referred for this.

Provocation tests

- Provocation tests are used to identify arrhythmias thought to be produced by problems with the electrical functioning of the cardiac conduction system.
- An anti-arrhythmic drug (e.g. flecainide or adenosine) is given IV under closely monitored conditions.
- The procedure carries a risk of inducing potential life-threatening arrhythmia, so resuscitation equipment needs to be available.

Cardiac catheterization

Cardiac catheterization is a generic term used to refer to percutaneous insertion of a fine, flexible, radio-opaque catheter into one or more chambers of the heart. The procedure can be used to visualize the heart structures by means of a radio-opaque substance under X-ray control (referred to as angiography). The procedure normally takes about 30 minutes.

- Cardiac catheterization can confirm the presence of a clinically suspected heart condition, such as coronary artery disease, ventricular wall ischaemia caused by infarction, or mitral and aortic valve defects or disease.
- It can also identify abnormal cardiac anatomy and physiology and, in some cases, can be used to perform therapeutic procedures.
- The invasive procedure is performed under sterile conditions in a cardiac catheterization laboratory.

- Cardiac catheterization is usually performed via the femoral artery, although the radial and brachial approaches can also be used.
- It is normally carried out as a day-case investigation for diagnostic purposes and as a first-response treatment for confirmed STEMI.

Angioplasty and stents

- As a treatment intervention, cardiac catheterization is used to widen narrowed or obstructed coronary arteries (angioplasty) or to insert a stent.
- During the catheterization procedure, an empty, collapsed balloon catheter is passed over a wire into the narrowed coronary arteries and then inflated to a fixed size. The balloon forces expansion of the artery muscular wall and is then deflated and withdrawn.
- A coronary stent may be inserted at the time of ballooning to ensure the vessel remains open.

Electrophysiological studies (EPS)

- EPS are tests that map the electrical conduction system of the heart. They are used to assess arrhythmias, to identify abnormal patterns of conduction, and to monitor the effectiveness of treatments. The test normally takes between 1 and 4 hours.
- Wires are placed in the heart, via cardiac catheterization, to record electrical activity and to induce arrhythmias in a controlled situation.
- After the procedure, cardiac function should be monitored via telemetry or a continuous cardiac monitor.

Radionuclide myocardial perfusion imaging

- Radionuclide myocardial perfusion imaging is a non-invasive method of assessing myocardial perfusion by IV injection of a radioisotope (usually thallium or technetium).
- Once injected, the isotope is distributed throughout the myocardium in proportion to blood flow and then observed through a gamma camera.
- The test can provide useful information on coronary artery blood flow, ventricular size, and ventricular wall movement.
- These investigations are normally carried out as outpatient or day cases, and in specialist imaging or nuclear medicine departments.

Magnetic resonance imaging (MRI)

- MRI uses powerful magnetic field and radiofrequency pulses to obtain images of the internal structures of the heart.
- MRI can be used to examine various cardiac abnormalities but cannot be used for people with implanted cardiac pacemakers and defibrillators.

Positive emission tomography (PET)

- PET is a specialist scanning technique used to quantify cellular biological activity.
- It is carried out in specialist units and is useful for determining myocardial viability and for distinguishing between normal, infarcted, and hibernating myocardium.

Whilst these clinical investigations may be carried out on people who are hospital inpatients, many can also be completed as outpatient, day-case, or post-discharge follow-up appointments.

Key nursing considerations in acute cardiac conditions

All people admitted to hospital with an acute cardiac episode can be expected to be in a state of heightened distress and anxiety. In a medical emergency situation, it is rarely the case that people are prepared for the disruption caused to their health and well-being, their lifestyle, or their family.

Nurses working with people with acute cardiac complaints have to deal with an urgent clinical condition, and also with all the psychological, socio-cultural, and emotional associations people have with 'the heart'. Irrespective of the acute coronary event and any heightened fear, stress, and anxiety, the patient's well-being can be further compromised by the anxiety of family and significant others.

In these situations, nursing decision-making and practices are framed by professional knowledge, values, and teamwork, and grounded in respectful, empathetic communication skills.

A lot of nursing practice in acute cardiac care is now the domain of specialist and advanced nurse practitioners, but for all people with acute cardiac conditions, key nursing considerations include the following.

Taking a history

- First observe the person's condition, noting any significant factors affecting their haemodynamic state.
- Identify urgent cardiovascular problems such as severe chest pain, breathing difficulties, cyanosis, or altered blood pressure and pulse, and treat as a priority.
- Wherever possible, explore the person's history. Through focused questioning and informed observation, vital information can be gained, even before any diagnostic clinical tests are undertaken.
- Wherever possible, use the opportunity for the person to re-live their experience and tell their 'story'.

A–F clinical assessment

Effective reperfusion therapy for an acute MI is dependent on the treatment being initiated early, ideally within 60 minutes of the onset of symptoms. Therefore, the clinical assessment should be immediate, brief, and focused:
- AIRWAY.
- BREATHING.
- CIRCULATION.
- DISABILITY.
- EXPOSURE.
- FAMILY.

ABCDE(F) assessment

The ABCDE(F) assessment is fundamental to nursing practice in any environment. The acronym should be used when making an assessment of a person's general condition, e.g. on admission to hospital, and always in clinical emergency situations.

The UK Resuscitation Council's ABCDE system allows nurses to make a global judgement about a person in their care, and we also add an 'F' for Family. When a person is unwell, whether in hospital or outside, it may well be that the nurse is the person who assumes, or is given, the task of informing or comforting the family or significant others.

- **A–Airway**: assess airway patency, which should be established prior to moving on to the next part of the assessment. In people who have suffered a trauma, it is important to be aware of the risk of a potential injury to the cervical spine with some airway manoeuvres.
- **B–Breathing**: assess the efficacy of breathing. Any life-threatening conditions, such as asthma, tension pneumothorax, or pulmonary oedema, should be treated immediately.
- **C–Circulation**: assess circulation, and if impaired, treat the cause. Ensure that IV access has been established, in case emergency drug administration or fluid replacement is needed.
- **D–Disability**: assess the level of consciousness (LOC) through noting alertness, voice, pain, and unresponsiveness (AVPU). Aim to establish the cause of any loss of consciousness, as this may require reassessment and urgent treatment of ABC.
- **E–Exposure**: assess the patient's overall condition and any injury by exposing the body for inspection, whilst maintaining the patient's dignity at all times.
- **F–Family**: candour and effective communication with the family and significant others are an important nursing responsibility, particularly when dealing with people in clinical emergency situations.

The outcome of the ABCDE(F) assessment will provide a baseline for risk assessment and monitoring, and determine the next steps to be taken.

ABCDE(F) assessment in clinical emergencies

All healthcare organizations will have their own policies and procedures for responding to clinical emergencies, and these should always be followed.

Most local protocols and procedures will incorporate the UK Resuscitation Council's recommended approach, and the guidelines for basic and advanced life support (www.resus.org.uk/resuscitation-guidelines/abcde-approach/).

The principles of the ABCDE approach to the critically unwell or injured person allow for systematic assessment of both the person and the situation. Each element is assessed and any life-threatening problem corrected, prior to moving on to the next step in the assessment.

The ABCDE approach facilitates early recognition of the need for help, promotes a team approach to emergency interventions and care, and supports ongoing reassessment and evaluation of the person and the situation.

In the community or outside a clinical environment, it may not be possible to correct all the immediate clinical problems, but nonetheless the ABCDE(F) approach should be used to guide assessment and facilitate an accurate 'handover' to the emergency services.

(See also ➔ Chapter 12, Risk assessment and ➔ Chapter 26, Clinical emergencies).

Care and monitoring

In the first instance, nursing care and interventions for a person admitted to hospital with an acute cardiac condition would follow the routine procedures and practices of the organization.

Subsequent nursing decision-making and practice would be determined by the nature of the clinical diagnosis, the needs of the person and their families, and the decisions of the MDT. In a critical or coronary care environment, additional time may be needed to orient the patient and their family to the place of care.

- Accurately measure and record vital signs
- Record ECG, and commence continuous cardiac monitoring according to local protocols.
- Timely and accurate administration and recording of prescribed pain relief, symptom relief, and other medications.
- Ensure IV access, and obtain blood samples (FBC, U&Es, CRP, LFTs, TFT, coagulation screen, and the local cardiac enzyme indicator).
- Administer oxygen, if required, to maintain oxygen saturation at >95% and a comfortable respiratory rate.
- Monitor fluid input/ urine output.
- Continually assess the effects of treatment.
- Accurately monitor and record all observations of the patient's condition, and report any changes to the MDT.
- Clearly explain all actions and interventions to the patient and any family or carers present.
- Give accurate explanations of likely events and investigations such as cardiac angiography.
- Maintain a safe and calming environment for recovery.
- Seek to honestly allay patient and family anxieties.
- As far as possible, ensure physical comfort.

Heart failure

Heart failure is the inability of the heart to pump enough blood through the venous and arterial circulation to meet the body's metabolic needs.

The term congestive cardiac failure is also sometimes used to describe ineffective heart pumping.

Heart failure may involve the right or left ventricle, either independently or together. Although it is a serious long-term condition, people can live a limited, but satisfying, life, supported by medications and lifestyle changes.

Heart failure is normally classified according to the New York Heart Association (NYHA) classification (see Table 15.1).

Left ventricular failure (LVF)

Failure of the left ventricle causes an accumulation of blood in the left ventricle and atria, causing pulmonary oedema in the lungs.

Right ventricular failure (RVF)

Failure of the right ventricle prevents deoxygenated blood from being transferred effectively to the pulmonary circulation. The deoxygenated blood accumulates in the systemic circulation, with corresponding systemic symptoms.

Causes of heart failure

- Coronary heart disease/ACS.
- Cardiac valve disease.
- Arrhythmia.
- Chronic hypertension.
- Cardiac myopathy.
- Certain drugs (β-blockers, anti-arrhythmics, and alcohol).

Table 15.1 New York Heart Association (NYHA) classification of heart failure

Class I	No limitations on physical activity. No fatigue, palpitations, or dyspnoea	
Class II	No symptoms at rest, but ordinary physical activity, such as climbing stairs, results in symptoms	Mild
Class III	Comfortable at rest, but marked limitations in physical activity	Moderate
Class IV	Symptoms at rest and unable to undertake any physical activity without discomfort	Severe

Data sourced from Dolgin M, Association NYH, Fox AC, Gorlin R, Levin RI, New York Heart Association. Criteria Committee. *Nomenclature and criteria for diagnosis of diseases of the heart and great vessels*. 9th ed. Boston, MA: Lippincott Williams and Wilkins; March 1, 1994.

Dyspnoea

- Dyspnoea is a common presenting problem in people with heart failure. Failure of the left ventricle causes pulmonary oedema, which then causes lung rigidity and decreased oxygen transfer.
- Dyspnoea may be associated with exertion but may also occur at rest. In some people with heart failure, shortness of breath may be positional and be brought on when the person is not in an upright position.

Oedema

- Oedema is a common manifestation of heart failure and is characterized by abnormal accumulation of fluid in the interstitial tissues.
- Oedema will collect preferentially in tissues of the limb extremities, and the distribution of fluid is determined by mobility.
- In most people with heart failure, fluid will collect in the legs and feet, but in immobile people, it will collect over the sacrum. The skin classically 'pits' when pressure is applied.
- In acute decompensation episodes of heart failure, oedema can accumulate rapidly and affect the whole of the lower extremities, the torso, and eventually the face. This requires urgent diuretic therapy.

Other symptoms of heart failure

- Limited ability to mobilize or exercise.
- Weight gain due to fluid retention.
- Palpitations.
- Fatigue.

Non-invasive treatment of heart failure

- Diagnosis by echocardiogram is vital to identify the type of heart failure and guide prescription of appropriate medicines.
- Medication to improve cardiac function and reduce accumulation of fluid.
- Oxygen therapy to improve myocardial contractility.
- Fluid and weight management.
- Rest and activity management to reduce cardiac workload.

Invasive treatment of heart failure

- Valve replacement or repair.
- Revascularization.
- ICD.
- Pacemaker (biventricular pacing).
- Intra-aortic balloon pump support.
- Cardiac transplantation.

Lifestyle modifications in heart failure

- Smoking cessation.
- Reduced alcohol intake.
- Reduced salt and fat intake.
- Exercise.
- Fluid restriction.
- Drug therapy.

Common clinical procedures in heart failure

- Clinical history.
- Physical examination and assessment.
- Respiratory examination.
- CXR.
- ECG.
- Respiratory function tests.
- Echocardiogram.
- Blood tests (BNP or NT-proBNP, plasma glucose, creatinine, estimated glomerular filtration rate (eGFR), serum total cholesterol, HDL cholesterol, U&Es, serum calcium, fasting lipid profile, TFTs, plasma glucose, FBC, blood gas analysis).
- Fluid restriction and monitoring.
- Urinary catheterization.
- Daily weighing.
- Regular monitoring of vital signs.

(Details of specific clinical procedures and processes can be found in ➲ *Oxford Handbook of Clinical Skills in Adult Nursing*.)

Key nursing considerations in heart failure

As in all nursing decision-making and practice, nursing care is framed by professional knowledge, values, and teamwork, and grounded in respectful, empathetic communication skills.

Many people who live with heart failure are supported by specialist nurses operating in the community and people's homes. However, on some occasions, people may need to be admitted to hospital. In any environment, nursing practice and decision-making should follow the routine procedures and practices of the organization.

The person admitted to hospital with heart failure may be experiencing an episode of sudden onset or an exacerbation of a long-term condition. Care and treatment would be determined by their clinical condition, the needs of the person and their families, and the decisions of the MDT. Nursing considerations include:

- Accurate measurement and recording of vital signs.
- Accurate measurement and recording of weight.
- Assessing the extent of any oedema and condition of the skin.
- Recording ECG and commencing continuous cardiac monitoring according to local protocols.
- Accurately recording respiratory rate, rhythm, and ease of breathing.
- Recording pulse oximetry.
- Regularly monitor and record all observations of the person's condition.
- Promptly report any changes in the person's condition to the MDT.
- Administering and recording prescribed oxygen therapy, diuretic therapy, and any other medications prescribed for symptom relief.
- Securing IV access and obtaining relevant blood samples.
- Restricting fluid intake (normally between 1.5 and 2L/day) and accurately recording fluid input/urine output.

- Restricting salt intake (avoid replacing with low-salt substitutes which are high in potassium).
- Pay particular attention to areas susceptible to the development of pressure sores.
- Maintain a safe and calming environment for recovery.
- As far as possible, ensure physical comfort.
- Clearly explain all actions and interventions to the patient and any family or carers, allowing time for questions.
- Seek to honestly allay patient and family anxieties.
- Facilitate an understanding of lifestyle management within the limitations of heart failure and/or dyspnoea.

Hypertension

Hypertension (high blood pressure) is defined as a consistent elevation of the blood pressure above 135/85mmHg (℗ www.nice.org.uk). Essential hypertension accounts for >90% of cases and the cause is unknown. Secondary hypertension is due to an identifiable cause such as renal disease, endocrine disease, and rare conditions such as coarctation of the aorta.

Blood pressure can also be raised in normal pregnancy. Hypertension in pregnancy may be associated with the condition pre-eclampsia, which can be fatal to both mother and child (see ➲ *Oxford Handbook of Midwifery*).

- Hypertension is often associated with age, race, culture, heredity, obesity, smoking, high salt intake, excess alcohol use, and emotional stress.
- It is often asymptomatic and may only be discovered on routine examination.
- Hypertension is one of the most important preventable causes of premature morbidity and mortality in adults.
- It is a major risk factor for stroke, MI, heart failure, kidney disease, cognitive decline, and premature death.
- The procedure of measuring blood pressure can itself give rise to extremely high readings, sometimes referred to as 'white-coat' hypertension.

Common clinical procedures in hypertension

- Manual or electronic blood pressure measurement and recording.
- 24-hour ambulatory blood pressure monitoring (ABPM).
- Continuous measurement via (invasive) arterial lines.
- Measurement of albumin:creatinine ratio in urine (laboratory test).
- 24-hour urine collection.
- 12-lead ECG.
- Blood testing (plasma glucose, creatinine, eGFR, serum total cholesterol, HDL cholesterol, U&Es, serum calcium, fasting lipid profile, TFTs, plasma glucose, and FBC).
- Eye examination (for hypertensive retinopathy).

(Details of specific clinical procedures and processes can be found in ➲ *Oxford Handbook of Clinical Skills in Adult Nursing*.)

Key nursing considerations in hypertension

Most people who live with hypertension will be monitored and managed in primary care or community settings. Admission to hospital may be associated with an acute illness episode, which may or may not be related to the pre-existing hypertension. An emergency admission to hospital may itself precipitate hypertension.

- Strive to create a calm and relaxing care environment.
- Accurately measure and record blood pressure.
- Seek to allay patient anxiety during the procedure of blood pressure measurement.
- Explain what the blood pressure measurements mean.

- Accurate and timely administration and recording of prescribed medication.
- Explain how any prescribed medication works, and the need for compliance and concordance.
- Explain the purpose of any blood tests or other clinical investigations.
- Advise people about ways they may manage hypertension.
- Advise and encourage lifestyle changes, diet, exercise, smoking, alcohol, and reduced salt intake.
- Encourage smoking cessation and referral to appropriate support.
- Dietetic referral or dietary advice.
- Annual review to monitor health, lifestyle, symptoms, and medication.

Cardiovascular surgery

People with cardiovascular disease may require surgical intervention at some point. Cardiac surgery is normally carried out in specialist centres or units and may involve cardiopulmonary bypass during the surgical procedure. In the immediate post-operative period, patients will normally be cared for in ICUs.

There are several types of cardiac surgery which vary in severity and risk, depending on the patient's underlying condition and symptoms.

Types of cardiac surgical procedures include, but are not limited, to the following.

Coronary artery bypass graft (CABG)

- This surgical procedure may be offered to people with ACS. The procedure surgically fashions an alternative blood supply to the myocardium.
- A graft is taken from the internal mammary artery or saphenous vein, and is used to bypass a blocked or narrowed coronary artery.
- Depending on the degree of atherosclerosis, one or more of the coronary arteries may be bypassed.

Valve replacement

- This is performed for congenital or acquired diseases of the cardiac valves. Over time, damaged heart valves can severely damage the ventricles and compromise cardiac function and output. Damaged valves are replaced with prosthetic valves.

Aortic aneurysm repair

- An aortic aneurysm is a localized dilation, swelling, or protrusion of the arterial wall and is classified according to location and shape. Aneurysms commonly occur in the aorta but can present in any artery of the body, and ruptured aneurysms can be fatal.
- People with an aneurysm may only become aware of their condition if the aneurysm 'leaks' or ruptures, which is a surgical emergency.
- The presenting signs of a leaking aortic aneurysm may sometimes be confused with the signs of an MI.
- Surgery aims to repair and reinforce the damaged arterial wall.

Embolectomy/thrombectomy

- This is often an emergency surgical procedure for acute arterial occlusion or critical limb ischaemia. It is performed when thrombolysis is not an option.
- The thrombus is removed using a balloon catheter, and the procedure is usually performed under general anaesthesia.

Endarterectomy

- This procedure involves opening the blocked artery and excising the atherosclerotic lesion on the arterial wall.
- With endarterectomy, there is a risk of emboli breaking away from the lesion and causing occlusion in another part of the circulatory system.

Reconstructive bypass surgery

- This may be performed if a person has severe ischaemic pain and ulceration or gangrene in their legs, and is an unsuitable candidate for angioplasty.
- Vascular bypass surgery is done under general anaesthesia and can use prosthetic grafts, or vein grafts taken from the person's saphenous or cephalic veins.

Key nursing considerations in cardiovascular surgery

- In the immediate post-operative period, people who have had cardiac surgery are cared for in an ITU environment. Mechanical ventilator support and invasive haemodynamic monitoring are normally required.
- Specific local care pathways for each condition will inform the organization of care delivery, and for people having cardiovascular surgery, these are likely to focus on:
  - Supporting patients through post-operative recovery.
  - Pain management.
  - Minimizing symptoms.
  - Preventing vasoconstriction and other complications.
- In the longer term:
  - Managing any other associated health conditions.
  - Assisting with mobility and resumption of activities.
  - Timely follow-up for prothrombin times (INR) measurement and regulation of warfarin dose if prescribed.
  - Where people who have received prosthetic valves or grafts, explaining the need for prophylactic antibiotics if dental work or other surgical procedures are necessary.
  - Referral to cardiac rehabilitation services.

People who have had cardiac surgery may not be permitted to drive for a time after their surgery and should seek guidance from the Driver and Vehicle Licensing Agency (DVLA).

The DVLA produces regularly updated medical guidelines on fitness to drive, which includes a comprehensive list of cardiovascular conditions which need to be notified. These can be found at ℘ https://www.gov.uk/guidance/current-medical-guidelines-dvla-guidance-for-professionals.

Useful sources of further information

- *Oxford Handbook of Cardiac Nursing*
- The Resuscitation Council UK ℛ www.resus.org.uk/resuscitation-guidelines/
- National Institute for Health and Clinical Excellence (NICE) ℛ www.nice.org.uk/guidance/conditions-and-diseases/cardiovascular-conditions
- British Heart Foundation ℛ www.bhf.org.uk

Drugs frequently prescribed for cardiovascular conditions

Common drugs used for cardiovascular disorders are listed in Table 15.2. *All drug doses in this table are adult doses only.* This table is only to be used as a guide, and the current *BNF* should be consulted for further advice. Nurses should involve themselves only in the administration of medications which fall within their sphere of competence.

Table 15.2 Drugs frequently prescribed for cardiovascular conditions

Diuretics	Dose	Common side effects
Bendroflumethiazide	Hypertension: 2.5mg each morning Oedema: initially 5–10mg each morning or on alternate days; maintenance dose 5–10mg 1–3 times a week	Postural hypotension, mild GI effects, hypokalaemia, hyponatraemia, hypomagnesaemia, hypercalcaemia, hyperuricaemia, hyperglycaemia, gout, altered plasma lipid concentration
Metolazone	Hypertension: 5mg each morning (maintenance 5mg on alternate days) Oedema: 5–10mg each morning (20mg daily in resistant oedema to a maximum of 80mg)	As above
Furosemide	Oedema: initially 40mg in the morning; maintenance 20–40mg daily, increased to 80–120mg daily in resistant cases	Hyponatraemia, hypokalaemia, hypomagnesaemia, hypocalcaemia
Bumetanide	1mg each morning, repeated after 6–8 hours if necessary; severe cases 5mg daily, increased by 5mg every 12–24 hours according to response; in elderly patients, 500 micrograms daily may be sufficient	As above
Potassium-sparing diuretics	**Dose**	**Common side effects**
Amiloride	Used alone: 10mg daily or 5mg twice daily, adjusted according to response, maximum 20mg daily With other diuretics: initially 5–10mg daily	GI disturbances, dry mouth, thirst, diarrhoea, rashes, confusion, postural hypotension, hyperkalaemia

(Continued)

Table 15.2 (Contd.)

Aldosterone antagonists	Dose	Common side effects
Spironolactone	Dose dependent on indication, but often starting at 100mg, although lower starting doses of 25mg are used in mild to severe heart failure. See BNF for further details.	GI disturbances, hepatotoxicity, confusion, drowsiness, dizziness, gynaecomastia, confusion, hyperkalaemia (discontinue), hyponatraemia

Anti-arrhythmic drugs	Dose	Common side effects
Amiodarone	200mg three times daily for 1 week, then 200mg twice daily for 1 week, then 200mg daily as maintenance or the minimum required to control the arrhythmia (should be initiated in hospital or under specialist supervision)	Nausea, vomiting, taste disturbances, raised serum transaminases (see BNF), jaundice, bradycardia, pulmonary toxicity, tremor, sleep disorders, hyper- or hypothyroidism, reversible corneal microdeposits, phototoxicity, slate-grey skin discoloration
Flecainide	Initially 100mg twice daily reduced after 3–5 days to lowest effective dose	Oedema, pro-arrhythmic effects, dyspnoea, dizziness, fatigue, fever, many more (see BNF)

Beta-blocker drugs	Dose	Common side effects
Atenolol	Hypertension: 25–50mg daily Angina: 100mg daily in 1–2 doses Arrhythmias: 50–100mg daily	Bradycardia, heart failure, hypotension, conduction disorders, bronchospasm, dyspnoea, headache, peripheral vasoconstriction, GI disturbances, fatigue, sleep disturbances, sexual dysfunction
Bisoprolol	Hypertension and angina: 10mg once daily (max 20mg daily) Heart failure: 1.25mg each morning for 1 week, then if well tolerated, stepped increases up to 5mg daily, then more slowly up to 10mg daily	As above
Carvedilol	5mg daily, increased to 25mg daily. May be increased at intervals of 2 weeks up to max of 50mg daily in single or divided doses In elderly people: 12.5mg may be sufficient to control symptoms	Postural hypotension, dizziness, headache, fatigue, GI disturbances, peripheral oedema, painful extremities, visual disturbances, flu-like symptoms

(Continued)

Table 15.2 (Contd.)

Nebivolol	5mg once daily, can be titrated up to 40mg daily	Fatigue, dyspnoea, chest pain, arrhythmias, dizziness, weight gain
Sotalol	Arrhythmias: initially 80mg daily in 1–2 divided doses, increasing to 160–320mg daily in two divided doses, gradually every 2–3 days. Higher doses may be used for life-threatening ventricular arrhythmias	As above, arrhythmias
α-blocker drugs	Dose	Common side effects
Doxazosin	Hypertension: 1mg daily, increased if necessary after 1–2 weeks to 2mg daily and thereafter to 4mg daily, up to a maximum of 16mg daily	Postural hypotension, dizziness, vertigo, headache, fatigue, asthenia, oedema, sleep disturbance, nausea, rhinitis
Prazosin	Hypertension: 500 micrograms 2–3 times a day for 3–7 days (initial dose taken *on retiring to bed*, increased to 1mg 2–3 times a day for 3–7 days, up to a maximum of 20mg daily in divided doses) Other indications: congestive heart failure, Raynaud's syndrome, and benign prostatic hyperplasia for which varying dosage schedules are used (see *BNF*)	Postural hypotension, dizziness, weakness, drowsiness, lack of energy, headache, nausea, and palpitation; urinary frequency, incontinence; and priapism also reported
Vasodilator drugs	Dose	Common side effects
Hydralazine	Hypertension: 25–50mg twice daily Heart failure: (initiated in hospital) 25mg 3–4 times daily, increased every 2 days, if necessary, to maintenance dose of 50–75mg four times daily	Side effects few if dose kept below 100mg daily but include tachycardia, palpitation, flushing, hypotension, fluid retention, GI disturbances, headache, dizziness, SLE-like syndrome after long-term therapy with doses over 100mg daily
Centrally acting anti-hypertensive drugs	Dose	Common side effects
Moxonidine	Hypertension: 200 micrograms once daily in the morning, increasing to 400 micrograms daily in one or two doses after 3 weeks. Maximum of 300 micrograms twice daily	Dry mouth, diarrhoea, nausea, vomiting, dyspepsia, dizziness, insomnia, back pain, rash, pruritus

(Continued)

Table 15.2 (Contd.)

ACE inhibitors	Dose—may need adjustment if diuretic also given (see *BNF*)	Common side effects (NB. Close observation of patient required if diuretic also given; see *BNF*)
Lisinopril	Hypertension: initially 10mg daily (2.5–5mg if used in addition to diuretic or in renal impairment), with usual maintenance dose of 20mg daily Heart failure and prophylaxis post-MI: doses vary, depending on blood pressure, but start low (2.5–5mg) and increased gradually to a maintenance dose of 5–20mg for heart failure and 5mg for post-MI prophylaxis	May cause rapid fall in blood pressure in patients taking diuretics; renal function (i.e. electrolytes) should be monitored before and during treatment; concomitant use of potassium-sparing diuretics increases the risk of hyperkalaemia; other side effects include profound hypotension, renal impairment, persistent dry cough, angio-oedema, rash, tachycardia, cerebrovascular accident, MI, dry mouth, blurred vision, confusion, mood changes, asthenia, sweating, impotence, and alopecia
Ramipril	Hypertension and heart failure: 1.25mg daily, increased at intervals of 1–2 weeks, usual range 2.5–5mg, maximum 10mg Prophylaxis after MI: started 3–10 days after infarction initially 2.5mg twice daily, increased after 2 days to a maintenance dose of 2.5–5mg twice daily Prophylaxis of cardiovascular events: initially 2.5mg once daily, increased after 1 week to 5mg once daily for 3 weeks, then 10mg once daily	As above
Perindopril erbumine	Hypertension and following MI, initially 4mg daily, increased slowly to a maximum of 8mg daily Heart failure: 2mg daily, increased after 2 weeks to 4mg daily, if tolerated	As above

(Continued)

Table 15.2 (*Contd.*)

Angiotensin II receptor antagonists	Dose	Common side effects
Losartan	Hypertension: 50mg once daily (elderly over 75 years, intravascular volume depletion: initially 25mg once daily); if necessary, increase after several weeks to 100mg daily Heart failure: 12.5mg daily, increased weekly to a maximum of 150mg daily	Symptomatic hypotension and dizziness (particularly in patients taking diuretics), hyperkalaemia, angio-oedema, diarrhoea, taste disturbance, cough, myalgia, asthenia, fatigue, migraine, vertigo, urticaria, pruritus, rash
Candesartan	Hypertension: 8mg once daily, (intravascular volume depletion 4mg), increased at 4-weekly intervals to 32mg once daily Heart failure: 4mg once daily, increasing to a 'target' of 32mg once daily	As above

Nitrates	Dose	Common side effects
GTN	Sublingually 300 micrograms–1 mg, repeated as required	Throbbing headache, flushing, dizziness, postural hypotension, tachycardia (paradoxical bradycardia has also occurred)
Isosorbide mononitrate	Initially 20mg 2–3 times daily or 40mg twice daily (10mg twice daily in those who have not previously received nitrates); up to 120mg daily in divided doses	As above

Calcium channel blockers	Dose (NB. Different versions of modified-release preparations may not have the same clinical effect; therefore, patients should normally be retained on the same brand)	Common side effects
Amlodipine	Hypertension or angina: initially 5mg once daily, maximum of 10mg once daily	Abdominal pain, nausea, palpitations, flushing, oedema, headache, dizziness, sleep disturbances, fatigue
Diltiazem	Angina: 60mg three times daily (twice daily initially in the elderly), increased if necessary to 360mg daily	Bradycardia, SA block, AV block, palpitation, dizziness, hypotension, malaise, asthenia, headache, hot flushes, GI disturbances, oedema

(*Continued*)

Table 15.2 (*Contd.*)

Nifedipine	Short-acting forms no longer recommended for angina prophylaxis or hypertension Long-acting preparations—see individual entry in *BNF* for details	Headache, flushing, dizziness, lethargy, tachycardia, palpitations; short-acting preparations may lead to exaggerated fall in blood pressure, and reflex tachycardia which may lead to myocardial or cerebrovascular gravitational oedema. Many more side effects (see *BNF*)
Verapamil	By mouth: Supraventricular arrhythmias: 40–120mg three times daily Angina: 80–120mg three times daily Hypertension: 40–480mg daily in 2–3 divided doses NB. It may be hazardous to give verapamil and a β-blocker together by mouth, unless myocardial function is known to be well preserved	Constipation, nausea, vomiting, flushing, headache, dizziness, fatigue, and ankle oedema
Anti-anginal drugs	**Dose**	**Common side effects**
Nicorandil	10mg twice daily (5mg if prone to headaches), increasing to maximum of 30mg twice daily	Nausea, vomiting, rectal bleeding, cutaneous vasodilation with flushing, increase in heart rate, dizziness, headaches, weakness
Anticoagulants	**Dose**	**Common side effects**
Low-molecular-weight (LMW) heparin, e.g. enoxaparin	For enoxaparin: prophylaxis of DVT in medical patients by SC injection 40mg (20mg if eGFR <30mL/min/1.73m^2) every 24 hours for at least 6 days until patient ambulant (maximum 14 days) Treatment of DVT or PE by SC injection: 1.5mg/kg (1mg/kg if eGFR <30mL/min/1.73m^2) every 24 hours for at least 5 days and until oral anticoagulation established UA and NSTEMI by SC injection: 1mg/kg every 12 hours (1mg/kg once daily if eGFR <30mL/min/1.73m^2) for 2–8 days (minimum 2 days) For other LMW heparins, see *BNF*	Haemorrhage, thrombocytopenia, urticaria, pruritus, erythema

(*Continued*)

Table 15.2 (*Contd.*)

Warfarin	Induction dose 10mg (less if baseline prothrombin time is prolonged, if LFTs abnormal, if patient is in cardiac failure or on parenteral feeding, less than average body weight, elderly, or receiving other drugs known to potentiate oral anticoagulants) daily for 2 days (see local protocol) Maintenance dose dependent on prothrombin time (expressed as INR) and usually 3–9mg *taken at the same time each day* See current *BNF* for more details	Haemorrhage, hypersensitivity, rash, alopecia, diarrhoea, drop in HCT, 'purple toes', skin necrosis, jaundice, hepatic dysfunction; also nausea, vomiting, and pancreatitis *NB. Many drugs interact with warfarin (see BNF Appendix)*
Non-vitamin K antagonist oral anticoagulants (NOACs) e.g. apixaban	Apixaban: stroke prevention in non-valvular atrial fibrillation 5mg twice daily (2.5mg in patients over 80 years with weight ≤60kg), following a discussion with the patient of the risks and benefits, compared with warfarin or other NOACs For other NOACs, see current *BNF* for more details	Nausea, haemorrhage, bruising, anaemia
Antiplatelet drugs	**Dose**	**Common side effects**
Aspirin	300mg as soon as possible after an ischaemic event, preferably given in water or chewed, followed by maintenance of 75mg daily	Bronchospasm, haemorrhage (mainly GI, but others also, e.g. subconjunctival)
Clopidogrel	ACS: 12 months (NSTEMI) or 4 weeks (STEMI) of treatment only—initially 300mg, then 75mg daily, in combination with aspirin Ischaemic stroke: 75mg daily Prevention of atherosclerotic events: treatment should be started within 35 days of MI or from 7 days to 6 months of ischaemic stroke	Dyspepsia, abdominal pain, diarrhoea, bleeding disorders (including GI and intracranial)

(Continued)

Table 15.2 (*Contd.*)

Thrombolytics	Dose	Common side effects
Streptokinase	MI: 1,500,000U by IV infusion over 60 minutes; different schedules for other thromboembolic events (see *BNF* or product literature)	Nausea, vomiting, bleeding, reperfusion arrhythmias, and hypotension; allergic reactions may occur, including rash, flushing, and uveitis; anaphylaxis has been reported
Reteplase	MI: IV injection of 10U over not more than 2 minutes, followed (after 30 minutes) by a further 10U	Nausea, vomiting, bleeding, reperfusion arrhythmias, and hypotension
Lipid-regulating drugs—statins		
Simvastatin	Dose range 10–80mg daily at night (most patients 40mg daily)	Reversible myositis is rare, but significant side effect of 'statins'; myalgia, myopathy, and rhabdomyolysis have also been reported; other side effects include headache, altered LFTs, peripheral neuropathy, alopecia, GI effects, jaundice, dizziness, anaemia, hepatitis, and pancreatitis
Pravastatin	Prevention of cardiovascular events: 40mg at night	As above
Atorvastatin	Dose 10mg once daily; may be increased at intervals of at least 4 weeks to a maximum of 80mg once daily	As above; also chest pain, angina, insomnia, dizziness, hypoaesthesia, arthralgia, and back pain

Neurological conditions

The nervous system

The nervous system's role in all human functions means that neurological disorders will impact on other body systems, so the management of neurological conditions is a complex and specialized area of nursing practice. People with neurological disorders will normally be cared for by specialist clinical teams working in neurological or neurosurgical units or spinal centres.

However, general adult nurses will come into contact with people who have a collection of symptoms suggesting a neurological disorder, and they are highly likely to encounter people who are living with dementia. It is therefore important that general adult nurses can recognize neurological changes and communicate effectively with people who have disorders of their brain or nervous system.

The nervous system includes the brain, the spinal cord, the cranial nerves, and the peripheral nerve pathways. These structures operate motor and sensory functions through voluntary, autonomic, and reflex actions, to control all human functions, sensations, cognition, and emotion.

Disorders of the brain, spinal cord, and nervous system may be manifest through observed changes in physical movements, sensory disorders, LOC, altered behaviour or language, and cognitive or emotional disturbances.

However, observed changes in a person may not always have a primary neurological origin but may be secondary to disorders in other body systems, and vice versa.

Conditions of the nervous system include infections, trauma, degenerative diseases, and malignancy, and in the majority of cases, people with brain, spinal cord, or neurological conditions will need specialist treatment in a neurology, neurosurgical, or spinal unit.

Headaches and brain injuries

Headache is a symptom which may be a transient experience associated with tiredness, hangovers, infections, colds, and flu. They can also be indicative of more serious conditions involving the eyes and ears, and toxicity arising from respiratory, renal, and GI disorders.

Headache is also a common symptom of many neurological conditions, and the type and duration of a headache which a person experiences is an important indicator of neurological disorders.

Primary headaches are those which are not associated with any known pathology and are normally described as migraine, tension, and cluster headaches. Secondary headaches are those related to an underlying pathology such as meningitis, tumours, or subarachnoid haemorrhage (SAH).

'Red flag' headaches

There are some headaches which may be indicative of an underlying neurological cause which requires urgent intervention.

- A sudden severe headache (sometimes known as 'thunderclap' headache).
- Any headache associated with loss of consciousness.
- Persistent headaches that have changed substantially in character.
- Headaches that are caused by coughing.
- Headaches with altered or abnormal pupil reactions.
- Headaches that are worse on lying down and improved by standing.
- Headaches associated with significant scalp tenderness.

Migraine

Migraine is a severe headache which can be accompanied by nausea and vomiting, and sensitivity to light, sound, or smell. The headache may be unilateral or bilateral, and is typically exacerbated by movement. Some people experience numbness and tingling on the face or arms, or, in rare cases, paralysis of an arm or leg on one side of the body. Prior to an episode of migraine, around 20% of people will experience a warning or aura, which can cause flashing lights or other disturbances of vision. Migraine can last between a few hours to several days.

The cause is not known, but migraine tends to run in families and may be associated with the menstrual cycle in women. Migraine may also be brought on by fasting, irregular meals, alcohol, exercise, dehydration, stress, and too much or too little sleep.

Cluster headaches

Cluster headaches are much less common than migraine and are more often seen in men and smokers. Each pain episode tends to be short and very severe. Episodes are usually clustered together in quick succession over several days or weeks, and each headache lasts anything between a few minutes to several hours.

People with cluster headache normally experience intense unilateral pain associated with feelings of agitation and restlessness. The eye on the affected side may water and become blood-shot.

Tension headaches

Tension headaches are usually mild, featureless, and bilateral, and have a variable duration. They are treated with common analgesics, relaxation techniques, and if chronic, amitriptyline may be prescribed (see Box 16.1).

Medication or caffeine headache

Regular or excessive use of any analgesic or caffeine and may produce symptoms similar to migraine or tension headaches. Treatment is withdrawal from the trigger substance, which may itself cause symptoms (see Box 16.1). In the absence of the stimulant, headaches will normally diminish over time.

Box 16.1 Useful treatments for primary headaches

- Regular hydration, food, and sleep.
- Avoiding excessive use of analgesics.
- Reducing caffeine intake.
- Analgesics or non-steroidal anti-inflammatory drugs (NSAIDs), with or without anti-emetics.
- For frequent or disruptive headaches, β-blockers may be useful.
- Biofeedback therapies.
- Relaxation therapies.
- Acupuncture.

Trigeminal neuralgia

Trigeminal neuralgia is irritation of the fifth cranial nerve. It creates brief spasms of very severe pain along the path of the trigeminal nerve in the face and/or jaw. It can be triggered by chewing, eating, speaking, touching the face, or even exposure to the wind. This type of facial pain is common in older people and is normally treated by anticonvulsants, tricyclic medications, or surgery.

Meningitis

Meningitis is an inflammation of the meninges, caused by viruses, bacteria, or fungi, which can affect people of any age. The symptoms of meningitis are headache, neck stiffness, and photophobia, and some people may also have nausea and vomiting, disorientation, and in some cases seizures.

In meningococcal meningitis, a rash is normally present, which does not blanch when pressed. The rash may sometimes appear as 'bruising' in the axilla and groin or around the ankles.

Where meningitis is suspected, a positive Kernig's sign is diagnostic. This is a simple test where the thigh (at the hip) and the knee are flexed at 90° angles, and then an attempt to extend the knee causes pain and resistance.

Treatment of meningitis will be determined by identification of the organism causing the inflammation, which is often made through lumbar puncture and microscopy of CSF.

(For lumbar puncture procedures, see ⟳ *Oxford Handbook of Clinical Skills in Adult Nursing*.)

Encephalitis

Encephalitis is a rare condition where the brain is inflamed, normally as a result of a viral infection. Encephalitis can be focal, affecting one part of the brain, or diffuse. People with encephalitis will typically experience a flu-like illness, followed by changed or abnormal behaviour, altered consciousness, or seizures.

Head injury

This may result in an altered LOC which can be associated with severe, or potentially life-threatening, complications.

The treatment of head injury will be determined by the nature of the injury itself and may necessitate surgery. Where a person has an altered LOC, they will require regular observation and monitoring, as determined by local policies, procedures, and guidelines.

However, common signs which may indicate a deteriorating condition following head injury include:

- Severe headache.
- Nausea and vomiting.
- Seizure.
- Amnesia.
- Irritability or abnormal behaviour.
- Altered pupil size.
- Asymmetrical pupil reactions.
- Glasgow coma scale score falling below 9 or by 2 points from a baseline measure.

(See the Glasgow coma scale in this chapter, p. 264.)

Stroke

Stroke is a source of significant morbidity and is the largest single cause of disability in adults. It is defined as a rapid onset of a focal neurological deficit of vascular origin lasting >24 hours, and there are two main types:

- *Ischaemic stroke*, which is the most common, is caused by atherosclerosis and/or thrombosis in the cerebral circulation. It accounts for between 80% and 85% of strokes. The functional and cognitive effects of the stroke will depend on the location of the compromised circulation and the associated tissue damage in the brain.
- *Haemorrhagic stroke* is less common, accounting for around 10–15% of strokes, and is sometimes referred to as intracranial haemorrhage. This is where a brain injury is caused by blood vessels bleeding into the brain and surrounding structures.

Risk factors for stroke include:

- Hypertension.
- Atrial fibrillation.
- Diabetes.
- Ischaemic or valvular heart disease.
- Increasing age.
- Obesity.
- Smoking.
- Alcohol.
- Diet.
- Family or previous history of stroke or transient ischaemic attack (TIA).

Stroke is most often a sudden event, which requires urgent treatment. Depending on the area of tissue damage in the brain, a person with a stroke may present with any of these symptoms:

- Numbness, weakness, or paralysis in the face or limbs.
- Uncoordination or general 'clumsiness'.
- Altered gait.
- Slurred speech, expressive or receptive dysphasia.
- Visuospatial defect.
- Visual field defect (hemianopia).
- Blurred vision, loss of vision, double vision.
- Confusion or disorientation.
- Difficulty understanding speech.
- Cognitive disorders.
- Severe headache.
- Altered LOC.

Stroke can be fatal, but prompt diagnosis and initiation of treatment can have an important impact on a person's eventual recovery and rehabilitation. In recognition of this, several screening tools have been developed and validated to aid rapid initiation of treatment where stroke is suspected.

These tools are most often used by pre-hospital services and in emergency departments.

- FAST (Face, Arms, Speech, Test) checks the face and arms for weakness and asymmetry, whilst assessing the speech for slurring.
- ROSIER (Recognition of Stroke in the Emergency Room) is a screening tool designed primarily for emergency department use. It builds on the FAST test through the addition of assessment of leg weakness and screening for any deficits in the visual field.

Active management in the initial hours after the onset of a stroke can prevent further infarction of brain tissue and enhance eventual recovery.

The UK NICE produce and update guidelines for stroke management (℞ www.nice.org.uk), and clinical investigations for people who have had a stroke may include:

- Blood pressure measurement and monitoring.
- Doppler carotid imaging.
- Magnetic resonance angiography.
- ECG (if there is a history of atrial fibrillation).
- Echocardiogram (to exclude a cardiac cause, particularly in young people).
- CT scanning of the brain and cerebral circulation.

The first-line treatment for an ischaemic stroke is thrombolysis, but this is only effective within a 4.5-hour window from the onset of symptoms. Thrombolysis is contraindicated in haemorrhagic stroke, so indications for immediate brain imaging in acute stroke include:

- People known to be taking anticoagulation therapy.
- People with a known underlying bleeding tendency.
- A Glasgow coma scale score below 13.
- Unexplained, progressive, or fluctuating symptoms.
- Papilloedema, neck stiffness, or fever.
- Severe headache at the onset of symptoms.

Consistent with NICE guidelines, all people with ischaemic stroke will normally be prescribed antithrombotics or anticoagulants, and statins.

The long-term care and treatment of people who survive a stroke is focused on rehabilitation and the restoration of optimum cognitive and physical functions. This may involve any or all of the following:

- Swallowing assessment and nutritional support.
- Speech and language therapy.
- Movement, mobility, and exercise.
- Continence management.
- Spatial awareness and vision science.
- Psychological assessment and support.
- Cognitive rehabilitation.

Some places have specialist stroke services where intensive multidisciplinary rehabilitation is offered to suitable people. Stroke rehabilitation is likely to involve physiotherapy, occupational therapy, speech and language therapy, dietetics, psychology, and mental health and medical services, both in hospital and the community.

Rehabilitation of people who have had a stroke is often a long-term health project which is challenging for the affected person, their significant others, and the health professionals working with them.

Transient ischaemic attack

A TIA is an episode of focal neurological deficit, which resolves within 24 hours. Symptoms of TIA are similar to those of stroke but normally resolve without treatment. TIA symptoms often subside within a few minutes but can last a few hours.

The risk of stroke for people who experience TIA is substantially increased, and normally the clinical investigations and treatments are the same as for a stroke.

- People with focal neurological symptoms should be treated as though they have had a stroke, until a stroke diagnosis has been excluded by clinical investigation.
- Those who have been diagnosed with TIA should have their ongoing risk for a subsequent stroke calculated using a validated risk assessment tool such as the ABCD2 score.
- The ABCD2 tool is validated to predict the short-term risk of stroke after TIA using five criteria (age, blood pressure, clinical features of TIA, duration of symptoms, and diabetic status), all of which are scored.
- People with an ABCD2 score >4 have a high risk of stroke and should be admitted to hospital for further investigations and possible surgery.
- People who are suitable candidates for surgery may benefit from a carotid endarterectomy.

Cerebral aneurysm

A cerebral aneurysm is a weakness in the wall of one of the blood vessels in the cerebral circulation. Aneurysms typically develop at points of bifurcation of the blood vessels, and the vessels of the circle of Willis are those most often affected. If an aneurysm ruptures, it bleeds into the subarachnoid space, which is known as a subarachnoid haemorrhage (SAH). Cerebral aneurysm can be a cause of sudden death.

People with a cerebral haemorrhage or SAH may have a history of intermittent severe headaches over a period of time (if the aneurysm has been leaking), or they may experience a sudden onset of a very severe headache.

The headache will often be described as a sensation like 'being hit on the back of the head' and is usually associated with neck stiffness, photophobia, and vomiting. The person may also experience loss of consciousness.

A diagnosis of a cerebral bleed is made by lumbar puncture showing blood in the CSF or by CT scan. In some people, a cerebral aneurysm may be repaired by neurosurgery.

Carotid endarterectomy

This is a surgical procedure to remove the sclerotic lining of the carotid artery, which can be carried out using either local[1] or general anaesthesia[2]. Local anaesthesia allows continual monitoring of brain function during surgery.

---

1 NHS Choices. *Local anaesthesia.* ℵ www.nhs.uk/Conditions/Anaesthetic-local/Pages/Introduction.aspx.

2 NHS Choices. *General anaesthesia.* ℵ www.nhs.uk/Conditions/Anaesthetic-general/Pages/Definition.aspx.

Epilepsy and seizures

A seizure is a sudden, excessive, disorderly discharge of electrical impulses in the brain, which causes a temporary alteration in the function of the CNS. A seizure may be an isolated occurrence, which may or may not be related to underlying conditions, and seizures may or may not result in unconsciousness.

Where a person has had more than a single seizure or has a pattern of recurring seizures, this is normally described as epilepsy. Epilepsy affects both adults and children, and onset can be at any time. There are different types, some of which last for a limited time and others which are life-long conditions.

Epilepsy and seizures are also referred to as convulsions or fits, and known causes of seizures include:

- Trauma to the brain.
- Tumours.
- Poisons.
- Drugs.
- High temperature.
- Hypoxia.
- Unknown cause.

Relative to how much of the brain is involved, seizures are either focal or generalized. Focal seizures affect a specific, localized part of one of the lobes of the brain, whilst general seizures affect all lobes.

Seizures can start in any of the cerebral lobes. What happens during a seizure will vary, depending on which lobe and in which part of the lobe the seizure originates. People's symptoms will also be different.

The disordered electrical activity that causes a focal seizure can sometimes spread through the brain and develop into a generalized seizure. In this case, the initial focal seizure acts as a 'warning' which is called an aura.

Auras are usually brief, lasting a few seconds, although some can last for much longer. An aura may manifest as an odd smell or taste, or a visual or perceptual disturbance.

Once the epileptic activity spreads to both hemispheres of the brain, it rapidly becomes a generalized seizure, which is normally manifest as a tonic–clonic, tonic, or atonic seizure.

- *Tonic–clonic seizures* are those most associated with epilepsy.
  - During the tonic phase, the person will lose consciousness, and their body will go stiff.
  - During the clonic phase, the limbs will jerk and there may be urinary or faecal incontinence and clenching of the teeth or jaw.
  - During the clonic phase, a person may stop breathing or have difficulty breathing, and show cyanosis around the mouth.
- *Tonic seizures* are when the person loses consciousness and their body goes stiff, but this will not be followed by the twitching of the clonic phase.
- *Atonic seizures* are where a person loses all muscle tone and drops heavily to the floor. These seizures are normally very brief and the person will often be able to get up again straightaway. However, people having atonic seizures are at risk for injury associated with the collapse.
- *Status epilepticus* occurs when a person has a seizure lasting longer than 30 minutes. This is a medical emergency requiring immediate treatment.

The recovery period following a seizure, known as the post-ictal phase, may be rapid or prolonged. During this period, a person may sleep or appear disoriented. They may also display odd or aggressive behaviour.

In the absence of any obvious underlying pathology, the triggers for many seizures are unknown, but some are:

- Not taking prescribed epilepsy medicine.
- Excessive tiredness.
- Stress.
- Alcohol.
- Drugs.
- Flashing or flickering lights.
- Menstruation.
- Hypoglycaemia.

(For more information on these triggers, see ℘ www.epilepsy.org.uk/info/.)

Paralysis

Paralysis refers to a complete or partial inability to move part of the body due to injury or disease of the brain, spinal cord, or the nerves supplying the muscles. Paralysis can result from stroke, brain tumour, brain abscess, or haemorrhage, spinal cord injury (SCI) or disease, nerve disorders or neuropathies, diseases such as multiple sclerosis and poliomyelitis, and muscle disorders such as muscular dystrophy.

- *Hemiplegia* is paralysis of half of the body.
- *Quadriplegia* is paralysis of all four limbs and the trunk.
- *Paraplegia* is paralysis of both legs, sometimes part of the trunk.
- *Paresis* refers to a significant weakening of affected muscles.
- Upper motor neuron damage causes an increased tightening of the muscles (*spasticity*).
- Lower motor neuron damage causes a reduction or loss of normal tone in the muscles (*flaccidity*).

Paralysis is at its most severe in the early stages after injury or disease, and recovery of function may occur over time. However, paralysis may also be permanent and there is not yet any known cure.

The impact of any type or degree of paralysis will be influenced by how the person and their families are able to adapt and develop coping strategies which allow them to continue living at a level of function and quality of life which is acceptable to them.

Spinal cord injury

An SCI is damage to the spinal cord that may result in temporary or permanent paralysis. An SCI will normally result in a loss of muscle function, sensation, or autonomic responses in all the organs and parts of the body below the level of the injury. Symptoms can vary widely, and people with spinal injuries are normally treated and helped to rehabilitate in specialist spinal units or centres.

Bell's palsy

Bell's palsy affects the seventh cranial nerve and causes paralysis of the facial nerve muscles on one side of the face and often results in 'drooping' of the face and inability to close the eye properly on the affected side.

The cause is not known, but the condition mostly affects adults and is usually reversible. There is no single treatment, although prednisone and aciclovir may be useful.

Dementia

Normal memory function can be affected by stress, tiredness, illness, and some medications, and as people get older, it is normal for them to experience some changes to their memory. However, as the number of older people in the population increases, there are inevitably more people living with more severe memory problems, and the Alzheimer's Society (⅏ www.alzheimers.org.uk) estimates that close to a million people live with dementia in the UK.

Dementia normally affects people over the age of 65 and is more common in women. It is a progressive neurological disorder and manifests as a collection of symptoms associated with an ongoing decline of the brain and its functions, which gets progressively worse over time. Early symptoms of dementia are often mild cognitive impairment, which may not always be recognized and can easily be attributed to a normal ageing process or 'personality' by people and their families and friends.

In the different types of dementia, the underlying structural brain changes may be associated with plaques, sclerotic changes in the cerebral circulation, atrophy, or ischaemia of brain tissue. Dementia may also be a result of head injury or brain tumours. The way symptoms develop and the speed of progression will depend on the underlying cause, as well as a person's general health or other co-morbid conditions. The different dementias are manifest in cognitive and behavioural changes which include:
- Memory loss.
- Reduced mental agility.
- Language and communication difficulties.
- Disorders of understanding and judgement.
- Loss of empathy.
- Compromised decision-making.
- Confusion.
- Apathy.
- Emotional lability.
- Hallucinations.
- Depression.
- Social withdrawal.
- Personality changes.
- Functional dependence.

Dementia is normally classified as Alzheimer's disease, vascular dementia, dementia with Lewy bodies, or frontotemporal dementia (FTD). The different dementias have many similar cognitive and behavioural symptoms, but there are differences, and although the progress of the dementias may be slowed or the symptoms controlled, there is no cure.

Alzheimer's disease

Alzheimer's disease is the most common cause of dementia, which is associated with the loss of neurons and build-up of amyloid plaques. The cause of Alzheimer's disease is unknown, although risk factors include:

- Age.
- Family history.
- Previous severe head injury.
- CVD.
- Lifestyle.

Medications which can temporarily improve some symptoms and slow the progression of Alzheimer's disease include acetylcholinesterase (AChE) inhibitor drugs such as donepezil, galantamine, and rivastigmine. Memantine may be prescribed for people with late-stage Alzheimer's disease.

Alzheimer's disease and vascular dementia often coexist and, in people with both conditions, is known as mixed dementia.

Vascular dementia

Vascular dementia is a disease of the small cerebral blood vessels, which may eventually result in infarction of brain tissue. Ischaemic changes in the brain normally cause processing dysfunctions, rather than memory and language impairment.

The symptoms of vascular dementia can develop suddenly and deteriorate very quickly, although symptoms can also develop gradually over time. People with vascular dementia may experience symptoms similar to stroke, including muscle weakness or paralysis on one side of their body. Predisposing factors for vascular dementia include:

- Age.
- Family history.
- Hypertension.
- Stroke.
- TIA.
- Known sclerotic disease.
- Smoking.
- Diet and exercise.
- High cholesterol.
- Obesity.
- Diabetes.
- Excessive alcohol consumption.
- Atrial fibrillation.
- Genetic predisposition.

The high rates of hypertension and diabetes in people of south Asian, African, or Caribbean ethnicity means they are often at increased risk for vascular dementia.

Medications prescribed to slow the progress of vascular dementia will be related to known co-morbidities and will often include prescription medicines such as ACE inhibitors, β-blockers, statins, antiplatelet drugs, anticoagulants, or diabetic medicines (see also ➲ Chapter 15, Cardiovascular conditions and ➲ Chapter 19, Diabetes).

People with vascular dementia may also be treated with antidepressants. The AChE medications often prescribed for people who have Alzheimer's disease are not useful for treating vascular dementia but may be prescribed in cases of mixed dementia.

Dementia with Lewy bodies

Dementia with Lewy bodies is a type of progressive neurodegenerative dementia closely associated with Parkinson's disease and damage to the substantia nigra tissue of the brain.

Dementia with Lewy bodies has many symptoms similar to Alzheimer's disease, but people with the condition will also usually experience fluctuating levels of confusion, drowsiness, visual hallucinations, and slowing of their physical movements.

The progression of dementia with Lewy bodies cannot normally be treated with medication, but the AChE inhibitors used in Alzheimer's disease may help reduce hallucinations. Other medications that may help control some of the symptoms of dementia with Lewy bodies include drugs used to treat Parkinson's disease, such as levodopa, and antidepressants.

Frontotemporal dementia

FTD is a type of non-Alzheimer's dementia which is characterized by progressive atrophy of the frontal or temporal lobes (or both) of the brain.

Early symptoms of FTD are usually seen as changes in emotions, personality, and behaviour, often with disinhibition. FTD can also result in language problems and word-finding difficulties. FTD is a type of dementia which can affect younger adults.

There is no medication specifically designed to treat FTD, and the AChE inhibitors often used for Alzheimer's disease are not effective. Selective serotonin reuptake inhibitor (SSRI) antidepressants can be used to help control disinhibited or compulsive behaviour, and in extreme cases, antipsychotic drugs may be prescribed if behaviour is putting the affected person or others at risk of harm.

Late-stage dementia

As dementia progresses, memory loss and difficulties with communication often become severe. People may no longer recognize close family and friends, or any details of their life, which can be extremely distressing for all involved.

In the later stages of the disease, people with dementia often need constant help and support in everyday functions such as mobility, continence, eating, and drinking. Some people may become immobile and totally dependent on others, which will put them at a high risk of developing chest or urinary tract infections, dehydration, weight loss, moisture wounds, and pressure ulcers.

Clinical investigations for dementia

Brain imaging

Brain scanning techniques can be used for diagnosing dementia once clinical investigations have excluded other conditions, such as stroke or brain tumour, and NICE (🖰 www.nice.org.uk) recommends MRI scanning for

confirmation of a dementia diagnosis. MRI is particularly useful to show detail of blood vessels where vascular dementia is suspected, or frontal or temporal lobe atrophy if the person may have FTD. Brain imaging techniques include:
- CT.
- MRI.
- PET.
- EEG (electroencephalogram).

The mini mental state examination (MMSE)

The MMSE is not a diagnostic test but is widely used to assess and measure the level of cognitive impairment a person with dementia may have. The test includes simple questions and problems in a number of areas such as orientation to time and place, understanding of words, arithmetic, use of language, comprehension, and basic motor skills.

Blood screening

Blood screening can be useful to assess a person's general health and to exclude other undiagnosed health disorders or conditions which may be giving rise to symptoms similar to those of dementia.

Supporting people with dementia

General nurses may encounter people with dementia who are living in their own homes, or when they are admitted to hospital for investigation or treatment of other health conditions.

There is no cure for dementia, but if detected early, the degenerative process can be slowed and, in some cases, symptoms relieved. Healthcare interventions will normally involve treatment for any underlying or associated health conditions, and lifestyle changes to diet, exercise, smoking, and alcohol consumption.

Care of people with dementia normally involves a multi-professional team approach. The aim is to help the affected person live as independently as possible, whilst supporting the family and significant others.

This may include advanced care planning or lasting power of attorney at the time of diagnosis. It may also involve the periodic use of specialist services such as those offered at day centres and specialist units. Other useful services include:
- Medicines management.
- Occupational therapy.
- Physiotherapy.
- Speech and language therapy.
- Psychological services.
- Cognitive stimulation.
- Art therapy.
- Reminiscence therapy.
- Music therapy.
- Relaxation therapies.
- Social care.
- Home modifications.

In helping people to live with dementia, the UK Alzheimer's Society suggests an extensive range of practical measures such as keeping diaries, labelling cupboards, and writing daily or weekly timetables.

However, if people with dementia are admitted to hospital, the change to their immediate environment can be extremely disorienting and distressing for them, so the way nurses communicate with people with dementia is of central importance (see also ➲ Chapter 7, Dignity and respect).

Degenerative conditions

Multiple sclerosis

MS is a long-term degenerative disease which damages the fatty myelin sheath of nerve tissue throughout the nervous system. There is no known cause, but environmental factors may trigger the condition in people with a genetic susceptibility.

MS is the most common neurological disease affecting young adults, and the peak incidence for onset is between the ages of 30 and 40. It is more common in women than men, and MS is described as one of three types:

- Primary progressive MS (PPMS)—where there is a gradual and continuous deterioration in a person's nervous system.
- Relapsing–remitting MS (RRMS)—deterioration with periods of complete or partial remission from the disease.
- Secondary progressive MS—where RRMS ceases to have relapse periods and the condition begins to deteriorate consistently.

The course and symptoms of MS vary from person to person and often result in increasing weakness and physical disability over time. However, some people may have a 'benign' form of MS and do not develop significant disabilities.

Symptoms of MS may be intermittent or more permanent, and may include any of the following:

- Fatigue.
- Loss of vision.
- Blurred or double vision.
- Limb weakness.
- Poor coordination.
- Balance problems.
- Numbness.
- Pins and needles.
- Bladder symptoms.
- Vertigo.
- Depression.
- Pain.

No single test or procedure can be used to diagnose MS, but lumbar puncture or MRI scanning may be useful. Corticosteroid drugs can be used to treat an acute phase of the condition, and other treatments will be directed to managing specific symptoms such as fatigue, pain, or depression.

Supporting people who are living with MS is likely to involve an MDT approach which may include medical personnel, specialist nurses, physiotherapists, continence advisors, psychologists, alternative or complementary therapists, and social and community care services.

Parkinson's

Parkinson's is a progressive degenerative disorder that damages the substantia nigra of the brain and results in a reduction in dopamine production. This, in turn, gives rise to the typical symptoms associated with Parkinson's disease of tremor, rigidity, and slowness of movement.

Every person with Parkinson's disease will have different degrees of impaired movement, and people with Parkinson's can find that other symptoms such as balance problems, speech difficulties, tiredness, pain, depression, and constipation also impact on their everyday lives. As the condition progresses, people may also experience cognitive difficulties.

The cause of Parkinson's disease is unknown and a curative treatment has not yet been identified. However, symptoms can sometimes be controlled using a combination of drugs, supportive therapies, and occasionally surgery. Medicines that replace dopamine and mimic its action or stop its breakdown, along with drugs that inhibit the action of acetylcholine, can be useful.

As Parkinson's disease progresses, an increased amount of physical care and support is often needed, although some people maintain a good quality of life with limited input from others.

Motor neuron disease

Motor neuron disease (MND) is an uncommon, but progressive, neurological disease that causes degeneration of the motor neuron system, leading to generalized weakness and wasting of the muscles.

The cause is unknown, but the extent of motor neuron involvement will determine the varying patterns of disability. People with MND will often experience stiffness and twitching, muscle cramps, general muscle weakness, respiratory muscle weakness, and speech and swallowing difficulties. Some people also experience emotional lability.

As with many degenerative neurological conditions, treatment is focused on controlling symptoms and supporting the person living with the condition. It includes drugs, physiotherapy, occupational therapy, and speech and language therapies. In some cases, people with MND may need assisted ventilation or parenteral nutrition.

Myasthenia gravis

Myasthenia gravis is a rare and long-term neurological disease which is caused by an autoimmune response that blocks the receptors at the neuromuscular junction.

People with myasthenia gravis experience intermittent periods of weakness and fatigue in selected voluntary muscles, and the severity of the condition depends on the number of neuroreceptors involved.

Depending on the type and severity of the condition, it can be treated by symptom control through medicine, surgery, plasmapheresis, or by IV immunoglobulin treatments. Occasionally periods of assisted ventilation may also be necessary.

Guillain–Barré syndrome

Guillain–Barré syndrome is a rare, but serious, condition of the peripheral nervous system. The exact cause of the condition is unknown, but it may be an autoimmune response to a viral or bacterial infection. The majority of people normally make a full recovery from symptoms, but not all do. Symptoms of Guillain–Barré syndrome include:

- Pain, tingling, and numbness.
- Progressive muscle weakness.

- Coordination problems and unsteadiness.
- Temporary paralysis of the legs, arms, and face.
- Temporary paralysis of respiratory muscles.
- Blurred or double vision.
- Difficulty speaking.
- Difficulty chewing or swallowing.
- Compromised digestion.
- Loss of bladder control.
- Alterations to heart rate or blood pressure.

Treatment will be individually determined by the symptoms the person is experiencing, and normal bodily functions may need to be supported for a period of time. People whose respiratory muscles are affected will need assisted ventilation until they are able to resume spontaneous breathing. Similarly, those people who are not able to swallow may need hydration and feeding support.

Huntington's disease

Huntington's disease is a chronic progressive dementia that causes involuntary movement abnormalities, cognitive deterioration, and affective disturbances. Huntington's disease is a genetic condition that begins to affect susceptible people from around 35–45 years and has no known cure.

People who have a family history of Huntington's disease are offered genetic screening and counselling.

Brain tumour

Brain tumours are classified as primary if they originate in the brain, or metastatic if they originate from a cancer in another part of the body. The most common primary tumours which metastasize to the brain are those of the lung, breast, stomach, and skin.

The most common primary brain tumour is a glioma (arising from the supporting glial cells). Gliomas can be classified as 'low grade' which often grow slowly over years, or 'high grade' which grow rapidly. A more benign type of brain tumour is a meningioma, which originates in the meninges.

The signs and symptoms of a brain tumour may be insidious but can also have a sudden, rapid onset. People with slow-growing brain tumours may show symptoms which are interpreted by family and friends as part of the 'personality' or a sign of a normal ageing process. People with brain tumours may experience some or all of the following symptoms:

- Recurrent headache.
- Drowsiness.
- Altered or fluctuating consciousness.
- Memory problems.
- Intermittent or increasing limb weakness.
- Sensory disturbances.
- Visual disturbances.
- Speech or language difficulties.
- Epileptic fits or seizures.
- Odd or unusual behaviour.

Depending on the site of the tumour, it may be possible to treat brain tumours with craniotomy, microsurgery, radiotherapy, or chemotherapy, and in the case of meningiomas, these can sometimes be removed completely. Steroid, anticonvulsant, and analgesic medicines may also be used.

Cerebral metastases are sometimes treated with palliative radiotherapy or surgery, and in some cases, people may have chemical implants inserted into the tumour cavity.

People who have had a diagnosis of a brain tumour have to inform the DVLA and may not be allowed to drive for up to 2 years after treatment (℘ https://www.gov.uk/government/organisations/driver-and-vehicle-licensing-agency).

(See also ➔ *Oxford Handbook of Cancer Nursing*.)

Craniotomy

A craniotomy is a surgical procedure to open the skull in order to access the brain and cerebral circulation. It is used to treat neurological disorders which need surgical intervention, including tumour removal, aneurysm repair, and treatment of trauma. People who need a craniotomy will be in the care of a specialist neurosurgical unit or centre.

Clinical investigations for neurological conditions

Many neurological conditions do not have an identifiable cause, and people with neurological disorders will manifest their symptoms in very different ways. Motor or sensory symptoms, moods, or altered behaviours can easily be attributed to other causes or disorders of body systems, which can serve to mask an underlying neurological disease.

Absent or abnormal neurological responses can provide useful information to help determine whether a symptom or behaviour is due to a specific neurological condition. Clinical neurophysiology is a specialist branch of clinical investigation which focuses on testing the electrical functions of the brain, the spinal cord, and the nerves in muscles where a neurological disorder is suspected. Clinical investigations often used in neurology include the following.

Lumbar puncture

A needle is passed into the lumbar spine, at L4–L5 or L5–S1 interspaces. A sample of CSF is collected for microscopic examination. (see ⊃ *Oxford Handbook of Clinical Skills in Adult Nursing*).

Electroencephalogram (EEG)

EEG is a recording of the electrical activity of the brain. Electrodes are placed on the person's scalp and a tracing is made.

Evoked potential tests

These are recordings of the electrical responses of the brain and spinal cord to direct stimulation of the senses through sight, hearing, and touch tests.

Electromyography (EMG)

EMG is a recording of the electrical activity of specific muscles, and nerve conduction studies can record the passage of electrical signals along nerves in the limbs.

Imaging techniques

- Plain X-rays of the skull and spine can be used to detect developmental, traumatic, or degenerative bone abnormalities.
- MRI scanning and CT record images and cross-sections of the brain, spinal cord, and soft tissues. Injection of contrast media may also be used in imaging techniques.
- Cerebral angiography involves injecting a contrast medium into the cerebral arterial circulation.
- PET scans are performed after the injection of a radioactive isotope.
- Myelography is the introduction of a radio-opaque liquid into the spinal subarachnoid space, following a lumbar puncture. The flow of the dye is then monitored by fluoroscopy.

Physical examination of people with neurological conditions

A physical examination of people with known or suspected neurological disorders is central to determining an appropriate course of treatment. Physical examination will include assessment of all body systems, but of particular relevance are:
- Motor disturbances and reflexes.
- LOC.
- Pupil size and reactions.
- Intracranial pressure.
- Headache and pain.
- Sensory disturbances.
- Cognitive and behavioural changes.

Motor disturbances and reflexes

Motor functions can be examined by observing a person's breathing pattern, gait, coordination, and movement and resistance in muscles of the arms and legs. Unusual or absent reflexes in the deep tendons of limb joints can also be indicative of neurological conditions (see Figure 16.1).

Level of consciousness

LOC describes people's awareness of self and sensory stimuli in their immediate environment. It is understood as a continuum, ranging from people who are fully aware and awake, through those with mild loss of awareness, to those with a complete lack of response to sensory stimuli.

In neurological conditions, regular assessment and monitoring of LOC are a crucial source of information to guide decision-making. For a rapid assessment of LOC, the AVPU scale can be used.

A = alert
V = responds to voice
P = responds to pain
U = unresponsive

An assessment tool in widespread use for a more detailed assessment of LOC is the Glasgow coma scale. This gives a total score for baseline and subsequent measurements and is useful for monitoring changes in a person's condition (see Table 16.1).

Assessment of LOC, together with observation of vital signs, should always be carried out according to local protocols.

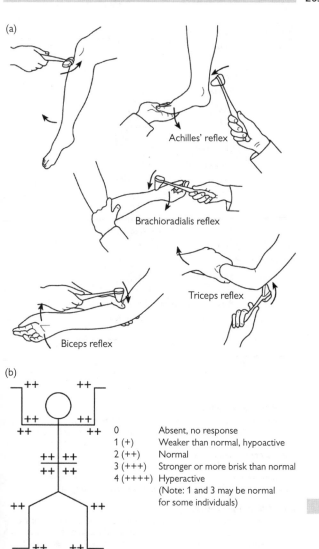

(a)

Achilles' reflex

Brachioradialis reflex

Triceps reflex

Biceps reflex

(b)

0	Absent, no response
1 (+)	Weaker than normal, hypoactive
2 (++)	Normal
3 (+++)	Stronger or more brisk than normal
4 (++++)	Hyperactive
	(Note: 1 and 3 may be normal
	for some individuals)

Figure 16.1 (a) Deep tendon reflexes. (b) Grading of reflexes.

Table 16.1 Glasgow coma scale

Test	Patient's response	Score
Eye opening		
	Spontaneously	4
	To speech	3
	To pain	2
	None	1
Motor response		
	Obeys verbal command	6
	Reacts to verbal command	5
	Identifies localized painful stimulus	4
	Flexes and withdraws from painful stimulus Abnormal flexion (decorticate position)	3
	Flexes and withdraws from painful stimulus Abnormal extension (decerebrate position)	2
	No response	1
Verbal response		
	Oriented and able to converse	5
	Confused or disoriented	4
	Random reply, inappropriate words	3
	Incomprehensible, moans, or screams	2
	None	1
Total score		

Reprinted from *The Lancet*, 2(7872), Teasdale G and Jennett B., Assessment of coma and impaired consciousness. A practical scale, Pages 81–4, Copyright (1974), with permission from Elsevier.

Pupil size and reactions

The size of the pupils and their responses to light can give a useful indication of neurological disorders. The pupils are typically an equal size, with an average diameter of 3.5mm. Maximum constriction should be around 1mm and maximum dilation 9mm. (See Figure 16.2.)

When a beam of light from a pen torch is shone into the eye, a normal pupil response will constrict quickly, and dilate when the light source is removed. Any abnormal reaction should be reported urgently.

Intracranial pressure

For people with head injury, infection, tumours, or other neurological conditions, there may be a small rise in intracranial pressure (ICP) which will affect neurological functions for a short time. However, increased ICP can also be life-threatening and will normally require urgent intervention to reduce ICP. This may be through a medical intervention such as IV dexamethasone or mannitol infusion, or burr-hole surgery.

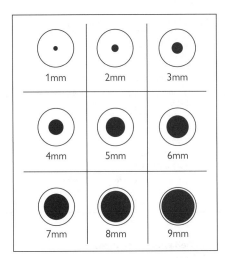

Figure 16.2 Pupil measurements.

In the absence of ICP monitoring devices, a pattern of a slowing heart rate and rising systolic blood pressure may suggest increasing ICP (see Table 16.2). Raised ICP also alters respiratory function and pupil responses.

Headache and pain

A person's experience or description of any headache should be carefully monitored, and particular attention paid to 'red flag' headaches (see also ➲ 'Red flag' headaches, p. 238). Carefully listening to people's descriptions, observing behavioural responses to pain, and the use of pain assessment tools can be useful to inform nursing decision-making.

Sympathetic nervous system responses associated with mild or moderate pain include pallor, elevated blood pressure, dilated pupils, muscle tension, dyspnoea, and tachycardia.

Parasympathetic responses which are associated with severe deep pain include pallor, decreased blood pressure, slow pulse, nausea, vomiting, dizziness, weakness, and loss of consciousness.

Sensory disturbance

Sensory disturbances of the nervous system are normally tested through peripheral stimulation using cotton wool and pinpricks on different parts of the body, which can identify numbness, or absent or unusual sensation.

Positioning of limbs can also be used to test for tremors and positional sense. People may also be able to describe any unusual sensations, numbness, tingling, weaknesses, muscle stiffness, aching, or cramps, indicative of sensory disturbances.

Table 16.2 Signs of increasing intracranial pressure (ICP)

	Early signs	Late signs
LOC	Not easily rousable Some orientation loss Restlessness and anxiety	Unrousable
Pupil reactions	One pupil constricts, then dilates Sluggish to light Unequal	Pupils fixed and dilated
Motor response	Sudden weakness Motor changes Profound weakness	Abnormal posturing
Vital signs	Rise in blood pressure Fall in pulse Change in breathing pattern	High systolic blood pressure Profound bradycardia Abnormal respirations

Cognitive and behavioural changes

Cognitive and behavioural changes in neurological conditions may be very subtle, and unless a person is well known to a healthcare team, it can be difficult to assess or monitor these. Listening to the person's or family's accounts and descriptions provide an important source of information to guide nursing decision-making.

Key nursing considerations

When working with people with neurological disorders, their families, and significant others, all nursing decision-making and practice is framed by professional knowledge, values, and teamwork, and grounded in respectful, empathetic communication skills.

For effective clinical decision-making, it is important to engage with both the person and their family, interpret any information they give within the framework of professional nursing knowledge, and be guided by local policies and procedures to determine an appropriate course of nursing action.

For all people with neurological conditions, these may include:

- Observing and accurately noting the person's general condition and completing all necessary risk assessments.
- In a hospital environment, calculating EWS and adjusting care in accordance with local track and trigger escalation plans.
- Regular and repeated observation and measurement of LOC, pupil reactions, reflexes, and vital signs according to local protocols.
- Ensuring timely and accurate reporting of any observations, clinical measurements, or changes in the patient's condition.
- Maintaining timely and accurate administration of any prescribed medicines, oxygen, fluid replacement, or other therapies.
- Informing the person of any procedures or investigations which are being carried out, even if the person is unresponsive.
- Clearly explaining all actions and interventions to any family or carers present.
- Seeking to clearly and honestly allay patient and family anxieties.
- Maintaining a safe and calming environment for recovery.
- As far as possible, ensuring physical comfort.

(For details of specific clinical procedures, see ❯ *Oxford Handbook of Clinical Skills in Adult Nursing*.)

People having a seizure

- Protect the person by clearing the immediate environment of hazardous objects which may cause injury.
- Protect their head with hands or soft padding.
- Do not move the person unless they are in immediate danger.
- Do not restrain the person or put anything in their mouth.
- Stay with the person to maintain their safety.
- Observe and accurately note the person's general condition.
- Measure and record the LOC according to local protocols.
- When possible, measure blood pressure, heart rate, oxygen saturation, temperature, respiratory rate, and LOC.
- Manage any investigations ordered as part of local care protocol.
- Safely and accurately administer any prescribed IV fluids, and accurately record fluid balance.
- Safely and accurately administer and record any prescribed medications, including anti-epileptic drugs or oxygen therapy.
- Reassess and record vital signs as the clinical condition dictates.

- Ensure timely and accurate reporting of any observations, clinical measurements, or changes to the patient's condition.
- Clearly explain all actions and interventions to the person and any family or carers present.
- Seek to clearly and honestly allay patient and family anxieties.
- Maintain a safe and calming environment for recovery, and as far as possible, ensure physical comfort.

People with long-term neurological conditions

Where people have a long-term neurological condition, the goal of treatment and rehabilitation is, wherever possible, to help the person and their family manage their physical symptoms and achieve a level of function and quality of life which is acceptable to them.

- *Muscular weakness.* Many neurological conditions cause muscular weakness and the associated restrictions on mobility, general movement, or eye–hand coordination. This can result in increasing dependence on others and profound frustration. Physiotherapy and mobility aids may be useful, along with psychological or complementary therapies.
- *Fatigue.* In many neurological conditions, fatigue often worsens as the day progresses. It can be exacerbated by extreme temperatures, poor sleep, pain, stress, inability to exercise, and medications.
- *Visual or hearing disorders.* People with neurological conditions may have hearing or visual disturbance secondary to their underlying neurological condition. These can seriously impact on quality of life, and specialist ophthalmic or audiology services may be needed. (See also ➲ Chapter 21, Conditions of the eyes, ears, nose, and throat.)
- *Vertigo and balance disturbance.* Where a neurological condition has affected balance mechanisms, then a person is likely to be at increased risk of falling and associated injury. Medication or mobility aids may be useful.
- *Bladder dysfunction.* Long-term bladder problems may require the use of catheters or other continence aids. Drug therapy can be useful, and some people may benefit from surgery.
- *Dysphagia.* People who have difficulty swallowing may need support from speech and language services, particularly if there is a risk of aspiration. Dietetic or nutritional services may also help people with dysphagia to maintain an adequate food and fluid intake.
- *Cognitive and emotional disorders.* These may be directly associated with a neurological condition but may also be a consequence of a person learning to live with a physically disabling condition.

Cognitive disorders can affect memory, concentration, abstract thinking, or problem-solving, as well as speech, language, and verbal fluency. Emotional problems may be manifest as depression and anxiety, both of which can be very distressing for people and their families. They can also include extreme mood swings, including anger, irritability, and euphoria.

Cognitive or emotional disorders which are associated with a neurological condition are likely to benefit from referral to specialist psychological or mental health services. Medications may also be useful.

Lifestyle modifications and living aids

Whether people have an acute neurological disorder or a longer-term degenerative condition, rehabilitation to achieve optimum function and quality of life can be a long and difficult project. Some people may never resume their previous level of function, and some will become progressively dependent on others.

Many people and their families will have to learn how to live with and manage a potentially disabling health condition. These people and families should normally be supported by an MDT approach to rehabilitation. People who have a neurological disorder may be entitled to disability living allowance or mobility transport (℅ www.gov.uk/dla-disability-living-allowance-benefit).

In many cases of neurological disease, especially following craniotomy or seizures, the DVLA will need to be informed and a person's driving licence suspended for a period of time (℅ www.gov.uk/government/organisations/driver-and-vehicle-licensing-agency). Air travel may also be restricted.

Living aids which may be useful to people living with neurological disorders include:
• Bath and shower seats and handrails.
• Powered beds and armchairs.
• Handrails and ramps.
• Stair-lifts.
• Wheelchairs.
• Walking sticks and frames.
• Remote controls for electrical equipment.
• Personal alarms.
• Computers, pads, and mobile telephones.
• Adapted cars.

Useful sources of further information

- Alzheimer's Society UK ✍ www.alzheimers.org.uk
- Alzheimer's Disease International ✍ www.alz.co.uk
- Brain and Spine Foundation ✍ www.brainandspine.org.uk
- Dementia UK ✍ www.dementiauk.org
- Spinal Injuries Association ✍ www.spinal.co.uk
- Stroke Association ✍ www.stroke.org.uk
- MS Society ✍ www.mssociety.org.uk
- Epilepsy Action ✍ www.epilepsy.org.uk
- Parkinson's UK ✍ www.parkinsons.org.uk
- DVLA ✍ www.gov.uk/government/organisations/driver-and-vehicle-licensing-agency
- NHS ✍ www.nhs.uk/Conditions
- Disability living allowance ✍ https://www.gov.uk/dla-disability-living-allowance-benefit

Drugs frequently prescribed for neurological conditions

Common drugs used for neurological disorders are listed in Table 16.3. *All drug doses listed in this table are adult doses only.* This table is only to be used as a guide, and the current *BNF* should be consulted for further advice. Nurses should involve themselves only in the administration of medications which fall within their sphere of competence.

Table 16.3 Drugs frequently prescribed for neurological conditions

Control of epilepsy	Dose (NB. Plasma monitoring of blood levels is used to adjust dose)	Common side effects
Levetiracetam	Granules or tablets—up to 1500mg twice daily	Rash, anorexia, nausea, vomiting, diarrhoea, drowsiness, unsteadiness, headache, tremor, amnesia, agitation, aggression, anxiety, blurred or double vision
Phenytoin	Initially 150–300mg daily as a single dose (or two divided doses) with or after food. Usual dose range 200–500mg (dependent on plasma level)	Nausea, vomiting, constipation, paraesthesiae, headache, tremor, transient nervousness, anorexia, and insomnia are common; ataxia, slurred speech, nystagmus, and blurred vision are signs of overdose; gingival hypertrophy can also occur
Sodium valproate	Initially 600mg daily in 1–2 divided doses after food, increasing at 3-day intervals by 150–300mg to a maximum of 2.5g daily in divided doses; usual maintenance dose 1–2g daily	Gastric irritation, nausea, ataxia and tremor, diarrhoea, hyperammonaemia, increased appetite, transient hair loss (regrowth may be curly), oedema, thrombocytopenia and inhibition of platelet aggregation, impaired hepatic function—withdraw immediately; many more side effects (see BNF)
Migraine	Dose	Common side effects
Prophylaxis—use β-blockers (see ➔ Chapter 15)	Propranolol most commonly used at dose of 80–240mg daily in divided doses	See ➔ Table 15.2. Common drugs used for cardiovascular disorders: β-blocker drugs, p. 226
Treatment—use sumatriptan if simple analgesia is ineffective	50mg (some patients may require 100mg) as soon as possible after onset; dose may be repeated in not less than 2 hours if migraine re-occurs, but do not give second dose for *same* attack; maximum dose of 300mg in 24 hours	Sensations of tingling, heat, heaviness, pressure or tightness of any part of body (if intense in throat/chest—discontinue), flushing, dizziness, feeling of weakness, fatigue, nausea, and vomiting (see also BNF)

(Continued)

Table 16.3 (Contd.)

Parkinson's disease	Dose	Common side effects
Co-beneldopa and co-careldopa	Dose varies according to preparation used	Nausea, vomiting, taste disturbances, dry mouth, anorexia, reddish discoloration of urine; many more side effects (see *BNF*)
Cabergoline	Initially 1mg daily, increased by increments of 0.5–1mg at 7- to 14-day intervals to a maximum of 3mg daily	Nausea, constipation, headache, hypotension, drowsiness, abdominal pain
Selegiline	5mg each morning, increasing to 10mg after 2–4 weeks if tolerated	Nausea, constipation, diarrhoea, dry mouth, postural hypotension, mouth ulcers; many more side effects (see *BNF*)
Entacapone	200mg with each dose of co-beneldopa or co-careldopa. Maximum of 2g daily	Nausea, vomiting, abdominal pain, constipation, diarrhoea; urine may be coloured reddish brown

Alzheimer's disease	Dose	Common side effects
Donepezil	5mg once daily at bedtime, increased if necessary after 1 month to 10mg daily (maximum of 10mg daily)	Nausea, vomiting, anorexia, diarrhoea, fatigue, insomnia, headache, dizziness, syncope, psychiatric disturbances, muscle cramps, urinary incontinence, rash, pruritus
Galantamine	Immediate-release: 4mg once daily, increasing to 4mg twice daily, to maximum of 8mg twice daily. Modified-release: 8mg on alternate days to 8mg daily, maximum of 16mg daily	Nausea, vomiting, anorexia, diarrhoea, fatigue, insomnia, headache, dizziness, hypertension, syncope, bradycardia, hallucinations, psychiatric disturbances, muscle spasm, tremor, fatigue
Rivastigmine	Oral: 1.5mg twice daily, titrated to maximum of 6mg twice daily. Also transdermal patches	Nausea, vomiting, anorexia, diarrhoea, fatigue, insomnia, headache, dizziness, bradycardia, arrhythmias, agitation, tremor, confusion, incontinence, sweating
Memantine	5mg once daily to maximum of 20mg daily	Constipation, hypertension, dyspnoea, headache, dizziness, fatigue, vomiting, confusion, thrombosis, hallucinations, abnormal gait

(Continued)

Table 16.3 (*Contd.*)

Multiple sclerosis	Dose	Common side effects
Prednisolone	Dose and route of administration vary	Dyspepsia, oesophageal and peptic ulceration, and candidiasis, osteoporosis, adrenal suppression, weight gain, fluid/electrolyte disturbances, hirsutism, increased susceptibility to infection, ophthalmic disorders, impaired healing, bruising (see *BNF* for more complete list)
Baclofen	5mg three times daily with or after food, increased gradually to a maximum of 100mg daily; discontinue if no benefit within 6 weeks	GI disturbances, dry mouth, hypotension, respiratory and cardiovascular depression, sedation, drowsiness, confusion, dizziness

Gastrointestinal conditions

The gastrointestinal system

The structures of the GI system are normally delineated as upper and lower GI tracts, with the upper GI tract including the mouth, oesophagus, stomach, liver, pancreas, and gall bladder. The lower GI tract relates to the duodenum, small intestine, colon, rectum, and anus (see Figure 17.1).

The function of the GI system is to process all ingested materials, whether nutritious or toxic, and eliminate the by-products of the body's digestive processes.

GI conditions encompass all parts of the GI tract and can range from mild and transient disorders, such as nausea, unrelated to an underlying pathology, through metabolic disorders and obstructions, to life-threatening diseases such as pancreatic cancer or liver failure.

People with disorders of the GI system may be encountered in both hospital and community settings. In the community, people with long-term or other acute health conditions may experience disturbances in their eating patterns or bowel habits, and within hospital, people having treatment for other diagnosed conditions may develop associated GI disorders.

People with severe or long-term GI conditions will often be cared for by specialist nurses, but general adult nurses will encounter people with GI disorders in all areas of clinical practice, either as a primary complaint or as a secondary complication of other illnesses or treatments.

General adult nurses may work with people being treated for specific GI diseases in specialist areas such as those specializing in treatment of liver or pancreatic disorders. People with disorders of the mouth may be admitted to ear, nose, and throat (ENT) units or be cared for by dental practitioners or surgeons.

The nature of the essential functions of the GI system means that general nurses are likely to encounter people with GI disorders in all clinical environments and in the community. The symptoms people with GI disorders experience can be very distressing for them, and in some cases, they can also be socially embarrassing.

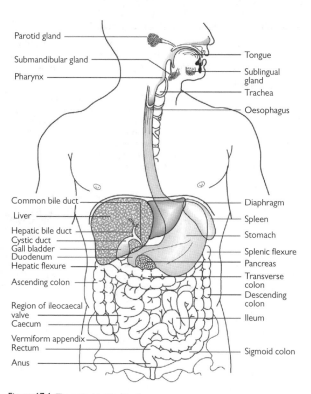

Figure 17.1 The gastrointestinal tract.

Reproduced from George Castledine and Ann Close, *Oxford Handbook of Adult Nursing*, (2009) with permission from Oxford University Press.

Conditions affecting the mouth

Conditions affecting a person's mouth may be a minor disorder but can also be indicative of other underlying diseases. An examination of the mouth can be a useful source of information about a person's general health state.

Dental disorders

Tooth decay and periodontal disease are the most common dental disorders, which often result in severe pain and problems with eating and speaking. Dental decay is normally associated with cavities, nerve damage, and sometimes dental abscess. Wearing ill-fitting dentures can cause mouth ulcers and give rise to yeast infections such as *Candida*.

Dental disorders can normally be prevented by good oral hygiene, regular dental checks, and restricted intake of sugary foods and drink.

Gingivitis

This is inflammation at the gum–tooth margin, which causes redness, swelling, and bleeding of the gums when brushing. Complications include periodontitis, pain, tooth loss, unpleasant tastes, halitosis, and problems with eating.

Glossitis

Glossitis is usually caused by nutritional deficit, and due to atrophy of the papillae, the tongue becomes smooth, sore, sensitive, and erythematous, which causes further problems with eating and drinking.

Stomatitis

Stomatitis is an inflammation of the mouth and can be infective, fungal or viral in origin. Stomatitis will often occur in people who are immunosuppressed or who have severe illnesses, and it may also affect the pharynx and oesophagus, causing dysphagia.

Bacterial stomatitis may be associated with streptococcal sore throat.

Fungal stomatitis is usually caused by *Candida*.

Viral stomatitis may be caused by herpes simplex (cold sores), hand, foot, and mouth disease, and herpes zoster (shingles), as well as glandular fever.

Non-infective stomatitis often has an unknown cause but may be part of other GI problems such as Crohn's disease. Stomatitis is also a feature of iron deficiency, vitamin B_2 deficiency, drug reactions, and Behçet's disease (a multi-organ disease with unknown cause).

Xerostomia

This is a dry mouth, most commonly caused by medication and often where multiple drugs are being used. It is also caused by malfunction of the salivary glands.

Halitosis

This is more commonly known as 'bad breath' and may be a result of dental problems or poor oral hygiene, or may be indicative of disease in other parts of the GI tract.

Mouth cancer

Cancer of the mouth may present in the first instance as a sore or ulcer that is slow to heal, warty lumps or nodules, or white, speckled, or pigmented patches on the oral mucosa. People may also have difficulty speaking and swallowing.

Specialist treatment is by surgery, chemotherapy, and radiotherapy, either alone or in combination, and is delivered by an MDT, normally at a specialist centre.

(See also ➲ *Oxford Handbook of Cancer Nursing*.)

Key features of oral hygiene

- Maintain a schedule of regular check-ups with a dentist.
- Brush teeth with fluoride-based toothpaste at least twice a day.
- Clean the gums as well as the teeth.
- Avoid sugary foods and drinks.
- Ensure an adequate daily fluid intake.
- Maintain a nutritionally balanced diet, with vitamins.

Key nursing considerations in mouth care

When people are unable to attend to their own oral hygiene, whether through GI disorders or other health conditions, nurses are able to make an important contribution to monitoring any underlying disease, and at the same time giving people considerable physical comfort.

Inspection of the mouth can help nurses' clinical decision-making if they suspect a person may be dehydrated and in need of oral or IV fluid replacement therapy.

The aim of oral care is to keep the mucosa and lips clean and moist, prevent infection, remove food debris, and ensure the person's mouth feels fresh and clean.

In the first instance, it is good practice to examine and assess the mouth, noting the general colour and condition and looking for any signs of abnormality, inflammation, infection, abnormal lesions, plaque, and the condition of gums and teeth.

With the tongue forward and down, the back and sides of the buccal cavity can be examined. With the tongue raised, the floor and sides of the buccal cavity can be seen.

- Wear gloves to prevent cross-infection.
- Ensure appropriate recording and reporting of any observations.
- Check for dehydration, and assess the person's ability and/or willingness to tolerate oral fluids.
- Agree a plan to ensure adequate hydration through monitored fluid intake, NG tube, and IV infusion.
- Encourage the person and their family or carers to avoid sugary drinks.
- Check nutritional status, and assess the person's ability and/or willingness to take food orally.
- Agree a plan to ensure appropriate nutrition, monitoring food intake, seeking dietetic advice, parenteral feeding, NG feeding, or percutaneous endoscopic gastrostomy (PEG) feeding.
- Ensure any dentures are removed, cleaned, and replaced.
- Ensure that food is not lodged or retained in the gums or cheeks.
- Use a soft toothbrush with fluoride toothpaste on all surfaces of the teeth, and brush the tongue and other tissues gently.
- Consider the use of chlorhexidine mouthwashes.
- Use soft paraffin to prevent dry lips.

Any local protocols or practice procedures for mouth care should always be followed.

Conditions of the oesophagus and stomach

Oesophageal varices

Varicosities in the veins of the lower oesophagus are normally due to portal hypertension. Oesophageal varices can bleed profusely, and this is an acute emergency.

Treatment is normally by endoscopy and ligation of affected vessels or sclerotherapy and vasoactive drugs (e.g. terlipressin IV). Sclerotherapy involves the injection of a solution (normally saline) directly into the vein. The solution irritates the lining of the blood vessel, causing it to swell and stick together, and the blood to clot.

Hiatus hernia

This is the protrusion of part of the stomach, through the oesophageal opening in the diaphragm. It is a common condition but is not necessarily pathological or symptomatic.

Where symptoms are present, these are normally due to oesophagitis or dysmotility and include dysphagia, peptic ulcer, and possible regurgitation of food at night, with the risk of aspiration pneumonia.

Hiatus hernia is more common in people over 40 and in women, and the condition is often managed conservatively. Conservative management includes dietary advice, eating small portions, not lying down before or after meals, and not eating immediately before bed. Other advice may include weight loss and smoking cessation. In some cases, a hiatus hernia may need to be repaired surgically.

Oesophageal reflux

Reflux occurs when gastric content enters the oesophagus due to relaxation of the lower oesophageal sphincter. It causes heartburn and an acid taste in the mouth.

It may cause oesophagitis, with or without inflammation and erosions of the oesophagus, and is normally treated with antacid medications. A small number of people may develop oesophageal strictures.

To manage the condition over the long term, diet and lifestyle changes are necessary, particularly reduction in alcohol intake and smoking cessation.

Oesophageal strictures

These are normally benign strictures, caused by persistent oesophageal reflux and subsequent scarring. If the stricture is severe, the regurgitation of food is common.

Treatments include controlled radial expansion (CRE) balloon dilatation, along with proton pump inhibitor drugs.

Oesophageal stricture may also be malignant, which would necessitate specialist treatment by surgery, chemotherapy, and radiotherapy, either alone or in combination, normally at a specialist centre.

Oesophageal cancer

Oesophageal cancers are most commonly squamous cell carcinoma, with a small percentage of adenocarcinoma in the distal end of the stomach. It has a poor prognosis because of the tumour's rapid growth, early invasion, and often late diagnosis.

Risk factors include long-term reflux, smoking, and excess alcohol consumption. Patients may feel unwell for a period, have progressive dysphagia, firstly with food and then with liquids, regurgitation, and weight loss. Hoarseness and cough may occur if the upper third of the oesophagus is affected.

Clinical investigations for oesophageal cancer include:
• Endoscopy and biopsy.
• CXR.
• CT scan.
• PET CT scan for staging of the cancer.
• Barium swallow.

Treatments for oesophageal cancer are limited, and radical resection of the tumour is undertaken only if cure is possible. It is therefore not suitable for many people. Oesophagectomy is the surgical removal of the oesophagus and reshaping of the stomach, and is normally undertaken at specialist upper GI surgical units.

Treatment may involve the insertion of a temporary feeding tube. Radiotherapy and/or chemotherapy may be used to shrink a tumour before surgery or for palliation. The insertion of mesh oesophageal stents via endoscopy can also be used to relieve obstruction (꿈 www.cancer-researchuk.org).

Peptic ulcers

Gastric ulcer

Usually occurs in the antrum area of the stomach to people in middle age and has a higher mortality rate than duodenal ulcers.

Risk factors include *Helicobacter pylori* (*H. pylori*), and 60% of gastric ulcers are associated with these bacteria. The use of NSAIDs, smoking, and steroid drugs are also risk factors for gastric ulcers. People with these ulcers normally have epigastric pain, especially after food, which is relieved by lying flat or taking antacids.

Duodenal ulcer

Normally occurs in the upper duodenal bulb of the stomach in middle-aged men. These ulcers are four times more common than gastric ulcers in patients over 40 years of age. More than 95% of non-drug-related duodenal ulcers are due to *Helicobacter*, and the other major risk factor is the use of NSAIDs.

People with duodenal ulcers are often overweight and have epigastric pain that is worse at night. These ulcers are rarely malignant, but they may perforate the wall of the stomach, which necessitates urgent treatment.

The treatment of peptic ulcers focuses on lifestyle changes to reduce symptoms such as eating little but often, reducing alcohol consumption, smoking cessation, and discontinuing the use of NSAIDs. *H. pylori* bacteria can be eliminated by proton pump inhibitor drugs and antibiotics. In some cases, surgery may be required, but this is rare.

Stomach cancer

Stomach cancers are usually adenocarcinoma, and the cause is not fully understood. The known associated risk factors are diet, excessive alcohol consumption, and smoking, and stomach cancer may also be associated with *H. pylori* infection.

Other risk factors include genetics, pernicious anaemia, gastric ulcers, and previous gastric surgery. People with stomach cancer often complain of feeling generally unwell, with anaemia, fatigue, weight loss, dyspepsia, and pain. Vomiting and melaena may also be present.

Clinical investigations for stomach cancer include:
- CT scans.
- MRI scans.
- Ultrasound scans.
- Gastroscopy and biopsy.
- Laparoscopy.
- Barium studies.

Treatment for stomach cancer is normally surgical. Gastrectomy is the surgical removal of part (partial gastrectomy) or all (total gastrectomy) of the stomach and would be offered on the basis of the size and location of the tumour and only if no metastatic disease was present.

Surgery may be combined with chemotherapy and/or radiotherapy, and chemotherapy alone may be offered for palliation if surgery is not an option. Stomach cancers which only involve the stomach lining can sometimes be safely removed by an endoscopy under sedation, known as endoscopic mucosal resection (EMR).

Common side effects of total and partial gastrectomy include reduced gastric capacity, dumping syndrome (rapid emptying of the stomach contents into the small intestine, causing transient hypovolaemia, weakness, faintness, palpitations, and nausea), diarrhoea due to intestinal hurry, vitamin B_{12} deficiency, resulting in anaemia, and iron deficiency anaemia.

(See also ➜ *Oxford Handbook of Cancer Nursing*.)

Key nursing considerations in common gastric conditions

It is often the case that people in hospital or the community, who may be suffering from another health condition, develop one or more of the common gastric disorders of nausea and vomiting, anorexia, or dyspepsia. These conditions may be transient, or they may be related to an underlying pathology. In decision-making and clinical practice, nurses should always ensure that they offer the person any physical comfort they can and also accurately observe, record, and report the person's symptoms.

Nausea and vomiting
- Support the patient during retching and vomiting.
- Remove used vomit bowls and replace with clean ones.
- Offer mouthwashes or oral care to help keep the mouth fresh.
- Help change clothing or bedding as necessary.
- Observe and record the characteristics, amount, and type of vomit.
- Observe for signs of dehydration and electrolyte imbalance (dry furred tongue, decreased urine output, inelastic skin).
- Identify any need for fluid replacement, by IV infusion if necessary.
- Administer any prescribed anti-emetics.
- Observe for signs of malnutrition if vomiting is prolonged.
- Reduce risks of possible complications such as supporting surgical wounds.
- Help position the person to prevent aspiration of vomit.

Anorexia
- Encourage small nutritious portions of food which can be tolerated.
- Administer any prescribed anti-emetics before meals.
- Help position the person to make eating comfortable.
- With prolonged anorexia, undertake a nutritional assessment and refer to a dietician if necessary.

Dyspepsia
- Assess pain and administer any prescribed analgesic, anti-inflammatory, and antacid drugs.
- Evaluate the effectiveness of any prescribed analgesia.
- Discuss strategies to manage pain and discomfort such as positioning after meals and sleeping elevated on pillows.
- Discuss dietary changes and refer to a dietician if necessary.
- Discuss and support smoking cessation and reducing alcohol consumption if relevant.

Gastric or oesophageal surgery

- People requiring stomach or oesophageal surgery may have been assigned an upper GI clinical nurse specialist who will have talked to them about the surgery itself and lifestyle changes that may be needed post-operatively.
- Preoperative dietary assessment is essential and will normally be carried out by a specialist dietician.
- Pre- and post-operative nutrition may involve the administration of high-protein high-calorie supplements, to maximize healing and support the function of the immune system.
- In the immediate post-operative period, patients having oesophageal or gastric surgery may be nursed on a high dependency or critical care unit.
- People having oesophageal surgery will normally have chest drains in place to allow the lung to fully re-inflate after surgery. Local guidelines for chest drain management should always be followed.
- Following stomach or oesophageal surgery, a period of fasting may be necessary, so fluid intake and nutrition will be managed by IV and central venous lines until oral intake can be tolerated. In some cases, jejunostomy feeding may be needed.

In the management of post-operative pain management, wound care, drains, NG tubes, mobilization, and nutrition, local policies and procedures should always be followed (see also ➲ Chapter 22, Surgery).

Liver conditions

The liver, gall bladder, and pancreas are organs of the biliary tract and have a central role in digestion. They are located on the right side of the upper abdominal cavity, and their anatomy is illustrated in Figure 17.2.

The complex functions of the liver include fighting infection and illness, removing toxins from the body, controlling cholesterol levels, facilitating blood clotting, and releasing bile to break down fats and aid digestion.

The liver is the only visceral organ that can regenerate with healthy cells, rather than scar tissue. However, repeated damage or disease will ultimately cause irreparable cirrhosis. Liver disease is now the fifth most common cause of death in the UK (⌘ www.nhs.uk/conditions/liver-disease). Prevalence has risen annually, and what was once thought to be a rare disease is becoming a major health problem. The main causes of liver disease are obesity, undiagnosed hepatitis, and alcohol. All types of liver disease may eventually lead to cirrhosis. Liver disease can be classified as:

- *Alcohol-related liver disease.*
- *Non-alcoholic fatty liver disease* (NFALD)—normally seen in overweight or obese people.
- *Hepatitis*—caused by a viral infection or alcohol.

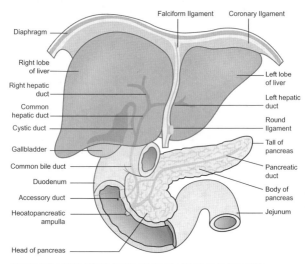

Source: Peate I, Wild K & Nair M (eds) Nursing Practice: Knowledge and care (2014)

Figure 17.2 The liver and biliary tract.

Reproduced from Peate I, *Anatomy and Physiology for Nurses: At a glance* (2015), with permission from Wiley.

- *Haemochromatosis*—a genetic disorder leading to a build-up of iron in the body, particularly around the liver.
- *Primary biliary cirrhosis*—a rare, long-term liver disease that damages the bile ducts in the liver.

Liver disease does not normally cause any obvious signs or symptoms until the condition is well advanced, but symptoms can include loss of appetite, weight loss, and jaundice.

Liver failure

Liver failure may occur suddenly in a previously healthy liver (acute liver failure), but more commonly it occurs as a result of the decomposition associated with chronic liver disease.

Acute liver failure (ALF) is classified as liver failure which has an onset within the previous 6–8 weeks and where encephalopathy is also present. Common causes include:

- Paracetamol overdose (the most common cause of ALF in the UK).
- Hepatitis A, B, and C.
- Drug reactions to NSAIDs, antibiotics (e.g. rifampicin), recreational drugs (ecstasy, magic mushrooms).
- Acute fatty liver of pregnancy.
- Rarer causes include yellow fever, cytomegalovirus, herpes simplex, biliary cirrhosis, haemochromatosis, autoimmune hepatitis, Wilson's disease, and liver cancer (primary or metastatic disease).

Signs and symptoms of acute liver failure include:

- Encephalopathy/cerebral oedema.
- Jaundice.
- Asterixis (hand-flapping tremor).
- Fatigue and lethargy.
- Acute kidney injury (AKI).
- Signs of chronic liver disease (ascites, variceal bleeding, pruritus).
- Signs of infection and fever.

Cirrhosis

Cirrhosis results from necrosis of liver cells followed by fibrosis and nodule formation. There is an irreversible loss of normal liver structure which interferes with liver blood flow and cell function.

The most common causes of cirrhosis are alcoholic liver disease and hepatitis C. Other rarer causes would include chronic hepatitis B, primary sclerosing cholangitis, metabolic liver disease, autoimmune hepatitis, and haemochromatosis.

A diagnostic liver biopsy is the traditional method of confirming cirrhosis. However, less invasive fibro-scans can also be used to assess fibrosis and monitor disease progression. Two types of cirrhosis are described:

- *Compensated cirrhosis*: refers to liver function where bilirubin, albumin, and PT may be normal and the person does not have ascites or hepatic encephalopathy. The aim of treatment is to prevent progression of liver disease (decompensation) and avoid complications.
- *Decompensated cirrhosis*: is normally indicated by the development of jaundice, hepatic encephalopathy, or ascites. The severity of a person's liver disease and cirrhosis, their risk of bleeding, and their overall prognosis can be estimated using the Child–Pugh assessment score (see Table 17.1).

Table 17.1 The Child–Pugh assessment score

Measure	1 point	2 points	3 points
Total bilirubin (micromole/L)	<34	34–50	>50
Serum albumin (g/dL)	>3.5	2.8–3.5	<2.8
PT (s)	<4.0	4.0–6.0	>6.0
Ascites	None	Mild	Moderate to severe
Hepatic encephalopathy	None	Grade 1–2	Grade 3–4
	Class A (Child's A)	Class B (Child's B)	Class C (Child's C)
Total points	5–6	7–9	10–15
Estimated 1-year survival	100%	80%	45c

Portal hypertension

Portal hypertension is a common complication of cirrhosis and occurs when the blood pressure in the hepatic circulation has risen to a dangerous level.

Portal hypertension can be classified according to the site of obstruction. Pre-hepatic obstructions are due to thrombosis in the portal vein. Intra-hepatic obstructions are commonly caused by cirrhosis, and post-hepatic obstructions may be caused by severe heart failure and pericarditis.

In portal hypertension, systemic venous return to the heart is through collateral vessels, normally around the intestines, the stomach lining, or the oesophagus, which are known as varices. Varices are susceptible to rupture, which is a clinical emergency.

Varices

Varices can occur in the lower oesophagus, in the stomach, around the umbilicus, and in the rectum. When the portal pressure gradient is >12mmHg, variceal bleeding may occur. The mortality associated with variceal bleeding is 30–50% per episode.

In this medical emergency situation, a person may become critically unwell in a very short period of time. They may also be very frightened by dramatic bleeding from their mouth or rectum.

First-line treatment is to restore haemodynamic stability with IV fluids and vasoactive drugs. Any clotting abnormalities will need to be corrected, and it may also be necessary to transfuse blood. Treatment may also include urgent endoscopy to establish and treat the source of bleeding.

Ascites

Ascites is the accumulation of fluid within the peritoneal cavity which can be a result of liver disease or advanced malignancy. The condition presents as abdominal swelling, with mild or severe abdominal pain. There may also be associated systemic oedema or pleural effusion.

Ascites can be treated with diuretic medicines but may need to be drained using a hollow trocar, cannula, or catheter in a procedure known as paracentesis.

Paracentesis is a specialist technique which may be carried out in a radiology department, using ultrasound guidance, or in a specialist clinical area.

Hepatic encephalopathy

Encephalopathy is a manifestation of liver disease which may be acute or chronic in nature. It is thought to be caused by neurotoxic substances bypassing the liver and irritating the brain, resulting in altered LOC, cognitive dysfunction, and behavioural changes.

Hepatocellular carcinoma (HCC)

HCC, also known as malignant hepatoma, is the most common type of primary liver cancer. Most cases are secondary to hepatitis B or C or cirrhosis. Treatment will depend on the size of tumour and its staging and would normally be determined by specialist liver services.

Treatment options include liver transplant, surgical resection (which offers the best long-term prognosis but is only suitable for a small number of people), or chemotherapy.

Liver transplantation

People with end-stage liver failure may be assessed at specialist centres to determine their suitability for transplant surgery. The MDT will include transplant coordinators, dieticians, pharmacists, religious representatives, social workers, and, if relevant, an alcohol or substance abuse specialist or counsellor.

Assessment will include consideration of a person's age, disease, prognosis, alternatives to liver transplantation, and physical suitability for surgery. Clinical investigations such as ultrasound, ECG, LFTs, U&Es, FBC, arterial pH, clotting, blood group, and virology will also be carried out.

As with other transplant surgery, liver donors may be cadaveric or living, but there is a general lack of available organ donors. In living donor transplants, a section of the liver is removed from the donor, and as the liver can regenerate, both the transplanted section and the remaining section of the donor's liver are able to re-grow into a normal-sized organ.

Clinical investigations for liver disorders

- LFTs.
- Coagulation screen (PT, APTT).
- Virology (for hepatitis B and C).
- Glucose and fasting lipid profile.
- Immunology.
- Tumour markers.
- Abdominal ultrasound.
- Ascitic tap.
- Abdominal X-ray.
- MRI with contrast to detect liver lesions.
- CT scan.
- Hepatic angiogram/venogram.
- Doppler flow studies of the portal and hepatic veins.
- Neurophysiological studies.
- Liver biopsy.
- Endoscopic retrograde cholangiopancreatography (ERCP).
- Magnetic resonance cholangiopancreatography (MRCP).

Gall bladder conditions

The primary function of the gall bladder is to store and concentrate the bile produced by the liver, and disorders often arise from inflammation or obstruction of the biliary tract.

Acute cholecystitis

Is an inflammation of the gall bladder and is usually caused by a gallstone that cannot pass through the cystic duct. Common signs and symptoms include pain in the right upper abdominal quadrant, vomiting, fever, positive 'Murphy's sign' (severe pain on palpation), local peritonitis, and flatulence.

Clinical investigations include physical examination, blood tests (CRP to assess for an inflammatory response), and ultrasound scanning. Treatment of acute cholecystitis normally requires hospitalization, for fasting, IV fluid therapy, pain relief, and antibiotics if infection is suspected.

Once the acute episode is over, people may be offered surgery to prevent symptoms from re-occurring. Surgery to remove the gall bladder (cholecystectomy) may be by laparotomy, but cholecystectomy can also be carried out laparoscopically. An alternative procedure is percutaneous cholecystostomy where a needle is inserted through the abdomen to drain any fluid that may have built up in or around the gall bladder.

Chronic cholecystitis

If acute cholecystitis is prolonged or a person suffers repeated episodes, it becomes chronic cholecystitis. Signs and symptoms would include vague abdominal pain, abdominal distension, nausea, flatulence, and intolerance of fats.

If chronic cholecystitis is not treated, then the condition can give rise to complications such as pancreatitis or impacted biliary stones.

Acute cholangitis

Acute cholangitis is infection of the bile duct, which is normally caused by a build-up of infected bile secondary to cholecystitis or a stone, tumour, or an infected ERCP stent.

Signs and symptoms would include pain in the right upper abdominal quadrant, jaundice, and rigors, and treatment would include antibiotic therapy and/or treating the underlying cause.

Cholestasis

Is a condition that results from an impairment of bile formation in the liver or obstruction in the flow of bile to the gall bladder. Cholestasis can lead to widespread liver disease and systemic illness. It can be caused by primary biliary cirrhosis (PBC) or primary sclerosing cholangitis (PSC). In both conditions, inflammation leads to progressive thickening, scarring, and destruction of bile ducts inside and outside the liver. Cholestasis may eventually cause cirrhosis or liver failure.

Cancer of the gall bladder

Gall bladder cancer is rare and is most often seen in people over 70 years of age, and the prognosis is usually poor.

Risk factors for gall bladder cancer include a history of gallstones, cholecystitis, gall bladder polyps, abnormal bile ducts, smoking, and obesity. Signs and symptoms include jaundice and right hypochondrium pain, and the diagnosis is often very difficult as symptoms can be mistaken for other diseases such as cholecystitis or cholangitis.

Treatment options depend on staging of the disease, and surgery is only offered if there is no metastatic spread and no vascular involvement.

(See ➲ *Oxford Handbook of Cancer Nursing*.)

Pancreatic conditions

As part of the digestive system, the pancreas has an endocrine function in the production of glucagon and insulin to regulate blood sugar levels. It also has an exocrine function in the excretion of enzymes for the breakdown of proteins, lipids, carbohydrates, and nucleic acids in food.

Acute pancreatitis

Acute pancreatitis is a condition where the pancreas becomes inflamed over a short period of time. It can be fatal in a small percentage of people. Common causes include gallstones and excess alcohol, and less common causes are trauma, use of certain steroids, mumps (rarely), autoimmunity, hyperlipidaemia, a complication following ERCP, or an idiopathic condition.

Signs and symptoms include epigastric or central abdominal pain (which often radiates to the back), vomiting, tachycardia, sometimes fever, diarrhoea, or jaundice.

Most cases of acute pancreatitis improve quickly and do not cause further problems. However, some complications can be severe and life-threatening. These include AKI, shock, poor diabetic control, pancreatic necrosis, pseudocysts or abscess, paralytic ileus, GI haemorrhage, ascites, and malnutrition.

Treatment focuses on supporting the functions of the body until inflammation has subsided, and treatment of the underlying cause. Normally this involves a period of time in hospital for IV fluid therapy, pain relief, nutritional support, and sometimes oxygen therapy.

In cases where there are severe complications, surgical intervention may be necessary, and patients will often be cared for in critical care areas or specialist pancreatic units.

Chronic pancreatitis

Chronic pancreatitis is where the pancreas becomes permanently damaged from inflammation, which is most often a result of excessive alcohol consumption. Chronic pancreatitis may also be idiopathic or genetic in origin.

Signs and symptoms include epigastric pain radiating to the back, which is normally associated with other symptoms such as steatorrhoea, due to an insufficiency of pancreatic enzymes. People with chronic pancreatitis have a higher risk of developing diabetes.

Treatment includes abstinence from alcohol, enzyme replacement therapy, and pain control. Specialist surgery may be necessary.

Cancer of the pancreas

Pancreatic cancer is the fourth leading cause of cancer death in the UK, with a 5-year survival rate of <5% (℗ www.cancerresearchuk.org). The vague signs and symptoms of the disease render it difficult to detect, frequently resulting in late diagnosis, often when metastases are present or a primary tumour is locally advanced. This means that only around 15% of people diagnosed may benefit from potentially curative surgical resection.

No definite causes have been identified, but risk factors are thought to include smoking, drinking alcohol in excess, and high fat intake. There is also a suggestion that the condition could be hereditary in families where two or more family members are affected by the disease.

Signs and symptoms depend on the site of the pancreatic tumour. Tumours in the head of the pancreas commonly present with painless obstructive jaundice. Tumours in the body and tail present with epigastric pain which typically radiates to the back and may be relieved by sitting forward. Either may cause anorexia, weight loss, acute diabetes, or change in bowel habits.

As most people are not suitable candidates for surgery, the majority will be referred for palliative chemotherapy. Palliation of jaundice through endoscopic or percutaneous stent insertion is often considered for tumours in the head of pancreas.

Pancreatic surgery will be carried out at specialist surgical units.

- *Pylorus-preserving pancreatoduodenectomy* (PPPD): this is now the most common surgery for cancer of the head of the pancreas. The procedure involves removing part of the pancreas, the duodenum, the gall bladder, and part of the bile duct.
- *Kausch–Whipple pancreatoduodenectomy* (KWPD): a traditional surgical procedure, similar to PPPD, but involves removing part of the stomach.
- *Total pancreatectomy*: involves removing the entire pancreas, the duodenum, part of the stomach, the gall bladder, part of the bile duct, the spleen, and many of the surrounding lymph nodes.
- *Distal pancreatectomy*: this is used to treat cancers of the body and tail of the pancreas and leaves the head of the pancreas intact. In specialist surgical units, this is now performed laproscopically.

(See also ➔ *Oxford Handbook of Cancer Nursing*.)

Clinical investigations for pancreatic conditions

- A full liver screen (especially if jaundiced).
- FBC.
- U&Es.
- Amylase and CRP.
- Clotting screen.
- Random glucose and/or HbA1c.
- Immunology.
- Genetic studies.
- Tumour markers.
- Abdominal ultrasound.
- CT scan.
- Contrast-enhanced CT.
- MRI scan.
- ERCP.
- MRCP.
- Endoscopic or endoluminal ultrasound (EUS).
- Laparoscopy.
- Faecal elastase.

Key nursing considerations in upper gastrointestinal conditions

There is a dedicated field of biomedical research focused on developing treatment interventions for liver, pancreas, and gall bladder disorders. Many people with these conditions are treated in specialist clinical units by MDTs that specialize in helping people to manage disorders of the upper GI tract.

When nurses encounter these people on general hospital wards, they may be helping them to prepare for surgery or for discharge from hospital. In community settings, they may be helping with rehabilitation or supporting people who are living with a life-limiting condition.

To a large extent, nursing responsibilities will be framed by local policies and procedures and will include:

- Ongoing clinical assessment and observations.
- Timely and accurate monitoring of the patient's condition.
- Timely and accurate record-keeping and reporting.
- Effective communication with the MDT.
- Liaison with specialist services (such as dieticians, pharmacists, clinical specialists).
- Completing any clinical investigations ordered.
- Timely and accurate administration of prescribed medicines.
- Pain management.
- Careful and accurate monitoring of fluid balance status, including daily weighing where indicated.
- Management of nutritional support regimes, including NG feeding.
- Supporting patients, families, and carers in understanding the condition and its implications.
- Working with patients' families and carers to address the psychological and social impact of their condition.

For people having upper GI surgery, local guidelines, as advised by individual surgical units, should always be followed. Post-operative care and management may involve the principles of enhanced recovery with early mobilization and introduction of diet (see also ➔ Chapter 22, Surgery).

Bowel conditions

Diarrhoea

The majority of people will experience diarrhoea at some time, and it can be very distressing and unpleasant until it passes, which can take up to a week. The most common cause of diarrhoea is gastroenteritis as a result of *viruses* (such as norovirus or rotavirus), *bacteria* (such *Clostridium difficile*, *Campylobacter*, and *Escherichia coli*), and *parasites*.

Diarrhoea can also be the result of anxiety, diet, food allergies, some medications, or a long-term condition such as irritable bowel syndrome (IBS). In hospitals or other clinical environments, people may suffer diarrhoea as a result of antibiotic or other medical treatments such as radiotherapy.

Treatment of diarrhoea aims to prevent dehydration, so in severe cases, IV fluids or oral rehydration solutions may be used. Antidiarrhoeal medicines, such as loperamide, can be useful in slowing down muscle movements in the gut, so that more water is absorbed from stools. However, loperamide should only be used when the diagnosis is clear.

Constipation

Constipation is a common condition that affects people of all ages, but which can be particularly distressing in older people. The severity of constipation varies, and it is normally a short-term condition. However, in some people, constipation can become a chronic condition that causes significant pain and discomfort and affects quality of life.

The exact cause of constipation is not known, but contributory factors include:
- A diet lacking in fibre.
- Insufficient fluid intake.
- A change in routine or lifestyle (such as hospitalization),
- Altered eating habits.
- Ignoring the urge to pass stools.
- Side effects of some medications (e.g. opioid analgesics).
- Anxiety or depression.
- Immobility.
- Neurological conditions (e.g. Parkinson's disease).
- Metabolic disorders (e.g. hypothyroidism).
- Pregnancy.

Dietary changes, increased fluid intake, and exercise are normally the first-line treatment for mild constipation. People who are hospitalized or are otherwise incapacitated or have chronic constipation may benefit from oral laxative treatments, suppositories, or micro-enemas.

People with long-term constipation are at risk of developing haemorrhoids, faecal impaction, or faecal overflow incontinence. Although constipation can be treated effectively, it may take several months before a regular bowel pattern is re-established.

Diverticular disease

Diverticulae are herniations in the mucosal lining of the colon, most commonly affecting the descending and sigmoid colon. It is a chronic disorder that is increasing in prevalence. The incidence increases with age and has the potential for complications that significantly impact on quality of life. There are two classifications of diverticular disease:

- *Diverticulosis*: a chronic condition of multiple diverticular formation that develops in middle age. It is typically discovered during routine colonoscopy screening and is often asymptomatic and requires no treatment.
- *Diverticulitis*: is an inflammatory complication of diverticulosis which is further classified as complicated or uncomplicated. People with uncomplicated diverticulitis typically complain of pain in the left lower abdominal quadrant. They may also experience abdominal distension, fever, elevated white blood cell count, nausea, vomiting, abdominal guarding, and urinary urgency with frequency.

Complicated diverticulitis manifests with similar clinical signs, but with the addition of symptoms suggestive of sepsis, GI bleeding, bowel obstruction, bowel abscess, fistula, or peritonitis.

The treatment of diverticular disease varies with the severity of symptoms and focuses on alleviating symptoms and preventing complications. It is often treated with antibiotics and a period of 'resting' the bowel, and people may be admitted to hospital for observation and treatment.

In the long term, the condition can be managed through a low-fat and high-fibre diet, drinking plenty of water, exercising regularly, avoiding the use of laxatives or enemas, and smoking cessation. Avoidance of foods or medications that could cause constipation are also recommended.

Crohn's disease

Crohn's disease is a chronic and incurable inflammatory bowel disorder with a relapsing, remitting, pattern. It can affect any part of the GI tract from mouth to anus, but usually affects the terminal ileum, the ileo-caecal area, or the colon.

It is more common in Western, developed countries and is associated with poor diet, smoking, stress, and infections (e.g. measles virus).

Symptoms commonly include diarrhoea, abdominal pain, rectal bleeding, anorexia, and weight loss. People with Crohn's disease are often susceptible to other inflammatory conditions of joints (arthralgia), skin (erythema), and eyes (uveitis, conjunctivitis).

Complications of the condition include strictures, a higher incidence of colorectal cancer, and fistulae. Clinical investigations include:

- Stool examination (for blood, mucus, consistency, and steatorrhoea).
- Blood tests for erythrocyte sedimentation rate (ESR), FBC, albumin, and CRP.
- Colonoscopy.
- MRI scan.
- CT scan.

People with Crohn's disease will most likely receive long-term care and monitoring by a specialist gastroenterology team. Treatments include the use of corticosteroids, aminosalicylates, antibiotics, immunosuppressive therapy, and anti-diarrhoeal agents. Although not common, the affected area of the bowel can be surgically resected, and people living with Crohn's disease may have other surgery to create a temporary stoma at some point in their illness.

Ulcerative colitis

Ulcerative colitis is also an inflammatory bowel condition, and the predisposing factors, symptoms, clinical investigations, and treatments are similar to those of Crohn's disease. The differentiating feature is that ulcerative colitis only affects the mucous membrane of the rectum and spreads proximally to involve the colon.

Diarrhoea and bleeding are often more frequent in ulcerative colitis, and abdominal pain and tenderness can be severe. In these cases, emergency surgical treatment may be necessary. For people who have severe uncontrolled symptoms, surgery may include subtotal colectomy, ileo-anal pouch, or pan-proctocolectomy.

Coeliac disease

This is a condition where gluten, found in wheat, barley, and rye, stimulates an immunological response which damages the small bowel mucosa.

People with coeliac disease are often asymptomatic but may have symptoms of IBS. In adults, stress seems to be commonly associated with the onset of symptoms. Strict concordance with a gluten-free diet is essential, as non-concordance may result in general ill health, growth retardation, and reproductive problems.

Colorectal cancer

Colorectal cancer is the third most common cancer worldwide, and the risk of developing the disease increases with age (℗ www.cancerresearchuk. org). In the UK, there is a national screening programme for bowel cancer. Risk factors include:
- A diet high in red meat and animal fat.
- Low intake of fibre, fruit, and vegetables.
- Genetic factors.
- Smoking.
- Alcohol abuse.
- Lack of exercise.
- Inflammatory bowel disease.

Presentation and symptoms will depend on the tumour site, and people often experience only vague symptoms such as changes in bowel habit, constipation, or diarrhoea. Other symptoms include:
- Rectal bleeding.
- Blood in the faeces.
- Anaemia.
- Lethargy.
- Unexplained weight loss.
- Abdominal distension.
- Increased flatulence.
- Tenesmus.
- Bowel obstruction or abdominal mass (late stages).

Different staging systems are used to describe the extent of the disease, to plan appropriate treatment, and to predict likely survival. Treatment options for colorectal cancer include surgery, radiotherapy, chemotherapy, or a combination of these interventions.

Surgery

The type of surgery will depend on the site of the tumour and often involves a resection of part of the colon. Some surgical procedures are performed laparoscopically, depending on the type of surgery needed and the specialty of the surgical unit.

For tumours of the colon and upper two-thirds of the rectum, a wide excision of the bowel is made, proximal and distal to the tumour, and an anastomosis of the remaining bowel is made, saving the anal sphincter muscle.

For tumours of the lower rectum, surgery often involves an abdominal perineal resection and creation of a permanent stoma on the abdominal wall.

Early rectal cancers can be treated by local excision through transanal endoscopic micro-surgery (TEM).

Radiotherapy

Is often used as part of the treatment of rectal cancer, either to shrink the tumour before surgery or to reduce the incidence of local recurrence post-operatively. A long course of radiotherapy (around 5 weeks), with or without chemotherapy, can be used as a treatment, whilst short-course radiotherapy (normally 1 week) is most often used palliatively. Single-dose radiotherapy can be used to treat bleeding.

Chemotherapy

Chemotherapy is also used to reduce the likelihood of metastasis, shrink tumour size, or slow tumour growth. It can be used after surgery (adjuvant), before surgery (neoadjuvant), or as the primary therapy in people who may not be suitable for surgery.

Stomas

In some cases of colorectal cancer, surgery may include the creation of a stoma on the abdominal wall. Other indications for a stoma include diverticulitis, Crohn's disease, volvulus, trauma, congenital abnormalities, faecal incontinence, radiation damage, and ischaemia.

A colostomy is formed from the colon and is normally sited in the left iliac fossa, and an ileostomy is formed from the small bowel and usually positioned in the right iliac fossa. A stoma may also be a temporary arrangement.

Stomas can have a considerable impact on self-esteem, sexual functioning, and body image, often leading to feelings of isolation (® www.colostomyassociation.org.uk). A wide range of appliances are available for stoma care and long-term management. People who live with permanent or temporary stomas are normally supported by specialist nurses in hospitals or the community. For general nurses working with people with an established or new stoma, the specialist nursing services should always be consulted.

(See also ➲ *Oxford Handbook of Cancer Nursing.*)

Other therapeutic interventions for bowel conditions

- Polypectomy.
- Balloon dilatation.
- Endoscopic mucosal resection (EMR).
- Stenting.

Clinical investigations for bowel conditions

Blood tests
- FBC.
- ESR.
- U&Es.
- CRP.
- LFTs.
- Serum iron, folate, and B$_{12}$.
- Clotting screen.
- Calcium, magnesium, phosphate, and elements (if malnutrition is suspected).
- Tumour markers if indicated.

Radiological imaging
- CT scan.
- MRI scan.
- Ultrasound imaging.
- CT colonography.
- Magnetic resonance enterography.
- Abdominal X-ray.
- Small bowel enema.
- Barium swallow.
- Barium enema.

Other clinical investigations
- Digital rectal examination.
- Microscopic faecal examination.
- Proctoscopy.
- Rigid sigmoidoscopy.
- Flexible sigmoidoscopy.
- Biopsy.

Key nursing considerations in bowel conditions

People with bowel disorders may be disturbed by alterations in their bowel habits, and very anxious about whether this is a transient disorder or indicative of an underlying pathology.

Many people are also socially embarrassed by bowel disorders and may find it difficult to discuss bodily functions. So, in order to deal with uncertainty and social distress, the key nursing considerations in decision-making and practice are grounded in professional knowledge and values and effective communication and interpersonal skills.

It is important to ensure that people's privacy and dignity are always respected when discussing their bowel condition and when helping them use the lavatory. This is particularly important if a person has to use a toilet, commode, or bedpan in a public space.

In the hospital environment, the effects of restricted mobility, altered diet, medications, and other treatment interventions often mean that people experience changes to their bowel habits, which can then become a focus for other concerns and anxieties.

Nurses should always treat any expressed concerns with respect and, if appropriate, ensure that the MDT are made aware and can prescribe appropriate medication where necessary.

Where indicated, other nursing responsibilities to people with bowel disorders include:

- Always following local policies and procedures for bowel preparation where patients are to have surgery.
- Liaising with specialist support and advice services, if necessary, such as stoma care specialists, cancer nurse specialists, dieticians, and social workers.
- Observing, monitoring, and recording nutrition and diet, and administering nutritional supplements or support where prescribed.
- Observing, monitoring, and recording bowel habits and output.
- Safe and timely administration, recording, and monitoring of pain relief and any other prescribed medicines.
- Maintaining physical comfort.
- Providing timely and accurate information to patients, family, and carers.

Useful sources of further information

- Liver disease ℘ www.nhs.uk/conditions/liver-disease
- Pancreatic conditions ℘ www.pancreasfoundation.org
- Cancer Research UK ℘ www.cancerresearchuk.org
- National Institute for Health and Care Excellence ℘ www.nice.org.uk
- Stomas ℘ www.colostomyassociation.org.uk
- Macmillan Cancer Support ℘ www.macmillan.org.uk/

Drugs frequently prescribed for gastrointestinal conditions

Drugs which are often prescribed for GI conditions are listed in Table 17.2. *All drug doses listed in this table are adult doses only.* This table is only to be used as a guide, and the current *BNF* should be consulted for further advice. Nurses should involve themselves only in the administration of medications which fall within their sphere of competence.

Table 17.2 Drugs frequently prescribed for gastrointestinal conditions

Anti-emetic drugs	Dose	Common side effects
Cyclizine	50mg three times a day	Drowsiness, urinary retention, dry mouth, blurred vision, GI disturbances, hypertension
Metoclopramide	10mg (500 micrograms/kg in three divided doses in adults under 60kg) three times a day. Maximum duration of treatment should be 5 days	Extrapyramidal effects, especially in children and young adults, hyperprolactinaemia
Prochlorperazine	By mouth for acute attack: initially 20mg, followed by 10mg after 2 hours Prevention: 5–10mg 2–3 times daily By IM injection: 12.5mg when required and then given by mouth after 6 hours	Extrapyramidal effects, particularly in children, elderly, and debilitated; drowsiness, dizziness, dry mouth, insomnia
Domperidone	10mg up to three times a day. Maximum of 30mg daily Maximum duration of treatment should be 1 week	Dry mouth, infrequently diarrhoea, drowsiness, malaise, headache. Reports of QT interval prolongation, ventricular arrhythmias, sudden cardiac death
Dyspepsia and gastro-oesophageal reflux drugs	Dose	Common side effects
Compound alginate preparations, e.g. Peptac®	See individual medicines in *BNF*. Taken after meals and at bedtime	Few reported; note some alginate preparations contain significant amounts of sodium

(Continued)

Table 17.2 (Contd.)

Antispasmodics	Dose	Common side effects
Hyoscine butylbromide	20mg four times a day	Constipation, dry mouth, transient bradycardia (followed by tachycardia, palpitations, and arrhythmias), reduced bronchial secretions, urinary urgency and retention, dilatation of the pupils with loss of accommodation, photophobia, flushing, and dryness of skin
Mebeverine	135mg three times daily 20 minutes before meals	Rarely allergic reactions (including rash, urticaria, and angio-oedema)

Ulcer healing drugs	Dose	Common side effects
Ranitidine	Dose and duration vary, depending on aetiology being treated; standard doses are 150mg twice daily or 300mg at night for 4–8 weeks. See BNF for more detail	Diarrhoea, headache, dizziness
Omeprazole	Dose and duration vary, depending on aetiology being treated; standard dose is 20mg once daily for 4 weeks in duodenal ulcer and for 8 weeks in gastric ulcer; maintenance dose for acid-related dyspepsia is 10–20mg once daily	GI disturbances (including nausea, vomiting, abdominal pain, flatulence, diarrhoea, constipation), headache, and increased risk of GI infections such as C. difficile
Lansoprazole	Dose and duration vary, depending on aetiology being treated; standard dose is 30mg once daily for 4 weeks in duodenal ulcer and for 8 weeks in gastric ulcer; maintenance dose for acid-related dyspepsia is 15mg once daily	As above

H. pylori eradication

A range of combination therapies are recommended in the *BNF*. These normally consist of a proton pump inhibitor, e.g. lansoprazole, plus two antibiotics, e.g. amoxicillin, clarithromycin, or metronidazole, for a total of 1 week. Choice of antibiotic will depend on recent antibiotics taken, allergies, and local sensitivity data.

(Continued)

Table 17.2 (Contd.)

Antidiarrhoeal drugs	Dose	Common side effects
Loperamide	4mg initially, then 2mg after each loose stool for up to 5 days (usual dose 6–8mg daily up to a maximum of 16mg)	Nausea, flatulence, headache, dizziness

Laxatives	Dose	Common side effects
Ispaghula husk (bulk-forming agent)	Dose varies with preparation but must be mixed with water before administration	Flatulence, abdominal distension, GI obstruction or impaction
Senna (stimulant agent)	15–30mg at night (initial dose should be low, then increased)	Abdominal cramps, diarrhoea
Docusate (stimulant agent)	Up to 500mg daily in divided doses	See senna
Bisacodyl (stimulant agent)	Oral: 5–10mg at night, increased if needed to 20mg at night Rectal: 10mg in the morning	See senna. Suppositories may cause local skin irritation
Lactulose (osmotic agent)	Initially 15mL twice daily, then adjust according to patient needs	Nausea, vomiting, flatulence, cramps, abdominal discomfort
Macrogol (osmotic agent), e.g. Movicol®	Dose varies with preparation but must be mixed with water before administration	Abdominal distension and pain, nausea, flatulence

Drugs for inflammatory bowel disease	Dose	Common side effects
Mesalazine	Site of action in the bowel and dose vary, according to brand and formulation of preparation used	Diarrhoea, nausea, vomiting, abdominal pain, exacerbation of symptoms of colitis, headache, hypersensitivity reactions
Sulfasalazine	Acute attack: 1–2 g four times a day until remission occurs, then 500mg four times a day	As above plus cough, insomnia, dizziness, fever, blood disorders, proteinuria, tinnitus, stomatitis; urine may be coloured orange; some soft contact lenses may be stained. See *BNF* for further details

(Continued)

Table 17.2 (*Contd.*)

Parasitic infections	Dose	Common side effects
Mebendazole	Threadworm: 100mg as a single dose (if re-infection occurs, a second dose may be needed after 2 weeks) Roundworm: 100mg twice daily for 3 days	Abdominal pain, diarrhoea, flatulence

Digestive enzymes	Dose	Common side effects
Pancreatin	Dose varies with preparation and is adjusted based on size, number, and consistency of stools. Dietary intake will influence dose required	Nausea, vomiting, abdominal discomfort, irritation of the perioral skin and buccal mucosa if product retained in the mouth Perianal irritation can occur with high doses

Stoma care

Enteric-coated and modified-release drugs are unsuitable for patients with stomas (particularly ileostomies), as there may not be sufficient release of the active ingredient. Laxatives, enemas, and washouts should not be prescribed for stoma patients, and antibacterials should not be given for an episode of acute diarrhoea. See the *BNF* for further information.

Preparations for anal and rectal disorders	Dose	Common side effects
GTN rectal ointment	Apply 2.5cm of ointment to the anal canal every 12 hours; maximum duration of use 8 weeks	Burning, itching, and rectal bleeding. See ➔ Table 15.2, Drugs frequently prescribed for cardiovascular conditions, p. 226

A variety of creams and ointments are available for treatment of haemorrhoids. Many contain soothing agents, and others are compound preparations including a steroid or local anaesthetic. Steroid-containing creams/ointments can cause atrophy of the anal skin and steroid-containing products can be absorbed through the rectal mucosa. Excessive application of such compound preparations should be avoided and duration of use limited to a few days only.

Drugs affecting biliary composition and flow	Dose	Common side effects
Ursodeoxycholic acid	Dissolution of gallstones 8–12mg/kg daily as a single dose at bedtime (or two divided doses) for up to 2 years; treatment continued for 3–4 months after stones dissolve	Nausea, vomiting, diarrhoea, pruritus

(Continued)

Table 17.2 (Contd.)

Bile acid sequestrants	Dose	Common side effects
Colestyramine	Pruritus: 4–8g daily in water (or other suitable liquid)	Constipation is common, but diarrhoea can occur; nausea, vomiting, and GI discomfort

Liver failure/ cirrhosis	Dose	Common side effects
Lactulose	30–50mL three times a day (dose adjusted to produce 2–3 soft stools a day)	Nausea, flatulence, vomiting, cramps, abdominal discomfort
Thiamine	Mild chronic deficiency: 25–100mg daily Severe deficiency: 200–300mg daily in divided doses	Few recorded
Vitamin B + C injection	Coma or delirium from alcohol: 2–3 high-potency pairs of ampoules IV every 8 hours	Anaphylaxis may follow injection

Hepatitis B	Dose	Common side effects
Pegylated interferon alfa		Influenza-like symptoms, lethargy, anorexia, nausea, ocular effects, depression
Lamivudine	100mg daily	GI disturbances, myalgia, arthralgia, fever, rash, urticaria, anorexia, nausea, vomiting, diarrhoea, pancreatitis, liver damage, blood disorders, dyspnoea, cough, headache, insomnia, fatigue, peripheral neuropathy, muscle disorders including rhabdomyolysis, nasal symptoms, alopecia

(Continued)

Table 17.2 (*Contd.*)

Transplantation	Dose	Common side effects
Prednisolone	Dose varies	Dyspepsia, oesophageal and peptic ulceration and candidiasis, osteoporosis, adrenal suppression, weight gain, fluid/electrolyte disturbances, hirsutism, increased susceptibility to infection, ophthalmic disorders, impaired healing, bruising (see *BNF* for more complete list)
Azathioprine	1–3mg/kg daily, adjusted according to response	Hypersensitivity reactions (malaise, dizziness, vomiting, diarrhoea, fever, rigors, myalgia, arthralgia, rash, hypotension, interstitial nephritis—calling for immediate withdrawal), dose-related bone marrow suppression, increased susceptibility to infections and many more (see *BNF*)
Tacrolimus	Dose varies according to transplant taken place, patient weight, and whether oral or IV (see *BNF* for details)	GI disturbances, inflammatory and ulcerative disorders, cardiomyopathy, hypertension, and many more (see *BNF*)
Mycophenolate	Dose varies according to transplant taken place (see *BNF* for details)	Taste disturbance, gingival hyperplasia, nausea, constipation, and many more (see *BNF*c

Renal and urinary tract conditions

Kidneys and the urinary tract

Renal conditions can be an acute health problem or a debilitating life-limiting condition. Kidney failure can present as a slowly progressing chronic disease chronic kidney disease (CKD) or as acute life-threatening medical emergencies known as acute kidney injury (AKI). People with chronic kidney failure will normally be cared for by specialist nurses and clinical teams working in hospital or community settings. General adult nurses will encounter people with kidney disease in all areas of clinical practice, either as a primary complaint or as a secondary complication of other disorders or treatments.

The kidneys have a number of critical roles in homeostasis, and functioning kidneys are essential to maintain the body's fluid balance, filter waste products, and produce erythropoietin.

The kidneys (see Figure 18.1) are located in the abdominal cavity, just below the rib cage, one on each side of the spine. They remove salt and other minerals from the blood, returning cleansed blood into the circulation. The glomerular filtration rate (GFR) is the amount of blood that passes through the kidney each minute and is a marker of how well the kidneys are functioning. A GFR rate of 90mL/min or more is the value for normal healthy kidney function. The body's excess waste and fluid are excreted from the kidneys, via the urinary tract (ureter, bladder, and urethra), in the form of urine.

Kidney failure occurs when this essential filtering function is compromised. It is described in stages which represent the decline in the kidney's ability to filter waste products from the blood and produce urine.

Kidney failure leads to a build-up of toxins in the blood and often disrupts the flow of urine. People with kidney disease will experience an alteration in urine output.

- Anuria <100mL of urine in 24 hours.
- Oliguria <400mL of urine in 24 hours.
- Polyuria >3L of urine 24 hours.

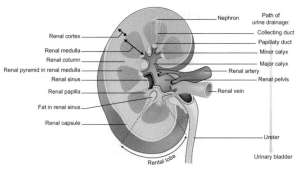

Source: Peate I, Wild K & Nair M (eds) Nursing Practice:
Knowledge and care (2014)

Figure 18.1 Diagram of a hemisected kidney to show its component parts.

Reproduced from Peate I, *Anatomy and Physiology for Nurses: At a glance* (2015), with permission from Wiley.

Renal conditions

Kidney stones

Kidney stones are usually formed following a build-up of calcium, ammonia, uric acid, or the amino acid cystine. They can be a result of an underlying medical condition, previous surgery, long-term dehydration, diet, and some medicines.

Small kidney stones are unlikely to cause symptoms and are often passed painlessly. Larger stones can cause severe pain if they obstruct the renal tract or give rise to a secondary infection.

Kidney stones larger than 6–7mm in diameter may need to be removed by means of procedures such as extracorporeal shock wave lithotripsy (ESWL), ureteroscopy, percutaneous nephrolithotomy (PCNL), or (rarely) open surgery.

Acute pyelonephritis

Is an acute inflammation of the kidney caused by an ascending UTI. Symptoms include pain, rigors, tachycardia, hypotension, urinary frequency, dysuria, cloudy and offensive urine, tenderness over the affected kidney, nausea, and vomiting.

General nurses working in hospital or community sectors may encounter people suffering from acute pyelonephritis, and treatment is normally with antibiotic therapy (% www.nice.org.uk).

Acute kidney injury (AKI)

AKI is common in hospitalized patients and is characterized by a rapid decline in kidney function that is often reversible, but occasionally leads to chronic kidney failure.

Blood plasma concentrations of waste products, including urea, creatinine, and electrolytes, are sampled to assess the level of kidney failure. The GFR is also measured to determine how well the kidney is filtering blood.

Causes of AKI include decreased blood flow to the kidneys (pre-renal causes), direct damage to kidney tissue and structures (renal causes), and obstructions of the urinary tract.

Pre-renal causes

- Hypotension.
- Shock.
- Haemorrhage.
- Sepsis.
- Thrombosis of the renal artery.

Renal causes

- Nephrotoxic drugs.
- Acute glomerulonephritis.
- Vasculitis.
- Multiple myeloma.

Obstructions in the urinary tract

- Cancers of the urinary tract.
- Kidney stones.
- Blood clots.

AKI can be life-threatening; therefore, urgent referral to specialist nephrology services are needed to help manage this condition.

Chronic kidney disease (CKD)

CKD is usually a long-term progressive disease that is characterized by a gradual decline in GFR. It can result in established kidney failure which requires renal replacement therapy in order to maintain life. CKD will show abnormal urinalysis results, with blood or protein present in the urine, and is classified in five stages, illustrated in Table 18.1 (⅏ www.kidneyresearchuk.org).

Causes of CKD

CKD has many causes, the most common being diabetic nephropathy. Other causes include, but are not limited to:

- Hypertension.
- Glomerulonephritis.
- Chronic pyelonephritis.
- Renal vascular disease.
- Polycystic kidney disease.

Symptoms of renal failure

With kidney stones, AKI, or other disorders of the kidneys, people may present with pain, nausea and/or vomiting, disordered urinary function, pyrexia, and abnormal blood and urinalysis results.

Table 18.1 Stages of CKD

Stage of CKD	GFR (mL/min)	Description
GFR 90mL/min or more = healthy kidney function		
1	>90	Normal or high GFR, with evidence of kidney damage
2	60–89	Evidence of kidney damage with a mild decrease in GFR
3	30–59	Moderately reduced GFR
4	15–29	Severely reduced GFR
5	<15	Established renal failure

Uraemic symptoms occur when excessive amounts of metabolic waste products, normally excreted by the kidneys, accumulate in the bloodstream. Uraemic symptoms include:
• Nausea, vomiting, taste changes, loss of appetite.
• Malnutrition.
• Lethargy, poor concentration, drowsiness, confusion, seizures.
• Headache.
• Breathlessness.
• Oedema.
• Skin irritation, itching.
• Bleeding due to platelet dysfunction.
• Anxiety, depression.

Clinical investigations

Where an infection is suspected, the clinical investigations will include microbiology screening of urine and blood to identify the responsible pathogen(s).

Many of the symptoms that people with kidney disease experience are directly related to the altered blood chemistry associated with their disordered kidney function.

For people with AKI, the clinical investigations can be an important part of diagnosis, so that the underlying cause can be effectively treated. For people with CKD, clinical investigations are central to the ongoing monitoring of their health condition and the efficacy of any renal replacement therapy. Clinical investigations include:
• Urinalysis.
• Creatinine clearance test.
• FBC.
• U&E profile.
• LFTs.
• Blood calcium screen.
• Parathyroid hormone screen.
• CRP.
• Abdominal X-ray.
• Renal ultrasound.
• IV urography (IVU) or pyelography (IVP).
• CT scan.
• MRI scan.
• Renal arteriography.
• Renal biopsy.

Treatment of renal conditions

The primary aim of treating renal disorders is to correct blood biochemistry and volume homeostasis, and to filter the waste products of metabolism effectively.

Most people with known kidney disease will need to be managed by specialist nephrology teams, either in hospital or the community.

Treatment of AKI

If a person with AKI is not already hospitalized, they will need urgent admission and review by renal specialists. The treatment of AKI will depend on the results of clinical investigations, and treatment may include fluid resuscitation or fluid restriction.

AKI can sometimes result in people receiving short-term renal replacement therapy until the kidneys have stabilized and an adequate level of function is restored.

Treatment of CKD

Treatment of CKD will depend on the stage of the disease.
- Stages 1 and 2 can often be managed conservatively with lifestyle changes and minimal disruption to everyday life.
- Stages 3–4 are usually managed by renal specialist services and include regular monitoring and control of blood biochemistry, blood pressure, and symptoms.
- Stage 5 patients are offered conservative management, renal replacement therapy, or transplantation.

Conservative management

Conservative management treats kidney failure without renal replacement therapy or transplantation. This is often the treatment option in early-stage CKD or when renal replacement therapy may not improve survival.

The focus of conservative treatment is individualized symptom management, preservation of remaining kidney function, and achieving the best possible quality life.

Renal replacement therapy

Renal replacement therapy is most often referred to as dialysis, which is the process of passing blood across a membrane to remove excess waste and fluid from the body when the kidneys have failed. Dialysis works by processes of diffusion, osmosis, and ultra-filtration.
- *Diffusion* is the movement of solutes from a high concentration to a lower concentration.
- *Osmosis* is the diffusion of water from a higher concentration to a lower concentration.
- *Ultra-filtration* is the process of solute removal using a pressure gradient.
- *Dialysate* is the solution used on the opposite side of a membrane (to blood) and is made up of electrolytes and other substances, including glucose.

Dialysis can be performed in hospital or at home, depending on the person's dialysis choice and clinical circumstances. There are two types of dialysis.

Peritoneal dialysis (PD)

The peritoneum lining the abdominal cavity is used as the membrane through which dialysis is achieved. A catheter tube is inserted into the abdominal cavity and dialysis fluid infused into the peritoneum, via the catheter, and is left for a period of time.

By means of the processes of diffusion and osmosis, waste products and water are removed from the blood. The dialysate fluid containing these waste products and excess water is then drained from the peritoneal cavity and discarded.

Peritoneal dialysis can be carried out as continuous ambulatory peritoneal dialysis (CAPD) or automated peritoneal dialysis (APD).

- *CAPD* is a manual process which allows a person to carry out their normal daily activities. Dialysate infused into the peritoneal cavity is left in the peritoneum for between 4 and 10 hours and then drained. This process is repeated at regular intervals during the day, and the final infusion of dialysate is left in the abdomen overnight.
- *APD* is performed overnight by a machine. It carries out the exchanges of dialysate automatically, whilst the person sleeps.

CAPD and APD can be carried out in non-specialist clinical areas or people's homes.

Haemodialysis (HD)

HD involves a person with renal failure being connected to a dialysis machine, usually for several days each week. This can be done in a specialist hospital setting or in an appropriately prepared environment at home.

In HD, the person's blood is transported via the machine through a semi-permeable membrane known as the artificial kidney. Waste products pass through this membrane into a dialysate solution, and excess water is pulled across the membrane using a preset pressure gradient in the dialysis machine. The 'clean' blood is then returned safely to the body.

This process is repeated throughout the dialysis session. Dialysis machines can also be used for haemofiltration (HF) and haemodiafiltration (HDF).

- HF is similar to HD but is often used for urgent or acute treatment. HF uses convection (pulling solutes across the membrane with water) to achieve blood clearance and fluid removal, and there is minimal diffusion.
- HDF is a combination treatment of both HD and HF.

For any of these HD treatments, direct access to the blood circulation is essential, and this can be through a central venous catheter or an arterio-venous fistula (AVF).

Central venous catheter

This is a narrow tube inserted into the jugular, subclavian, or femoral vein to gain access to the person's circulation. Central venous catheters can be secured under the skin if circulatory access is going to be needed for longer than 5 days.

Central venous catheters are usually a temporary measure until such time as an AVF can be created.

To minimize complications and infection, catheters inserted for dialysis therapy should only be used for dialysis and only accessed by health professional staff who are trained in their use.

Arteriovenous fistula (AVF)

An AVF is created by a surgical procedure where one of the arteries in the arm is re-routed to join a vein. An alternative to an AVF is the insertion of a synthetic polytetrafluoroethylene (PTFE) graft. See Figure 18.2.

Fistulae and grafts should only be used for dialysis access and never accessed by any staff who are not trained in their use. *Where a person has an AVF for dialysis, that arm should never be used for measuring blood pressure or any other clinical procedure.*

Complications of dialysis

For people having HD over a period of time, there are several potential complications associated with the procedure, which can seriously compromise well-being, and some of which will require urgent interventions.

- Infection.
- Hypotension.
- Needle dislodgement.
- Cramp.
- Dialysis disequilibrium syndrome.
- Acute reactions.
- Atherosclerotic vascular disease.
- Hypertension.
- Renal bone disease.
- Anaemia.

Transplantation

Kidney transplantation is often the desired treatment for people with CKD. However, there is a dearth of organ donors, and the average wait for a suitable kidney from a deceased donor is 2–3 years (🔊 www.nhs.uk). Many people wait much longer than this, and some become too ill to undergo transplant surgery, even when a suitable organ match is available.

Many countries operate organ donor registers, and in some places, the system is an 'opt out' where everyone is assumed to be a potential donor unless they specify otherwise. Other countries operate an 'opt in' system where people need to register their wish to be an organ donor (🔊 www. organdonation.nhs.uk).

Deceased donor organs are retrieved from people who have been certified as brainstem-dead. Consent can be given either as an advance directive from the donor or after death by their next of kin.

Live donor transplantation gives the transplanted kidney a greater chance of survival, and often waiting times are shorter. Live donors can be a relative (live related), or a partner, friend, or person unknown to the patient (live unrelated).

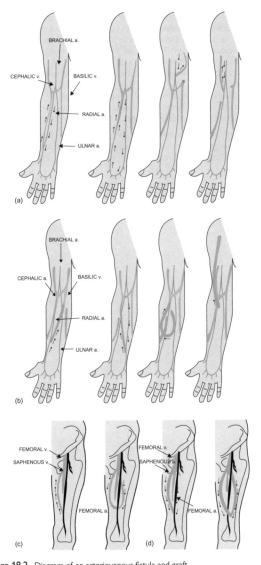

Figure 18.2. Diagram of an arteriovenous fistula and graft.

Reproduced from Nissenson A R and Fine R N, *Handbook of Dialysis therapy* 5e (2016), with permission from Elsevier.

For live donor transplants, both donor and recipient must undergo rigorous testing to ensure that they are both fit enough to undergo surgery and that there is an adequate tissue match to minimize the chances of rejection of the transplanted kidney. The risk of the donor or recipient developing renal problems in the future must also be considered.

Kidney transplant, whether from cadaveric or live donors, is not without risks. These include:
- Surgical risks related to the transplant procedure itself.
- Risks related to long-term use of immunosuppressant medicines.
- Rejection of the transplanted kidney.

Whilst complications of transplant surgery often occur in the period immediately following surgery, they can also develop many years later, and people living with a kidney transplant need long-term monitoring and support.

Key nursing considerations in renal conditions

When working with people with renal conditions, nursing decision-making and practice is focused on specialist knowledge and skills. It also relies on effective communication skills necessary for supporting the person and their family, who are living with a disruptive and potentially life-limiting condition.

The majority of people living with CKD will be supported by specialist renal nurses who have the advanced technical competencies to monitor blood biochemistry and fluid balance, control blood pressure, and deliver renal replacement therapy.

There are also some specific health problems to which people being treated for renal disorders are susceptible.

Anaemia

The kidneys release the hormone erythropoietin, which stimulates the bone marrow to produce red blood cells. In many stages of kidney disease, this process is disrupted, so all patients with renal disease need to have their Hb levels monitored regularly and they are often treated with erythropoietin-stimulating agents.

Iron deficiency

Many people with kidney failure are deficient in iron due to poor nutrition, poor absorption, and blood loss through HD. This is normally treated with IV iron therapy.

Calcium and phosphate imbalance

Calcium and phosphate imbalance may lead to renal bone disease, so it is important that a renal dietician is involved in agreeing a suitable diet and nutritional supplements. Phosphate and calcium medication can be prescribed.

Hyperkalemia

Hyperkalemia is common in people with progressive kidney disease, so dietary advice is an important aspect of expert care. Adequate medication, dialysis if necessary, and good vascular access are vital in ensuring that serum potassium levels remain within the normal range.

Infection

People having dialysis are at increased risk for infection from their central venous catheter or arteriovenous shunt, so particular care needs to be taken with standard precautions and aseptic techniques when working with these people.

People who have had a transplant will be taking immunosuppressant drugs to minimize the risk of organ rejection. This leaves them particularly vulnerable to systemic infections.

Malnutrition

May result from nausea, vomiting, anorexia, taste changes, dietary restrictions (protein, phosphate, and salt), restricted fluid intake, or infections. Thorough nutritional assessment and concordance are extremely important in renal disease. A specialist renal dietician must be involved in the long-term management arrangements for people with CKD.

Oedema and fluid restriction

Oedema results from fluid retention, so people with kidney failure often have their daily fluid intake restricted to the volume of the previous day's urine output plus 500mL. This is to maintain fluid balance and prevent the patient from becoming overloaded with fluid. Specialist dietetic advice is required for people who have a restricted fluid intake.

General nurses who care for people with renal disorders need to administer any prescribed diuretics, maintain accurate fluid balance records, and ideally weigh the person daily.

Anxiety, fear, and depression

Many renal diseases are chronic, and people often have concerns regarding their long-term prognosis, the effects of the kidney disease and dialysis treatment on personal, work, and family life, and their ability to cope.

In addition, the disrupted biochemistry associated with renal disease can affect a person's mood and emotional state. Psychological and social support is a very important aspect of helping people to live with their kidney disease.

(See also ⊖ *Oxford Handbook of Renal Nursing.*)

Urinary tract conditions

The urethra and bladder may be affected by pathology or injury, and both are prone to opportunistic infection, particularly in women. These disorders can be transient but very distressing, and occasionally they may be indicative of other more serious conditions such as bladder cancer.

The first indication of a disorder of the urethra or bladder may be observed by a person noting a change in the way they pass urine or in the characteristics of their urine:

* Haematuria.
* Dysuria.
* Nocturia.
* Hesitancy.
* Post-void dribbling.
* Urgency.
* Feeling of incomplete emptying.
* Frequency (>4–6 times per day).
* Incontinence.

Cystitis

Cystitis is an acute infection of the bladder, normally caused by bacterial infection, although it sometimes happens when the bladder is irritated or damaged for another reason. Cystitis is much more common in women than men.

Most infections are thought to occur when bacteria that live harmlessly in the bowel or on the skin enter the bladder through the urethra. Causes of cystitis include:

* Poor toilet hygiene.
* Sexual intercourse.
* Tampon use.
* Pregnancy.
* Menopause.
* Urinary catheter insertion.
* Incomplete bladder emptying.
* Diabetes.
* Chemical irritants (soap, perfumed toiletries).
* Bladder surgery.
* Radiotherapy (pelvic).[1]
* Some chemotherapy medicines.[2]
* Recreational drug use (ketamine).

Retention of urine

Acute retention of urine is the sudden painful inability to pass urine and is differentiated from anuria which may be associated with kidney failure.

Chronic retention of urine has a slower onset and may be associated with an obstruction of the urinary tract. It is often painless but may lead to overflow incontinence.

---

1 NHS Choices. *Radiotherapy*. ⏎ www.nhs.uk/conditions/Radiotherapy/Pages/Introduction.aspx
2 NHS Choices. *Chemotherapy*. ⏎ www.nhs.uk/conditions/chemotherapy/Pages/Definition.aspx

Bladder cancer

Bladder cancer can be non-invasive where the epithelial lining of the bladder is affected, or invasive where the tumour infiltrates the bladder wall or other structures.

It is more common in men than women, and known risk factors are smoking, age, gender, exposure to chemicals, recurrent infection, previous treatment, and family history.

The most common symptom of bladder cancer is haematuria, sometimes with dysuria or low back pain. Suspected bladder cancer is investigated by either flexible or rigid cystoscopy, and localized non-invasive cancers can be treated by cystoscopy to remove malignant cells. In these cases, the condition is managed by regular repeat cystoscopy under general anaesthesia.

Invasive or advanced bladder cancers can be treated by chemotherapy[3], or bacille calmette–Guérin (BCG)[4] vaccine inserted directly into the bladder. In some cases, treatment is surgical cystectomy and creation of a urostomy, normally by specialist oncology and urology services.

(See also ➜ Oxford Handbook of Cancer Nursing.)

3 Macmillan Cancer Support. Chemotherapy. ℘ www.macmillan.org.uk/information-and-support/bladder-cancer/non-invasive-bladder-cancer/treating/chemotherapy/chemotherapy-explained.

4 Macmillan Cancer Support. BCG treatment for non-invasive bladder cancer. ℘ www.macmillan.org.uk/information-and-support/bladder-cancer/non-invasive-bladder-cancer/treating/bcg-treatment/bcg-treatment-non-invasive-bladder.html.

Urinary incontinence

Incontinence is a common disorder of the urinary tract, and it is estimated that up to 5% of the general population are affected, including between 30 and 50% of older people. Urinary incontinence may be a transient or long-term disorder, and women are at greater risk than men of developing the condition (ℳ www.continence-foundation.org.uk).

Urinary incontinence is described as stress, urge, and mixed (a combination of stress and urge). Treatment and management depend on the type of incontinence suffered, and the management plan will normally need to be made with specialist continence services or an incontinence advisor.

In addition to physical discomfort, inconvenience, and restrictions in normal daily functions, urinary incontinence may result in emotional problems and social isolation due to embarrassment or anxiety about increased frequency, leaking, or smelling of urine.

Causes and contributory factors

Damage or deterioration of the pelvic floor muscles or nerves
- Childbirth.
- Menopause (due to hormonal changes).
- Uterine prolapse.
- Abdominal or pelvic surgery (e.g. prostatectomy).
- Disorders that affect nerve conduction (e.g. diabetes, stroke, Parkinson's disease, spinal disorders).
- Chronic cough.
- Constipation.
- Heavy lifting.
- Obesity.

Overactive or unstable bladder
- Hypersensitivity of unknown cause.
- Stroke.
- Parkinson's disease.
- Atrophic vaginitis.

Functional causes
- Urinary tract obstruction (which prevents normal voiding and may lead to lower UTIs or symptoms such as dribbling or increased frequency).
- Immobility.
- Inability to access facilities.
- Cognitive or behavioural problems or confusion.

Treatment of urinary incontinence

Conservative treatments
Helping people to manage and live with urinary incontinence is normally the remit of specialist continence services and advisors. A multi-professional specialist approach may include:
- Exercise to improve the function of pelvic floor muscles.
- Electrical stimulation of pelvic floor muscles.
- Bladder retraining.

- Medications, such as anticholinergic drugs, which may help prevent muscle contraction.
- Transcutaneous electrical nerve stimulation (TENS) to reduce symptoms of an overactive bladder.
- Pads and sheaths.
- Indwelling catheterization is sometimes used when intractable incontinence cannot be managed in any other way.

Surgical treatments
- In women, surgical 'sling' procedures which elevate the bladder neck (may be done laparoscopically).
- In men, transurethral resection of the prostate (TURP) may be used for chronic retention and overflow incontinence.
- Artificial urinary sphincters.
- Injection of bulking agents to tissues around the bladder neck.
- botulinium toxin injections (for incontinence secondary to neurological disorders).

Urinary catheterization
Where people have disorders of the urinary tract following general or urological surgery, or for accurate fluid balance measurement, urinary catheterization is often used. Urinary catheters can also be used for bladder function testing, irrigation, or drug administration.

Urinary catheters may be permanently, temporarily, or intermittently inserted and can be successfully managed by people with long-term health conditions in their own homes.
- *Intermittent self catheterization*—is normally used where a person has incomplete bladder emptying, or for urethral dilatation.
- *Urethral catheterization*—is most often seen in hospital environments, as a short-term measure following surgery, or to treat acute urinary retention. People with long-term health conditions may also live with a urinary catheter at home.
- *Suprapubic catheterization*—is used when it is not possible to access the bladder through the urethra, and the catheter is normally inserted through the abdominal wall under general anaesthesia.

(For details of specific clinical procedures and processes relating to urinary catheterization, see ➜ *Oxford Handbook of Clinical Skills in Adult Nursing*.)

Clinical investigations in urinary tract conditions

Urine dipstick test
This is useful as a routine first-line investigation for suggesting when further clinical investigations may be necessary.
- Protein—may indicate renal disease or UTI.
- Glucose and ketones—diabetes.
- Blood—bladder or renal cancer, bladder trauma, obstruction, or infection.
- Nitrites and leucocytes—UTI.
- Bilirubin—hepatobiliary conditions.

Midstream specimen of urine (MSU)

An MSU specimen is taken for microscopy, culture, and sensitivity if a UTI is suspected or to confirm the presence of red blood cells.

Blood tests

These include FBC, U&Es, blood culture, and blood glucose, all of which can be indicative of other disorders or infection. Raised levels of prostate-specific antigen (PSA) are an indication for further investigation of possible prostate cancer.

Flexible cystoscopy

A flexible cystoscope is introduced via the urethra into the bladder to identify lesions, stones, urethral stricture, or tumours. This is usually performed in an outpatient clinic, using local anaesthetic lubrication.

Rigid cystoscopy

This procedure uses a rigid cystoscope to examine the bladder, whilst the person is under general anaesthesia. Small pieces of the bladder urothelium may or may not be taken for histological analysis. A bladder biopsy may also be taken if bladder cancer is suspected.

Intravenous urogram (IVU)

IVU involves the injection of a contrast medium to view, through X-ray, the anatomy of the renal and urinary tract.

Urinary tract ultrasound

Ultrasound is a useful, non-invasive first-line investigation for a number of urological conditions. It may reveal hydronephrosis, bladder or renal stones, renal cysts or tumour, or bladder diverticulae.

CT and MRI scans

May be used to help in the diagnosis of a urinary tract condition, in staging urological cancers, or for monitoring the effects of treatment interventions.

Key nursing considerations in urinary incontinence

Nurses working with people with incontinence, either in hospital or the community, not only have a responsibility to help deliver any treatments, but also have to support the person in managing their symptoms.

Irrespective of the underlying cause, incontinence can be profoundly disruptive and socially embarrassing and have a damaging impact on a person's quality of life. In these circumstances, nursing decision-making and practice are focused not only on practical knowledge and skills, but also effective communication skills necessary for building trust with the patient and their family, to help them understand and effectively manage their condition. (See also → Chapter 5, Communication in a healthcare context.)

A lot of nursing practice in continence management is now the domain of specialist practitioners, and the contribution of general nurses will be determined by the nature of the clinical diagnosis and the physical, social, and emotional needs of the person and their family.

Useful sources of further information

- Continence ᔆ www.continence-foundation.org.uk/
- Renal ᔆ www.kidneyresearchuk.org
- Cancer ᔆ www.macmillan.org.uk/
- NHS Choices ᔆ www.nhs.uk/Conditions
- National Institute for Health and Care Excellence ᔆ www.nice.org.uk
- Organ donation ᔆ www.organdonation.nhs.uk

Drugs frequently prescribed for renal and urinary tract conditions

Drugs frequently used for renal and urinary disorders are listed in Table 18.2. *All drug doses listed in this table are adult doses only.* This table is only to be used as a guide, and the current *BNF* should be consulted for further advice. Nurses should involve themselves only in the administration of medications which fall within their sphere of competence.

Table 18.2 Drugs frequently prescribed for renal and urinary tract conditions

People with renal conditions are often treated with drugs commonly used for cardiovascular conditions such as diuretics (not potassium-sparing), β-blockers, α-blockers, vasodilators, ACE inhibitors, angiotensin II receptor antagonists, and calcium channel blockers. Information on these medicines can be found in ➲ Chapter 15, Cardiovascular conditions, p. 226.

Drug	Dose	Common side effects
Renal disease		
Erythropoietin	Many different erythropoietins are available. Dose and frequency of administration vary considerably, but all are aimed at increasing Hb concentration to a stable level of 10–12g/100mL	Dose-dependent increase in blood pressure and platelet count; influenza-like symptoms, thromboembolic events
Iron sucrose	Used to treat iron deficiency anaemia; dose varies	Taste disturbance nausea, hypersensitivity reactions (see *BNF*)
Calcium salts	Used as a phosphate binder; dose dependent on product used	GI disturbances, bradycardia, arrhythmias
Sevelamer hydrochloride	Used as a phosphate binder; dose dependent on product used	Nausea, vomiting, abdominal pain (see *BNF*)
Lanthanum	Used as a phosphate binder; dose dependent on product used	GI disturbance (see *BNF*)
Vitamin D, e.g. alfacalcidol	1 microgram daily (500ng in elderly), adjusted to avoid hypercalcaemia; maintenance normally 0.25–1 micrograms	Anorexia, lassitude, nausea and vomiting, diarrhoea, weight loss, polyuria, sweating, headache, thirst, and raised concentrations of calcium and phosphate
Sodium bicarbonate	3g in water every 2 hours until urinary pH exceeds 7; maintenance of alkaline urine: 5–10g daily	Belching, alkalosis on prolonged use

(Continued)

Table 18.2 (*Contd.*)

Drug	Dose	Common side effects
Urinary frequency, enuresis, incontinence		
Oxybutynin	5mg 2–3 times daily, increased to a maximum of 5mg four times daily. Elderly patients initially 2.5–3mg twice daily, increased to a maximum of 5mg twice daily	Dry mouth, GI disturbances, blurred vision, difficulty in micturition, palpitation, skin reactions; CNS stimulation and facial flushing (both more common in children); many more (see *BNF*)
Tolterodine	2mg twice daily	Dry mouth, GI disturbances, blurred vision, difficulty in micturition

Drugs used in nephritis or UTI: include penicillins, cephalosporins, tetracyclines, aminoglycosides, and macrolides.

Diabetes

Diabetes

Diabetes is an irreversible metabolic disorder of multiple aetiology ($\mathcal{S}$ www.who.int), which is characterized by hyperglycaemia (abnormally raised blood glucose). It is a progressive condition that, due to the inefficient metabolism of glucose, often results in long-term tissue damage to other organs and systems in the body. The incidence of diabetes is increasing globally, particularly type 2 diabetes which accounts for 90% of all diagnosed cases.

General adult nurses may encounter people with diabetes in a variety of circumstances and settings, but many people manage their own condition in the community, supported by specialist nurses.

- *Type 1* diabetes is an insulin insufficiency caused by the destruction of pancreatic β-cells, which secrete insulin.
- *Type 2* diabetes is a combination of reduced insulin secretion and insulin resistance (the ineffective utilization of insulin at cellular level).
- *Secondary diabetes* can result from other conditions such as pancreatic disease, CF, or trauma. It may also be a result of the long-term use of specific medications, primarily corticosteroid therapy. The clinical presentation of secondary diabetes will vary, depending on the degree of β-cell destruction in the pancreas.
- *Gestational diabetes* is a temporary rise in blood glucose levels due to pregnancy, which does not necessarily develop into a long-term condition.

Symptoms and presentation of diabetes

See Table 19.1.

The mean blood glucose measure in the general population is 5.5mmol/L, with a range of 3.5–7.0mmol/L. Blood glucose levels fluctuate throughout the day and are moderated by insulin produced by the pancreas. In the development of diabetes, there is a steady increase in the level of glucose in the blood as insulin secretion declines. There may also be a reduced effectiveness in insulin utilization in the cells of the body. This results in hyperglycaemia where blood glucose is above the normal range, and can manifest in some or all of these symptoms:

- Polyuria (excessive urination, different to frequency).
- Polydipsia (persistent and excessive thirst).
- Blurred vision.
- Unexplained or unintentional weight loss.
- Lethargy or fatigue.
- Localized skin infections.
- Delayed healing.
- Elevated blood glucose, urinary glucose, and ketosis.
- Diabetic ketoacidosis (DKA).
- Hyperosmolar hyperglycaemic state (HHS) (rare).

Table 19.1 Characteristics of diabetes

Characteristic	Type 1	Type 2
Genetic link	Weak	Strong—more prevalent in certain ethnic groups
Contributory factors	Thought to be a combination of genetic and environmental factors—of multiple origin	Lifestyle, raised body mass index (BMI), diet, inactivity, medication
Insulin status	Insulin secretion depletion often caused by autoimmune destruction of pancreatic β-cells	Reduced insulin secretion and/or insulin resistance
Age of onset	Usually under 30, but can be any age, including childhood	Prevalence increases greatly with age. Increasing presentation in children and young adults
Presentation	Rapid onset with acute hyperglycaemic symptoms	Slow onset with varying degrees of hyperglycaemic symptoms
Ketosis	Potential risk	Unlikely, but possible during acute illness and dehydration

Hyperglycaemia

This refers to a blood glucose level above the normal range, whether the result is consistently elevated or a single measurement. Possible causes of hyperglycaemia include:

- Undiagnosed diabetes.
- Under treatment of diabetes (i.e. insufficient insulin or oral agents).
- Excessive carbohydrate intake.
- Infection or illness.
- Medication that induces hyperglycaemia (e.g. steroids).
- Inactivity.

Prolonged hyperglycaemia increases the risk of long-term diabetes-related complications. These are caused through damage to both large and small blood vessels and result in increased mortality. The body systems specifically at risk are kidneys (nephropathy), eyes (retinopathy), nerves (neuropathy), and the cardiovascular system.

Treatment of hyperglycaemia requires the MDT to establish the underlying cause of hyperglycaemia and treating it as necessary. In type 1 diabetes, acute hyperglycaemia can lead to diabetic ketoacidosis (DKA), and in type 2 diabetes to hyperosmolar hyperglycaemic state (HHS). Both conditions are medical emergencies which require hospitalization.

Hypoglycaemia

Hypoglycaemia refers to a low blood glucose level (below 3.5mmol/L) and is the most common side effect of insulin and sulfonylureas in the treatment of all types of diabetes. Hypoglycaemia results from an imbalance between glucose supply, glucose utilization, and current insulin levels.

Although the majority of people living with diabetes self-manage their condition with support from community diabetic services, it is estimated that 15% of inpatients in England and Wales have known diabetes. The hospital environment presents additional obstacles to maintaining good glycaemic control and avoiding hypoglycaemia (🅫 www.diabetologists-abcd.org.uk/JBDS/JBDS.htm).

Hospitals and other clinical organizations will often have national guidelines or local protocols in place for the treatment of hypoglycaemia, and these should always be followed.

The common symptoms and treatments of hypoglycaemia are summarized in Table 19.2.

Regular and prolonged hypoglycaemic episodes can lead to a loss of awareness, and the symptoms themselves can have a major impact on an individual's quality of life.

Table 19.2 Symptoms and treatment of hypoglycaemia

Symptoms	Treatment
Lethargy	15g of quick-acting carbohydrate (e.g. five glucose tablets, five fruit pastilles, or 100mL of Lucozade®).
Severe tiredness	
Dizziness	
Weakness	Repeat after 10 minutes if symptoms have not resolved.
Sweating	
Palpitations	Followed by 15g of long-acting carbohydrate (e.g. a slice of bread or one digestive biscuit) or a regular meal
Tremor	
Headache	
Visual disturbances	
Confusion	
Impaired LOC or inability to swallow	Place in the recovery position and maintain airway. IM glucagon or IV dextrose solution may be given

Diabetic emergencies

DKA and HHS are both life-threatening complications of diabetes. Their clinical characteristics and treatment priorities are summarized in Table 19.3.

Table 19.3 Characteristics of diabetic emergencies

Characteristic	DKA	HHS
Occurrence	Type 1 (also possible in type 2 and secondary diabetes)	Type 2 and secondary diabetes
Plasma glucose	>11mmol/L	>40mmol/L
Blood ketones	>3	<1.5
pH	<7.3	>7.3
Bicarbonate	<15	>15
Plasma osmolality	N/A	>320mOsm/kg
Hydration status	Variable (mild to severe dehydration)	Severe dehydration
U&Es	Deranged potassium (K⁺)	Severely deranged K⁺
Treatment—according to local practice protocols or guidelines	Urgent restoration of: • Hydration • Electrolyte balance • Blood glucose • Reversal of ketoacidosis Treatment of underlying cause	Urgent restoration of: • Hydration • Electrolyte balance • Blood glucose Treatment of underlying cause

Clinical procedures associated with diabetes management

- Measurement of blood glucose levels.
- Measurement of fasting plasma glucose level. This should be <6.9mmol/L, but if the person is symptomatic, two results are required.
- A 2-hour plasma glucose screen.
- Random plasma glucose test.
- Fasting oral glucose tolerance test (OGTT).
- Glycated haemoglobin (HbA1c) measurement.
- Blood chemistry profile.
- U&E status.
- Liver and renal function tests.
- Measurement of blood cholesterol levels.
- Laboratory urinalysis—albumin:creatinine ratio.
- Diabetic eye screening.
- Foot examination and chiropody treatment.

(For details of specific clinical procedures, see ➲ *Oxford Handbook of Clinical Skills in Adult Nursing*.)

Treatment of diabetes

Type 1 diabetes

The aim of clinical treatment of diabetes of all types is to normalize metabolism, particularly that of carbohydrate and glucose, so as to enable the body to utilize glucose effectively at a cellular level.

- Type 1 diabetes normally requires treatment with insulin.
- There are many different types of insulin, which vary in duration of action. An individual insulin regime will be prescribed by the clinical team.
- Insulin is administered by SC injection using insulin syringes (used mostly within institutional settings), insulin pen devices (these can be pre-loaded or reusable), and insulin pumps.
- Insulin management is monitored by regular capillary blood glucose testing (at least daily), which may be carried out by the person, their family, or designated members of the healthcare team.
- People with type 1 diabetes will also have regular measurement of their blood glucose levels and blood biochemistry profiles, along with annual diabetic eye screening (retinal photography), foot examination, and testing for peripheral neuropathy.

Type 2 diabetes

- Although the incidence of type 2 diabetes is increasing globally, it is estimated that there may be large numbers of the population living with the condition who are undiagnosed. Many people may only have mild symptoms of hyperglycaemia or, in some cases, no symptoms at all.
- For some people, a diagnosis of type 2 diabetes is made incidentally as a result of routine screening or health checks.
- Type 2 diabetes may also be identified only when the condition is established and the person is admitted to hospital with a complication of undiagnosed diabetes such as MI or foot ulcer.
- Initial clinical management of type 2 diabetes is focused on addressing lifestyle interventions involving changes to diet and activity patterns.
- For people with a high BMI, lifestyle modifications will include weight reduction strategies.
- Smokers should be advised and supported in smoking cessation.
- Type 2 diabetes is a progressive condition. If lifestyle changes are insufficient to maintain blood glucose levels, hypoglycaemic drug therapies can be used to support lifestyle adjustments.
- Over time, some people with type 2 diabetes may eventually require treatment with insulin therapy.
- Type 2 diabetes is associated with an increased risk of atherosclerotic cardiovascular disorders, particularly hypertension and hyperlipidaemia. Regular monitoring of blood pressure and blood cholesterol levels is necessary.
- People with type 2 diabetes will also need regular laboratory measurement of their blood glucose levels and blood biochemistry profiles.

Monitoring the effectiveness of diabetes treatment

The efficacy of clinical treatment for type 1 and type 2 diabetes is monitored primarily through HbA1c measurement and capillary blood glucose measurement.

HbA1c

This is the test which measures long-term glycaemic control. It reflects the blood glucose levels over the preceding 3 months and is usually measured every 3–6 months. The target range should be set individually, but NICE guidelines (℅ www.nice.org.uk) advise 48–60mmol/L.

Capillary blood glucose monitoring

It is normal for blood glucose levels to fluctuate throughout the day. A capillary blood test, performed at different times of the day, will reveal individual patterns in response to medications, diet, and exercise.

Capillary blood glucose monitoring can be used to support decisions regarding changes to oral medications and insulin doses. Frequency of blood glucose monitoring is normally determined by individual need and may be subject to local practice policy, protocols, or guidelines.

Long-term monitoring

As diabetes is a long-term and progressive health condition, people living with diabetes are usually offered regular clinical investigations and support in the management of their well-being.

Individual responses to treatment for diabetes are regularly monitored by laboratory measurement of blood glucose levels, along with annual diabetic eye screening (retinal photography), foot examination, and testing for peripheral neuropathy.

In the UK NHS, long-term support and monitoring are normally carried out by specialist diabetic nurses in the hospital or the community, practice nurses in GP surgeries, or through specialist hospital outpatient clinics.

If blood glucose levels are not well controlled, and there is a risk of hypoglycaemia, a person with diabetes may not be able to drive or operate dangerous machinery. DVLA driving regulations stipulate the minimum legal requirement for a safe blood glucose level for people using insulin or any medication that can potentially cause hypoglycaemia (℅ www.gov.uk/guidance/current-medical-guidelines-dvla-guidance-for-professionals).

People hospitalized with diabetes

Undiagnosed diabetes

People may be hospitalized as a result of a medical event or episode which is subsequently found to be undiagnosed diabetes. In this case, the care and treatment offered would be determined by the results of any diagnostic clinical investigations.

In the first instance, nursing care and interventions for a person admitted to hospital with a case of undiagnosed diabetes would follow the routine procedures and practices of the organization.

Subsequent nursing decision-making and practice would be determined by the type of diabetes diagnosed, the needs of the person and their families, and the decisions of the MDT.

Diabetic emergencies

People who live with type 1 or type 2 diabetes may be admitted to hospital as an emergency with an episode of DKA or HHS. Both DKA and HHS are life-threatening conditions, and the aim of treatment, in accordance with local practice policy and protocols, is urgent restoration of hydration, electrolyte balance, blood glucose levels, and reversal of ketoacidosis.

Once the person's condition has been stabilized, nursing decision-making and care will focus on treatment of the underlying cause of the diabetic emergency and restoration of the diabetic management regime.

People with diabetes having surgery

Where people with diabetes are to have elective or emergency surgery, optimal glycaemic control is essential to enhance immediate post-operative recovery, promote wound healing, and reduce the risk of surgical or diabetic complications.

If possible, surgery should be performed in the early morning, to minimize disruption to normal diabetes treatment and reduce the need for IV insulin therapy.

- Prior to surgery, the degree of glycaemic control should be established (HbA1c <69mmol/L, with stable blood glucose levels).
- During surgery and post-operatively, blood glucose levels should be monitored regularly, so that, wherever possible, hyperglycaemia and hypoglycaemia are avoided.
- Acceptable blood glucose levels can be maintained by the use of IV insulin therapy.
- After recovery from anaesthesia and discontinuation of any treatments introduced during surgery, the usual diabetes therapy can be re-introduced.
- Post-operatively, it may be necessary to review the person's diabetic management regime, so a referral to the local diabetes specialist team could be helpful.

(See also Joint British Diabetes Societies Inpatient Care Group at ℅ http://www.diabetologists-abcd.org.uk/JBDS/JBDS.htm and ➔ Chapter 22, Surgery.)

Key nursing considerations in diabetes

As diabetes is a long-term health condition, effective healthcare requires an MDT approach, of which nurses in hospitals and the community have a central role.

Nursing decision-making and practice are founded on professional knowledge and values, and extend beyond the person with diabetes to the family, carers, and significant others. The cornerstone of the nursing role in this health condition is effective communication to support and empower people, so that they can confidently manage their diabetic condition in the long term.

The type and duration of the diabetic condition will determine the nursing interventions when working with people with diabetes, but at different stages, these will include:

- A comprehensive nursing assessment, consistent with local policy and procedures, to help determine the information and support needed to facilitate informed decision-making about living with diabetes.
- Effective communication with all other members of the MDT involved in the individual's care.
- Awareness of the effect of concurrent illness on glycaemic control in people with diabetes.
- Awareness of the relationship between diabetes and mental health.
- Recognition and timely reporting of hypoglycaemic and hyperglycaemic episodes.
- Accurate measurement and reporting of all routine and specialist clinical observations and investigations.
- Safe and accurate measurement and reporting of blood glucose levels.
- Safe administration of injectable and oral diabetic therapies.
- Providing timely and relevant information to individuals and their families about the safe management and administration of diabetic medications.
- Explaining and supporting individuals, and their families, who are learning to self-inject and self-monitor blood glucose levels.
- Encouraging compliance and concordance with oral antihyperglycaemic agents.
- Providing timely and relevant information to individuals and families in relation to lifestyle, activity, and diet.
- Signposting dietary information or local diabetic support services.
- Encouraging positive changes to lifestyle, including exercise.
- Supporting the individual in setting and achieving realistic lifestyle goals.
- Encouraging access to annual diabetes screening.

Useful sources of further information

- World Health Organization ⚬ www.who.int
- Diabetes UK ⚬ www.diabetes.org.uk
- Joint British Diabetic Societies for Inpatient Care Group ⚬ http://www.diabetologists-abcd.org.uk/JBDS/JBDS.htm
- National Institute for Health and Care Excellence ⚬ www.nice.org.uk
- NHS Choices ⚬ www.nhs.uk

Drugs frequently prescribed for diabetes

Drugs often used in people with diabetes are listed in Table 19.4. *All drug doses listed in this table are adult doses only.* This table should only be used as a guide, and the current *BNF* should be consulted for further advice. Nurses should involve themselves only in the administration of medications which fall within their sphere of competence.

Table 19.4 Drugs frequently prescribed for diabetes

Insulin—The aim of treatment is to achieve the best possible control of blood glucose concentration, whilst avoiding troublesome hypoglycaemic reactions. The duration of action of a particular type of insulin varies from one patient to another and needs to be assessed individually. Insulin regimens usually consist of one or a combination of the insulin groups below. Although many of the insulins are readily available as 100U/mL, there are a number of new insulins of different concentrations, e.g. 200U/mL. It is important to check not only the correct insulin is selected, but also the correct strength.

	Dose—always expressed in units	Common side effects
Short-acting insulin, e.g. soluble insulin, insulin lispro, insulin aspart, insulin glulisine	Usually injected SC 15–30 minutes before meals—soluble insulin onset of action is 30–60 minutes, with a peak at 2–4 hours and a duration of up to 8 hours; if given IV (and can be given IM), the peak effect is very quick (within minutes) and effectively disappears within 30 minutes Other short-acting insulins have a quicker onset and a shorter duration of action, making them a suitable choice for patients prone to hypoglycaemia or who wish to inject shortly before a meal or even shortly after	All types of insulin have the potential to cause hypoglycaemia and can also cause transient oedema, local reactions, and fat hypertrophy at the injection site; rarely, hypersensitivity reactions (e.g. urticaria) and rash, though insulin-containing protamine may cause allergic reactions
Insulin of intermediate duration of action, e.g. isophane insulin, insulin zinc suspension	When given by SC injection, intermediate- and long-acting insulin has an onset of action of 1–2 hours, with maximal effect at 4–12 hours and duration of 16–42 hours	
Insulin whose onset of action is slower and lasts for long periods, e.g. insulin glargine, insulin detemir		

(Continued)

Table 19.4 (*Contd.*)

Oral antidiabetic drugs are used for patients not adequately controlled by diet and exercise. They should be used to augment the effects of diet and exercise, not replace them. These agents generally fall into one of three types—sulfonylureas, biguanides, and a group of miscellaneous agents such as the thiazolidinediones.

	Dose	Common side effects
Sulfonylureas, e.g. glibenclamide, gliclazide, tolbutamide, glipizide, glimepiride	See individual agent in *BNF* Used in patients who are not overweight or where metformin is contraindicated; glibenclamide and chlorpropamide are best avoided in the elderly because they may cause hypoglycaemia, even at normal doses	Nausea, vomiting, diarrhoea, and constipation; excessive dosage causes prolonged hypoglycaemia
Biguanides, e.g. metformin	Used in patients who are overweight, unless contraindicated 500mg with breakfast for at least 1 week; then 500mg with breakfast and evening meal for at least 1 week; then 500mg with breakfast, lunch, and evening meal; maximum dose of 2g daily in divided doses	Anorexia, nausea, vomiting, diarrhoea (usually transient), abdominal pain, metallic taste; rarely lactic acidosis but can occur in patients with renal impairment and is an indication for withdrawal of biguanide
Dipeptidyl peptidase-4 inhibitors, e.g. saxagliptin, sitagliptin, and vildagliptin	See individual agent in *BNF*	GI disturbance, peripheral oedema See individual agent in *BNF*
Meglitinides (stimulate β-cell production of insulin), e.g. repaglinide, nateglinide	See individual agent in *BNF* As they are taken within 30 minutes of a meal, they can be very useful for patients who miss meals	Abdominal pain, diarrhoea, constipation, nausea, and vomiting
Glucagon-like peptide-1 (GLP-1) agonists, e.g. exenatide, liraglutide	Given by SC injection. See individual agent in *BNF*	Nausea, vomiting, diarrhoea, dyspepsia See individual agent in *BNF*

(*Continued*)

Table 19.4 (Contd.)

Thiazolidinediones	Pioglitazone—initially 15–30mg once daily, increased to 45mg daily, according to response. Start with lowest effective dose and increase slowly in the elderly	GI disturbances, weight gain, oedema, anaemia, headache, visual disturbances, dizziness, arthralgia, hypoaesthesia, haematuria, impotenceIncreased likelihood of heart failure when used alongside insulin
Hypoglycaemic emergency	**Dose**	**Common side effects**
Glucose injection	75–100mL of 20% glucose injected IV over 15 minutesor 150–200mL of 10% glucose injected IV over 15 minutes	
Glucagon injection	Administered by SC or IM injection: 1mg if body weight over 25kg; 500 micrograms if body weight under 25kgNB. If no response within 10 minutes, IV glucose must be given	Nausea, vomiting, abdominal pain, hypokalaemia, hypotension

Chapter 20

Musculoskeletal conditions

The skeleton, skeletal muscles, and connective tissues

The skeleton is the framework of the human body, which in adults is made up of 206 bones, providing protection for the internal organs, a support system for the limbs, and the mechanics for human movement.

The vertebral column, rib cage, skull, and associated bones are known as the axial skeleton. The appendicular skeleton is made up of the shoulder girdle, the pelvic girdle, and the bones of the limbs. The skeletal muscles, joints, tendons, and ligaments facilitate movement. Cartilage within the bone surfaces of joints acts as a cushion to absorb impact on the skeleton.

Musculoskeletal (MSK) and orthopaedic conditions refer to any dysfunction of the bones, joints, muscles, tendons, and ligaments, and how well they function with regard to effective movement and mobilization.

Disorders of the MSK system will often be the result of trauma or long-term degenerative conditions, which can affect people of any age, although older people are at increased risk. Many people with MSK conditions will be treated by specialist orthopaedic and rheumatology services, but general adult nurses will come into contact with many people who are suffering from a range of MSK disorders.

Whether these are muscle sprains, people living with a long-term arthritic conditions, or those who have suffered a potentially life-threatening traumatic injury, all will have some degree of compromised movement. It is important that general adult nurses can work with people to help restore function and reduce risk from the many complications which can arise from immobility or disability.

Regardless of the cause or extent of MSK damage, the consequence will normally be some reduction in the movement of joints and limbs or, in some cases, temporary or permanent immobility.

Many MSK conditions can be treated with rest, immobilization, drug therapy, or surgery. Where a MSK disorder is the result of trauma, this will often require emergency surgery, but in degenerative conditions any surgical intervention is more likely to be elective, such as in joint replacement surgery.

Musculoskeletal trauma

MSK trauma is one of the main causes of disability in adults. It can range from a simple muscle strain to multiple fractures and soft tissue damage. Trauma may also be life-threatening, place a limb at risk, or compromise an eventual return to full function and mobility. The most common causes of MSK trauma are:

- Road traffic accidents.
- Industrial or work-related accidents.
- Sports injuries.
- Falls (particularly in older people).

MSK injuries may not themselves be immediately life-threatening, but in some cases, a complication of trauma or bone fracture may give rise to life-threatening conditions such as:

- Arterial damage.
- Haemorrhage.
- Compartment syndrome.
- Wound infection or contamination (with open fractures).
- VTE.
- PE.
- Fat embolism.
- Sepsis (gangrene, tetanus).

Fractures

A fracture is defined as any break in a bone, which may be open or closed. A closed fracture is where the skin is intact, and an open fracture is where the skin has been punctured, which increases the risk for infection in bone and surrounding tissues. Other descriptive classifications of fractures are:

- Transverse—a fracture occurring at a right angle to the long axis of the bone.
- Spiral—the fracture line twists along the long axis of the bone.
- Oblique—the fracture line is diagonal.
- Comminuted—the bone has fragmented into many pieces.
- Impacted—fragments of bone are compressed into each other.
- Greenstick—incomplete fracture that is found in children.

See Figure 20.1.

Fractures can affect any bones in the body, but the aim of fracture management is to reduce the fracture, promote optimum bone healing, and restore function.

Depending on the site and type of fracture, the presence or likelihood of complications, and the general health and condition of the person, all fractures are treated either surgically or conservatively.

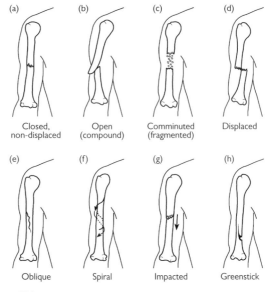

Figure 20.1 Types of fracture.

Reproduced from George Castledine and Ann Close, *Oxford Handbook of Adult Nursing*, (2009) with permission from Oxford University Press.

Some fractures of joints and long bones can be manipulated manually, splinted, and immobilized without surgery, whilst others will need surgical reduction and fixing. The five key principles of fracture treatment are:

- *Resuscitation*: as many people presenting with fractures will have suffered a traumatic injury, they may have a degree of bleeding or shock, so it is important that their haemodynamic status is stabilized before the fracture is treated.
- *Reduction*: although some fractures may remodel without reduction, significant displacement of broken bones will require reduction or realignment of bone ends, so that effective healing can take place. This can be achieved by traction or by surgical reduction.
- *Restriction*: a fractured bone normally takes between 6 and 12 weeks to heal, depending on its type and position. Throughout the healing period, the bone ends need to be aligned and kept in a good position. This can be achieved by traction, a cast, and external or internal fixation. Immobilization of the fracture aids the healing process.
- *Restoration*: refers to the methods used to treat the fractures, so that optimum bone healing can take place. Treatment can be through external devices such as casts, or internal methods such as plates and screws.
- *Rehabilitation*: the consequences of fractures for movement and mobility mean that restorative exercises or physiotherapy will be necessary at some point to help restore function to the affected limb or joint. However, rehabilitation also includes helping maintain function in other joints and limbs not affected by the fracture.

Surgical fixation

- *Internal fixation* involves the surgical insertion of nails, plates, wires, screws, or rods to provide stability for a fractured bone. The benefit of internal fixation methods is that people can normally mobilize more quickly and therefore reduce their risk for developing the complications of immobility.
- *External fixation* involves inserting skeletal pins into the bone on either side of a fracture and holding it in alignment by a scaffold or ring fixators. External fixation can be used in injuries with severe soft tissue damage that prevents internal fixation, poor tissue condition due to underlying co-morbid pathology, or for the gradual correction of a bone deformity. However, external fixation necessitates periods of severely restricted movement for anything from 6 weeks to a year or more, and so increases the risk for developing the complications of immobility.

Fractured neck of femur

A fractured neck of femur predominantly occurs in older people following a fall. It is more prevalent in women, as osteoporosis is a significant risk factor, and surgical repair is normally carried out within 24 hours of injury.

- A fractured neck of femur can be either intracapsular (within the femoral head) or extracapsular (below the femoral head).
- A common complication of intracapsular fracture is a significant reduction in blood supply to the femoral head, which can lead to avascular necrosis.

- The normal treatment options for fixing a fractured neck of femur are hemiarthroplasty, total hip replacement, proximal femoral nail, or dynamic hip screw. The method of fixation is dependent on the position of the fracture.
- Hemiarthroplasty replaces the femoral head, but not the acetabulum of the joint. There is a risk for dislocation with hip hemiarthroplasty.
- Total hip replacement includes both the femoral head and the acetabulum of the joint.
- With extracapsular fractures where there is little or no fragmentation, a dynamic hip screw will normally provide adequate fixation.
- Treatment options for fractured neck of femur will be influenced by the age, fitness, and mobility of the person. Where people have long-term health conditions, poor mobility, limited life expectancy, or cognitive impairment, then the fracture may be fixed by hemiarthroplasty.
- Conservative non-surgical treatment is also an option for fractured neck of femur and may be considered if people are too frail or unwell for surgery. However, conservative treatment necessitates prolonged bed rest, which increases the risk for pressure ulcer development, chest infection, and UTI.
- After fixation of a hip fracture, people can usually begin full, partial, or non-weight-bearing mobilization the day after surgery.

Fractured shaft of femur

A fractured shaft of femur is usually caused by high-impact injuries such as those sustained in road traffic accidents, falls from a height, and crushing injuries. Osteoporosis and metastatic bone disease are also causes of fractures to the shaft of femur. Depending on the age and general health of the person and the position of the fracture, treatment may be surgical or conservative.

- Fractures in the shaft of the femur are commonly displaced, angulated, or shortened due to the skeletal muscles in the upper leg.
- Surgical fixation of a fractured shaft of femur is normally by open reduction internal fixation (ORIF) with intramedullary nails. Internal fixation does not necessitate traction and allows early mobilization.
- In heavily contaminated open fractures, external fixators may be used.
- Conservative treatment of a fractured shaft of femur may be considered for older people or others deemed unsuitable for surgery. This involves alignment of the bone by skin traction or skeletal traction, normally with a Steinman pin (see Figure 20.2).
- Immobilization necessitates a lengthy period of bed rest.

Fractures of the tibia

These fractures are generally the result of major-impact injuries to the lower leg, such as occur in contact sports. They can also occur following low-impact injury, torsion, repeated stress, and minor trauma to bones which are pathologically weakened.

- Tibial fractures are commonly open fractures due to the low amount of tissue and skin covering the bones in the lower leg.
- Spiral fractures are also common in the tibia, and tibial fractures frequently involve the ankle or knee joints.

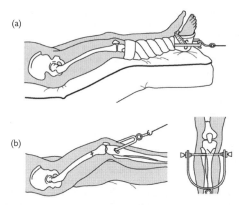

(a)

(b)

Figure 20.2 Traction. (a) Skin traction (b) Skeletal traction

- Swelling and neurovascular complications are often associated with tibial fractures, which can delay surgical intervention.
- Early elevation, ideally on a Braun's frame, in order to minimize swelling is recommended before reduction and fixation of the fracture.
- For tibial fractures which are not displaced, treatment will normally be a long leg cast.
- For displaced tibial fractures, treatment will be either a long leg cast with ORIF with intramedullary nails or external fixation with a circular frame.

Tibial plateau fractures

These fractures are caused by high-impact compressive forces such as road traffic collision or falls. If the fracture is minimally displaced, then it can normally be treated with a cast for 6–8 weeks.

- Tibial plateau fractures may also damage the cruciate and collateral ligaments and menisci of the knee joint.
- Tibial plateau fractures are commonly comminuted fractures with haemarthrosis of the knee.
- If the fracture is unstable, it will require ORIF with cannulated screws, plate, and screws, or external fixation.

Ankle fractures

Ankle fractures generally involve the distal fibula (medial malleolus) and the distal tibia (lateral malleolus), as well as the talus, and they are classified as single malleolar fracture, bi-malleolar fracture, or tri-malleolar fracture.

- Ankle fractures are usually caused by rotational forces, and inversion and eversion of the foot whilst walking or running.
- Stable fractures with minimal swelling can be treated with a below-knee cast for around 6 weeks, with non-weight-bearing for the first few days post-injury, followed by heel walking.

- With unstable ankle fractures which have swelling and bruising, ORIF with wires, screws, and plates may be required. Back slab or removable casts are also often used to prevent foot drop, with non-weight-bearing for at least 6 weeks.
- Neurovascular complications and ligament and tendon damage are common with ankle injuries, and so substantial rehabilitation therapy may be needed.

Foot fractures

- *Talus fractures* are normally associated with a fall from height or a foot on a pedal during a traffic collision.
  - These fractures can be managed conservatively, and for fractures which are not displaced, they can be treated with a below-knee cast and non-weight-bearing for 3 months. Conservative options for displaced fractures normally include reduction with plantar flexion of the foot in a below-knee cast, and non-weight-bearing for 3 months.
  - Unstable and displaced talus fractures require ORIF with K-wires, screw, or pins. Avascular necrosis is common with talus fractures due to poor blood supply. The development of osteoarthritis is also common as a long-term consequence.
- *Calcaneal fractures* usually occur following a fall from height onto the heels and are often associated with spinal damage. If the fracture is simple, it can be treated with bandage and elevation and non-weight-bearing movement until pain reduces. Chronic heel pain is common in the long term.
  - Displaced and unstable calcaneal fractures require ORIF with a below-knee cast for 6 weeks.
- *Metatarsal fractures* are commonly caused by crushing injuries to the foot. Conservative treatment includes a wool and crêpe bandage below-knee cast for 6–7 weeks. Unstable and comminuted fractures may require ORIF with K-wire.

Arm fractures

- *Proximal humerus fractures* are commonly associated with pathological or fragility fractures, which, in older people, may result from a fall on an outstretched hand. In younger people, humeral fractures are normally associated with high-energy trauma, excessive rotation of the arm, and/or direct violence.
- Minimally displaced fractures of the humerus can be treated conservatively with a broad arm sling or collar and cuff. Closed reduction with traction in line with the humerus is another option. ORIF or external fixation is used for severely displaced proximal fractures.
- *Humeral shaft fractures* have a similar mode of injury to proximal humerus fractures, with a risk of neurovascular impairment through damage to the radial nerve.
  - If treated conservatively, a U-slab or hanging cast with a collar and cuff is normally used, or a functional brace may be considered.
  - Surgical interventions include ORIF with plates and/or screws or intramedullary nails, or external fixation.

Scaphoid fractures are a very common type of fracture associated with punching or a fall on an extended arm. Poor blood supply means non-union, delayed healing, and avascular necrosis are common. Stable scaphoid fractures can be treated conservatively with short arm cast for 8–11 weeks. Alternatively, K-wire fixation with a cast for 8 weeks can be used.

Smith's fracture of the distal radius is commonly caused by a fall on an outstretched hand. Displaced fractures require reduction, then a cast with the wrist in supination for 3–4 weeks. Smith's fracture can also be treated with plate and screws or external fixation.

Colles' fracture is a fracture of the radius within 2.5cm of the articular surface of the wrist joint. It is normally the result of falls onto hands and is common in people in the age groups 5–14 and 60–69. Colles' fractures can result in tendon rupture or damage to the medial nerve. Undisplaced fractures can be managed in a short arm cast for 5–6 weeks, but if displaced, closed reduction is required before a cast is applied. If closed reduction is unsuccessful, then ORIF may be used.

• *Galeazzi fracture* is a fracture of the shaft of the radius with dislocation of the radio-ulnar joint, usually caused by falls on outstretched hands. Treatment is normally by ORIF with screws and plates, together with closed reduction of the dislocated radio-ulnar joint, with a long arm cast for around 6 weeks.

• *Monteggia fracture* is an unstable fracture of the ulna with dislocation of the head of the radius, usually caused by high-energy trauma. This normally requires ORIF with an above-elbow cast.

• *Isolated radial or ulnar fractures* commonly occur following direct force injuries. These fractures can often be treated by manipulation under anaesthesia, back slab and broad arm sling, or long arm cast. Internal or external fixation may also be used.

Hand fractures

• *Metacarpal fractures* can be sustained at the head, neck, shaft, or base of the metacarpal bones, or any combination of these sites. They are largely associated with punching injuries and are normally treated by splinting to another finger (neighbour strapping) for 3–4 weeks.

• *Bennett's fracture* describes a fracture dislocation at the base of the carpometacarpal joint of the thumb, normally caused by shearing force. This is often associated with basketball or skiing. These fractures are reduced with traction and placed in a cast to the tip of the thumb for around 4 weeks. If reduction is unsuccessful or the injury is unstable, then percutaneous pinning may be considered.

• *Phalangeal fractures* can involve the base, shaft, neck, or tuft of the phalanges and are associated with falls, or crushing, machinery, or sporting injuries. Conservative treatment is neighbour strapping, but unstable fractures may require ORIF with screws, plate, and wires.

Pelvic fractures

These are commonly sustained in road traffic accidents, falls, or sporting injuries and may cause heavy blood loss and damage to pelvic organs, the bladder, and bowel. Stable pelvic fractures are normally treated with bed rest, but unstable fractures may require internal or external fixation and are generally treated in specialist units or centres.

Spinal fractures

Spinal fractures and injuries may result from any activities or accidents which cause whiplash, compression injuries, axial loading damage, and hyperflexion or hyperextension of the spine.

Damage to the spinal vertebrae can be confined to bone or ligament injury but may also involve the spinal cord or spinal nerves. People with spinal fractures or injuries are at considerable risk for spinal cord damage.

A spinal cord injury causes temporary or permanent loss of muscle function, sensation, or autonomic nervous function in the parts of the body below the level of the cord lesion. Whilst fractures of spinal vertebrae may heal uneventfully, spinal cord damage can be a life-changing event for both the affected person and their family.

Spinal cord damage can be the direct result of trauma but can also be a consequence of moving and handling a person after their initial injury.

People who have spinal injuries will normally be treated in specialist units or centres (see also ➲ Chapter 16, Neurological conditions).

Muscle and tendon injuries

Fractures often have associated muscle or neurovascular damage, and muscles, tendons, and ligaments can also be torn or damaged without a fracture.

For muscle injuries, the principles of rest, ice, compression, and elevation (RICE) are normally used to control any haemorrhage and haematoma, along with pain relief.

Tendon and ligament injuries may be immobilized and rested or surgically repaired.

Degenerative bone diseases and disorders

Osteoporosis

Osteoporosis is a systemic skeletal disease characterized by low bone density and deterioration of bone tissue that causes skeletal fragility and increases the risk of fracture.

Osteoporosis can affect the whole skeleton but is most common in the wrist, hip, and spine. Bone loss is part of a normal ageing process, so the condition affects both men and women, but post-menopausal women are at increased risk. Known causes of osteoporosis include:

- Smoking.
- High alcohol intake.
- Lack of exercise.
- Family history.
- Low BMI.
- Inflammatory arthritic conditions.
- Thyrotoxicosis.
- Primary hyperparathyroidism.
- Menopause.
- Early menopause.
- Amenorrhoea.
- Hypogonadism.
- Malabsorption disorders.
- Liver disease.
- Multiple myeloma.
- Long-term steroid use.

Osteoporosis is not necessarily painful, and many people only become aware of the condition when they suffer a fracture, often of their wrist or hip, and are admitted to hospital for emergency treatment.

However, the development of osteoporosis can be prevented or delayed by means of lifestyle modifications such as ensuring adequate calcium intake, limiting alcohol consumption, smoking cessation, and physical activity. Clinical investigations where osteoporosis is suspected include:

- Spinal X-rays.
- Bone densitometry (dual-energy X-ray absorptiometry (DEXA) scan).
- Serum calcium, alkaline phosphatase, parathyroid hormone, and creatine.
- Serum biochemical profile.
- Serum protein electrophoresis.
- TFTs.
- Serum testosterone levels in men.

Treatment for osteoporosis aims to reduce the risk of fracture and may involve prescription of anti-resorptive agents such as bisphosphonates, calcium, and vitamin D, and selective oestrogen receptor modulators.

Parathyroid hormone may be used to stimulate bone formation. NICE also produces and regularly updates guidelines for the treatment of osteoporosis and the reduction of falls and fracture risk (℞ www.nice.org.uk).

Osteomalacia

This is a reversible metabolic disease in which there is a disorder in mineralization of bone. It is a rare condition but may occasionally be seen in older people and people who have a vitamin D deficiency or liver disease. The condition can be treated with dietary intake of vitamin D and calcium, careful exposure to sunshine, and vitamin supplements.

Osteomyelitis

Osteomyelitis describes an infection of bone, which may be an acute or long-term condition. A person with acute osteomyelitis will have symptoms of general fever, swelling and heat around the affected area, reddening of the skin, tenderness, and pain. In more long-term osteomyelitis, people may develop skin ulceration, sinus tract formation, and discharge from the affected area.

Osteomyelitis is normally treated by IV antibiotic drug therapy, infection control measures, and possibly surgery to drain pus or abscesses.

The condition can occasionally develop into septic arthritis where the infection tracks into a joint and causes severe pain and reduced joint movement. Treatment includes IV antibiotics, arthroscopy, or open surgery to clean and drain the joint.

Tuberculosis (TB)

TB usually occurs in the lungs but may spread, particularly to the vertebral column. TB in the skeleton develops slowly and symptoms may only be manifest as local tenderness. Clinical investigations for suspected TB involve blood screening, X-ray, and MRI scanning.

Treatment is with drug therapy. In some cases, spinal fusion surgery may be necessary, as TB can cause vertebral collapse and paralysis.

Benign bone tumours

Benign bone tumours are often asymptomatic and only discovered incidentally on routine X-ray examination or following a fracture. The cause is unknown, and the tumours are classified according to the type of tissue involved such as osteochondroma from cartilage or osteoblastoma from bone. Treatment includes drug therapy and possibly surgical excision.

Bone cancers

Malignant tumours in the skeleton may originate in the bone such as osteosarcoma, Ewing's sarcoma, and chondrosarcoma. Bone tumours may also be the result of metastatic spread from other primary cancers. Metastatic bone disease puts people with cancer at high risk of pathological fractures.

Primary bone tumours are diagnosed by bone biopsy, X-ray, and CT scan. Treatment normally involves reducing the size of the tumour by chemotherapy and radiation or, in some cases, by cryosurgery. If surgery is a feasible option, this may be reconstructive surgery and allografts or amputation. Intractable pain in bone cancers can be treated surgically with cordotomy.

(See ➲ *Oxford Handbook of Cancer Nursing*.)

Carpal tunnel syndrome

This is a common condition of the hand, occurring in both men and women. The carpal tunnel is the canal lying between the carpal bones and flexor muscle of the wrist. In carpal tunnel syndrome, the median nerve becomes compressed, causing pain, tingling, and numbness of the fingers. Treatment includes analgesia, wrist splints, and corticosteroid injection. The condition can also be treated by carpal tunnel release surgery.

Dupuytren's contracture

Is a slowly progressive deformity of the palmar fascia in the hand, resulting in flexion of the fourth and/or the fifth digits. The condition is more common in men, but the cause is unknown. It is treated surgically.

Hallux valgus

The common name for hallux valgus is a bunion, and it is where the big toe deviates laterally at the base. It is often congenital but can occur as a result of arthritis. Women are affected more than men, and it is normally treated by splinting or surgery.

Back pain

It is estimated that around 80% of people will experience back pain at some point in their lives (℘ www.nhs.uk). Back pain can be a short-term or intermittent disorder, but in some people who suffer from persistent back pain, it can be a seriously debilitating condition.

Back pain can be associated with an identifiable cause such as bending, lifting, trauma, or disease, but in many cases, it will be non-specific. Known causes of back pain include:

- Trauma.
- Repetitive lifting.
- Obesity.
- Lack of exercise.
- Congenital spinal conditions.
- Scoliosis.
- Posture.
- Prolapsed or herniated ('slipped') intervertebral disc.
- Vascular disorders.
- Tumours.
- Chronic degenerative conditions.

Damage or degenerative changes to the intervertebral discs in the cervical, thoracic, or lumbar spine will normally result in compression of spinal nerves, giving rise to pain, numbness, or tingling sensations in the areas supplied by those nerves.

Pain in the cervical vertebrae of the neck is often related to general muscle tension or stiffness but can also be caused by 'whiplash' injuries. Back pain in the thoracic vertebrae is not common but is normally associated with posture, muscular strain, or direct injury.

The most common type of back pain is in the lumbar vertebrae of the lower back, and whilst low back pain is often non-specific, it may also be related to compression of the sciatic nerve through prolapsed or herniated (slipped) intervertebral disc. Sciatic nerve compression causes severe pain in the back, buttocks, and legs and can result in compromised mobility. Treatments for back pain include:

- Analgesia.
- Local application of heat or ice packs.
- Exercise and stretching.
- Physiotherapy.
- Manual manipulation.
- Surgery.

Lumbar decompression surgery

Where non-surgical treatments for back pain are not effective, then surgery to treat compressed nerves in the spine may be recommended. Spinal surgery is normally carried out in neurosurgical units or specialist centres.

- Laminectomy—removal of a section of vertebral bone.
- Discectomy—removal of damaged intervertebral disc tissue.
- Spinal fusion—fusion of two or more vertebrae.
- A combination of these surgical techniques.

'Red flag' back pain symptoms

Back pain may also be indicative of a serious disorder of the MSK system, the spine, or the nervous system, an example of which is the compression of spinal nerve roots seen in cauda equina syndrome. Although this condition is rare, if not treated promptly, it can result in permanent incontinence or paralysis. So where back pain is one of a collection of any of the following symptoms, these need to be investigated and treated urgently.

- Unrelieved back pain.
- Pyrexia.
- Loss of bladder or bowel control.
- Incontinence or inability to pass urine.
- Numbness or altered sensation in the genitals or perianal region.

Arthritic conditions

Osteoarthritis

Osteoarthritis (OA) is a localized, degenerative condition of the synovial joints and is the most common type of arthritis in the UK (ℜ www.arthritis-researchuk.org). OA most often develops in people over 40, particularly where there is a family history. It is more common in women, and the joints mostly affected by OA are those in the hands, knees, spine, and hips.

The condition may have an unknown cause or be associated with other joint-related conditions such as gout or rheumatoid arthritis (RA). In some cases, OA can be a long-term consequence of an injury.

Risk factors for developing OA include congenital joint abnormalities, ageing, obesity, high levels of impact sport, and repetitive movements such as those associated with some types of work.

In OA, there is gradual destruction of the joint cartilage, with incomplete repair and formation of new bone. The degenerative changes put an excessive burden on tendons and ligaments and often lead to the formation of bony spurs. Where cartilage loss is severe, it can lead to bone-on-bone friction and alterations to the shape of the joint. These processes make movement more difficult in the affected joint(s) and give rise to pain and stiffness.

OA is a major cause of disability and symptoms include:
- Joint pain and stiffness.
- Compromised movement and mobility.
- Bony enlargement.
- Bony deformity.
- Loss of function.
- Inflammatory symptoms.
- Muscle wasting.
- Development of nodes in interphalangeal joints (see Figure 20.3).

Clinical investigations for OA will involve identification and mapping of structural changes in the joint. Imaging techniques may show loss of cartilage, narrowing of the joint space, osteophytes, and sclerosis. Although there is no cure for OA, treatment to relieve symptoms can include:
- Analgesic regimes.
- NSAIDs.
- Corticosteroid medicines.
- Mobilization.
- Exercise.
- Diet and lifestyle modifications.

OA can become so severe that functionality and quality of life are affected. In these cases, joint surgery may be offered such as joint replacement (arthroplasty), joint fusion (arthrodesis), or realignment of affected bones (osteotomy).

Hip and knee joints are those most commonly replaced, but elective surgery for elbow, ankle, and shoulder joints can also be offered.

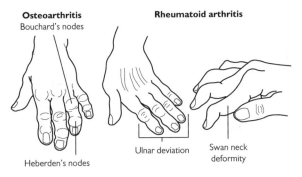

Osteoarthritis
Bouchard's nodes

Rheumatoid arthritis

Ulnar deviation

Swan neck deformity

Heberden's nodes

Figure 20.3 Joint deformities in osteoarthritis and rheumatoid arthritis.
Reproduced from Hoeman, S, *Rehabilitation Nursing* 3rd edition (Mosby: 2001), with permission from Elsevier.

Rheumatoid arthritis

RA is an autoimmune disorder that affects the synovial joints, particularly the hands, fingers, and shoulders. It is characterized by intermittent periods of inflammation and latency. The condition is chronic, progressive, and systemic.

The cause of RA is unknown, but there is a genetic link, and infection, stress, trauma, and smoking can act as triggers to a period of inflammatory activity. RA often starts when a person is between 40 and 50 years old, and the condition is more common in women.

In RA, the synovial lining of the joint capsule becomes inflamed and congested with lymphocytes. This ultimately leads to erosion of cartilage and bone and manifests as swelling, pain, and tenderness of the peripheral joints of the hands and feet. As the condition progresses, other joints can also become affected.

Over time, people with RA can develop characteristic deformities of the joints (see Figure 20.3) and may also develop autoimmune problems with other tissues and organs in their body.

When RA is in an active phase, symptoms are likely to be intense and may include:

- Pain.
- Stiffness of affected joints.
- Fatigue.
- Joint inflammation.
- Swelling.
- Extra-articular features such as anaemia, subcutaneous nodules, dry eyes and mouth, and vasculitis.
- Systemic symptoms such as raised temperature and nausea.
- Cognitive, mood, or emotional disorders.

There is no single diagnostic test for RA, but along with clinical history and examination, high serum ESR and CRP levels can be indicative of inflammation. Imaging techniques may be used to map the extent of erosion in the joints, and synovial fluid can be aspirated for analysis. (See also ➲ Chapter 13, Physiological measurements.)

Long-term treatment and support of people with RA will normally involve a multidisciplinary approach which focuses on maximizing physical, psychological, and social function within the constraints of the disease.

Drug treatment will often involve analgesics and NSAIDs to modify symptoms and also disease-specific drugs such as sulfasalazine and methotrexate used in combination. In some cases, intra-articular and IM steroids may be prescribed for relief of active symptoms (ℜ www.nice.org.uk). In the long term, helping people to live with RA may involve:

• Lifestyle modifications.
• Joint protection devices, splints, and immobilizers.
• Physiotherapy and exercise.
• Occupational therapy.
• Household and personal aids.
• Surgery.

Ankylosing spondylitis

This is a long-term inflammatory condition that affects the bones, muscles, and ligaments of the spine. Ankylosing spondylitis (AS) more commonly affects men and has a genetic precursor.

The inflammation in the axial skeleton causes bone erosion and fusion, resulting in pain, stiffness, and reduced movement in the spine. As the condition progresses, body posture alters and it becomes more difficult for affected people to straighten their spine. As a result, mobility may be affected. People with AS may also experience inflammatory symptoms in their eyes such as iritis and conjunctivitis. If the condition is aggressive, it can result in pulmonary fibrosis and aortic incompetence.

NICE guidelines for treatment of AS suggest drug therapy with NSAIDs, disease-modifying drugs, and possibly biological agents (ℜ www.nice.org. uk). Regular exercise is also important to maintain movement of the spine and hips.

Systemic lupus erythematosus

SLE is a complex, multisystemic autoimmune disorder, in which antibodies are developed and attack healthy organs, tissues, and skin. The cause is unknown but may be genetic. SLE can be associated with some medications and is more common in women and black people.

SLE can affect any body system, including the chest, heart, nervous system, and kidneys. Where the kidneys and CNS are involved, long-term prognosis is usually poor. Symptoms range from mildly distressing to life-threatening, and SLE is normally characterized by intermittent periods of latency and activity. General symptoms include:

• Fatigue.
• Skin rashes.
• Scaly plaques on the skin.
• Hair loss.

- Arthritis.
- Joint pain.
- Muscle pain.
- Mouth ulcers.
- Raynaud's phenomenon.
- Weight loss.
- Pleurisy.
- Vasculitis.
- Depression.
- Paranoia.
- Seizure.

Treatment of SLE will depend on which body systems are affected and may require specialist interventions. Treatments can include:
- Topical cortisone creams.
- Analgesia.
- NSAIDs.
- Steroid therapy.
- Immunosuppressive agents (such as azathioprine).

Gout

Is a type of arthritis caused by excessive uric acid in the body, which is deposited in the joints. Although gout normally affects the big toe, it can develop in any joint and causes intense pain, redness, and swelling. Gout often affects men over 40 and may also affect older women. Acute attacks of gout present suddenly with severe pain in the affected joint, which may be in the feet, ankles, knees, wrists, or hands. Known causes of gout include:
- Acute illness or infection.
- Trauma.
- Excessive alcohol intake.
- Obesity.
- Hypertension.
- Drugs that alter plasma urate concentration (such as salicylates, thiazides, furosemide, and pyrazinamide).
- Starvation.

The symptoms of gout normally include red, swollen joint(s), with constant and severe pain. In some cases, nodular swellings may develop on the fingers, toes, and ears.

The condition is normally episodic, but symptoms can be controlled through reduction in alcohol intake, prescribed medication, and treatment of other pain and symptoms in acute episodes. Affected joints can sometimes be injected with steroids.

Psoriatic arthritis

This is a chronic inflammatory arthritis and normally has an early onset. It is characterized by inflammation of the finger and toe joints or the spine in people who have psoriasis. Some people will also have eye inflammation.

Treatment is similar to that used for RA and includes NSAIDs to reduce pain and stiffness, and disease-modifying drugs to reduce arthritic activity. Specialist treatment for the primary psoriasis condition may involve dermatology services.

Enteropathic arthritis

Is a form of chronic inflammatory arthritis associated with existing inflammatory bowel disease (IBD). The areas commonly affected by enteropathic arthritic inflammation are the limb joints and spine.

Reactive arthritis

Reactive arthritis is normally secondary to a bowel, genital tract, or less frequently a throat infection. The arthritic symptoms are inflammation of the joints, eyes, and urethra. Men and women are equally affected, and symptoms generally resolve over 3–6 months. However, reactive arthritis can develop into a long-term condition.

Fibromyalgia

Fibromyalgia is a tissue disorder which causes widespread pain in the body's muscles, ligaments, and tendons. The cause of fibromyalgia is unknown, but the condition has been linked to CNS disorders, biochemical imbalances, stress responses, sleep problems, and genetic causes. The onset of symptoms may be triggered by physical, psychological, or social stressors.

Symptoms vary widely between different people, and fibromyalgia may be mistaken for myalgic encephalopathy (ME) or MS. People who suffer from fibromyalgia can experience any of the following symptoms:

- Widespread pain.
- Hypersensitivity.
- Hyperalgesia.
- Allodynia.
- Stiffness.
- Muscle spasm.
- Fatigue.
- Poor sleep quality.
- Cognitive problems (memory, information processing, speech).
- Headaches.
- Nausea.
- Dizziness[1] and clumsiness.
- Restless legs syndrome.
- Paraesthesiae.
- Extremely painful menstrual periods.
- Anxiety.
- Depression.

There is no cure for fibromyalgia, and treatment is focused on relief of symptoms, which will include analgesia and lifestyle support. It may also include specialist investigations and treatment by rheumatology, neurology, or psychology services.

---

1 NHS Choices. *Dizziness (lightheadedness)*. ℛ www.nhs.uk/conditions/dizziness/Pages/Introduction.aspx.

Juvenile arthritis

Arthritis can also affect young people (<16 years of age), in which case it is known as juvenile arthritis. This inflammatory condition is normally systemic and affects both boys and girls. Juvenile arthritis commonly affects the large joints, and treatments will include symptom control, physiotherapy, rest, and exercise.

There is no cure for the arthritic disorders, but there are many interventions that can slow down degenerative conditions and relieve acute symptoms. The main treatments for arthritis include lifestyle measures, diet and exercise, pain relief, and supportive therapies. There are also practical aids to help people living with arthritic conditions to maintain an acceptable level of function and quality of life.

Elective joint replacement surgery

Joint replacement surgery can be carried out as an emergency or elective procedure. Elective arthroplasty is normally offered to people with degenerative or arthritic conditions, whose symptoms can no longer be controlled by conservative management, or those who have severely limited function in the affected joint(s). People who have joint replacements are often older, and the purpose of the surgery is to:

• Relieve pain.
• Improve the function of the joint.
• Improve mobility.
• Enhance quality of life.

Joint replacement surgery excises the damaged joint tissues and replaces these with a prosthetic device. Arthroplasty is most commonly performed on the hip and knee joints, with the expectation that prostheses should last around 10–15 years. Elbow, shoulder, and ankle joints can also be replaced.

People having elective joint replacement surgery will normally have a preoperative assessment some time before the scheduled surgery. This is likely to involve physical and clinical examinations, X-ray or other imaging of the joint, and VTE screening and prophylaxis. (See also ➲ Chapter 22, Surgery.)

The surgery itself can be carried out under general or epidural anaesthesia, depending on the person's general condition and the clinical decisions of the surgeon and anaesthetist.

Post-operative care and rehabilitation of people who have had joint replacement surgery will normally involve an MDT of medical staff, nurses, physiotherapists, and occupational therapists. Other specialist services may also be involved such dietetics and social care.

Healthcare organizations will normally have local protocols or care pathways for joint replacement surgery, and these should always be followed. It is often the case that people who have a total hip or knee replacement will be encouraged to mobilize as soon as is feasible. In some cases, people will be able to get up and walk on the same day as their surgery.

In the post-operative period and during rehabilitation, people will also be given advice and support on caring for their new joint, including the types and extent of exercise, walking, standing, and lying down safely.

In elective joint replacement surgery, discharge planning often commences at the preoperative assessment. As large numbers of older people have joint replacements, it may be that those who live alone or do not feel able to cope independently may need a supported discharge. This can be through involvement of social services, intermediate care rehabilitation packages, private care, or discharge to a rehabilitation facility.

Dislocation and peri-prosthetic fractures

In total hip replacements, there is a risk for dislocation of the prosthetic joint. Although this is not common, the risk is greatest in the first 3 months after surgery. If a prosthetic joint dislocates, it can normally be corrected by closed reduction, without the need for further surgery.

Following joint replacement surgery, there is also a risk for peri-prosthetic fractures, particularly in very old people or those with other co-morbid conditions. Causes include loosening of the prosthesis or deterioration in an osteoporotic or other pathological condition. Peri-prosthetic fractures may also occur due to falls.

Treatment options for peri-prosthetic fractures will depend on the position and displacement of the fracture and may include protected weight-bearing, fixation with wires, and bone grafting.

Amputation

Amputation can be traumatic or surgical, and the fingers, toes, arms, or legs may be removed. In surgical, rather than traumatic, amputation, parts of the legs and feet are amputated more frequently than other body parts. Conditions and circumstances which can lead to amputation include:

- Diabetes.
- Circulatory disease or disorders.
- Severe chronic infection.
- Bone cancer.
- Traffic accidents.
- Industrial accidents.
- Armed combat.

Whether an amputation is traumatic or part of the treatment of a disorder or health condition, people are at risk of haemorrhage, infection, and other post-operative complications. Amputation will also affect a person's functional movements and/or their mobility.

- People who have had a body part amputated may report phantom pain where they experience sensations as if the amputated limb was still intact.
- Where a limb has been amputated, people may also experience severe disturbance of their body image or personal identity, sometimes with a profound loss or grief reaction.
- With limb amputations, physiotherapy interventions will be needed to assist with restoring mobility and functional movement.
- Prosthetic limbs can be designed and fitted at specialist centres.
- Rehabilitation after limb amputation may involve occupational therapy, physiotherapy, and social services to help restore an acceptable level of mobility, function, and quality of life.
- This may include assessment for driving and mobility aids, invalidity or carer support, re-employment, or retraining.

Complications of musculoskeletal trauma and surgery

Compartment syndrome

Compartment syndrome occurs when pressure builds in one or more of the sheaths of inelastic fascia that support and partition muscle, blood vessels, and nerves. It is most commonly caused by a direct or indirect trauma to a limb, usually the lower leg or forearm. It can also occur in people with severe oedema from burns.

Compartment syndrome can arise at any point before or after MSK trauma or surgery due to bleeding within the compartment, or as a result of external compression such as a cast or the use of a tourniquet during surgery. If undetected or untreated, it can lead to irreversible damage to nerves and blood vessels, resulting in loss of function in the affected limb. Compartment syndrome should be considered if a person has:

- Pain—particularly on passive movement which appears disproportionate to the injury.
- Paraesthesiae.
- Paralysis.
- Pallor.
- Pulselessness.

Compartment syndrome is a medical emergency, and in the first instance, any limb elevation should be discontinued, any casts split down to the skin, and any bandages or dressings removed.

Surgical treatment for compartment syndrome is fasciotomy where the inelastic fascia is cut to allow expansion of the compartment. The wound may be left open, whilst the compartment swelling reduces and may require frequent dressing changes. There are also devices for measuring pressures in the compartment which can be employed.

Venous thromboembolism (VTE)

VTE is the general term used to describe any thrombus that has formed within the venous system. In the orthopaedic and trauma environment, the risk for DVT and PE is increased as a result of the immobility normally associated with MSK conditions.

DVT most commonly occurs in the calf, and predisposing factors include:

- Venous stasis, due to reduced mobility.
- Increased blood viscosity (hypercoagulability).
- Traumatic or surgical damage to veins.

People with lower limb injuries are likely to have all three predisposing factors and therefore have a greater risk for developing DVT. VTE risk assessments need to be completed on admission to orthopaedic or trauma units, and local policy and procedures should always be followed. Preventative management plans may include:

- Anticoagulation medication.
- Anti-embolic stockings or calf pumps.
- Earliest possible mobilization.

DVT can be asymptomatic, with no presenting signs or symptoms, but signs of a DVT include redness, heat, and swelling in the calf, and pain on passive movement.

PE occurs if a DVT dislodges and travels along the circulatory system to the pulmonary circulation. People with PE may be asymptomatic, but signs of PE include:

- Breathlessness.
- Confusion.
- Chest pain.
- Tachycardia.

If a PE is suspected, the medical team should be called immediately, as high dependency or intensive care interventions may be needed. (See also ➲ Chapter 12, Risk assessment.)

Fat embolism syndrome (FES)

Fat emboli are associated with long bone fractures, such as those of the femur or tibia, but can also occur following elective surgery. Risk factors include younger people, closed and multiple fractures, and conservative treatment of long bone injuries, as well as operative procedures such as intramedullary nailing.

Clinical features of fat emboli often develop around 24–72 hours after trauma or surgery. Although the cause is not clearly understood, it is likely that FES occurs when fat globules are released from the bone into the circulatory system and small vessels of the lungs and brain at the time of fracture or surgical intervention.

FES is rare but presents in a similar manner to PE, with the added signs of a petechial rash on the upper body, particularly the axillae, and cerebral dysfunction. Treatment of FES will be similar to that of PE.

Dementia

It is relatively common for older people who have suffered a MSK trauma to have an existing diagnosis of dementia, and their injury is often sustained following a fall.

It may be useful to conduct MMSEs, as part of an admission procedure, and assess whether the person has the mental capacity to consent to surgery or other interventions.

It may also be useful for an appropriate health professional to complete a capacity assessment and possibly a best interest consent form. A deprivation of liberty protocol may need to be completed in accordance with local policies and guidelines.

For people who have dementia, being in an unfamiliar environment, together with the pain of a fracture or surgery, may serve to considerably disorient and distress them.

All possible steps should be taken to reduce anxiety and create a safe and comfortable environment for recovery. This may involve talking and listening to the family, relatives, or care home staff, using appropriate analgesia and other medications, or employing non-pharmacological treatments such as music therapy.

Delirium is also often seen in people who have dementia but can also be an acute problem for post-operative patients generally. A useful tool to assess people and help manage delirium is the PINCH ME assessment of:
- Pain.
- Infection.
- Nutrition.
- Constipation.
- Hydration.
- Medication.
- Environment.

(See also ➔ Chapter 16, Neurological conditions and ➔ Chapter 7, Dignity and respect.)

Moisture-associated skin damage and pressure ulcers

Moisture-associated skin damage is an inflammation and erosion of the skin caused by prolonged exposure to moisture, which can cause superficial loss and damage to the epidermis and/or dermis. Risk factors which compromise the skin's moisture barrier include:

- Old age.
- Immobility.
- Obesity.
- Poor nutrition.
- Urinary and faecal incontinence.
- Perspiration.
- Wound exudate.
- Mucus/saliva.
- Cognitive impairment.
- Friction/shear injuries.
- Some medications.

Moisture-associated skin damage can occur to people of any age, but it is more prevalent in older people due to the increased fragility of their skin. A large number of people who sustain a MSK injury are elderly and are therefore at a significantly higher risk for developing moisture-associated skin damage and/or pressure ulcers.

The most common type of moisture-associated skin damage found in people with MSK conditions is incontinence-associated dermatitis (IAD).

- Moisture lesions result from prolonged moisture exposure to intact skin of the perineum, buttocks, groins, inner thighs, natal cleft, skinfolds, and where skin is in contact with skin.
- They are usually painful, and the skin will either present as excoriated, superficial broken skin which is red and dry, or macerated.
- Skin damage is usually uneven, apart from on the natal cleft where the damage presents as a linear vertical split in the skin.
- Moisture can also damage the skin to such an extent that it is more susceptible to bacterial infection and physical damage, e.g. shearing and friction injury whilst moving in bed.
- Moisture lesions are not usually associated with a bony prominence of the skeleton, but they may be found alongside a pressure ulcer of any grade.
- Moisture lesions are commonly misdiagnosed as pressure ulcers, but it is important to recognize the difference so that they can be treated appropriately.

Pressure ulcers

A pressure ulcer is an area of skin and its underlying tissues which are damaged as a result of direct pressure and impaired blood supply. Pressure ulcers are localized and normally have a regular shape, and the wounds can vary in depth and can become necrosed. Pressure ulcers are often, though not always, associated with bony prominences. Risk factors for pressure ulcers include:

- Serious illness.
- Neurological conditions.
- Impaired mobility.
- Poor nutrition.
- Poor posture.
- Old age.

The European Pressure Ulcer Advisory Panel (ℜ www.epuap.org) publishes universal classifications of pressure ulcer grades, along with guidelines for treatment (see Figure 20.4).

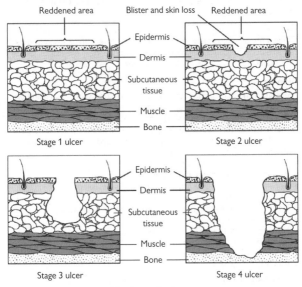

Stage 1: ulcer presents as a defined area of redness.
Stage 2: superficial ulcer with some skin loss, blister appearance, and a shallow crater.
Stage 3: full-thickness skin loss, damage to subcutaneous tissue, and deep crater.
Stage 4: full-thickness skin loss, damage extends to muscle and bone with tunnelling and sinus.

Figure 20.4 Grades of pressure ulcer

Reproduced from George Castledine and Ann Close, *Oxford Handbook of Adult Nursing*, (2009) with permission from Oxford University Press.

Grade 1

Grade 1 pressure ulcers have intact skin but will show non-blanching erythema, skin discoloration, warmth, induration or hardness relative to surrounding skin, pain, or itching.

Grade 2

Grade 2 ulcers will show partial-thickness skin loss involving the epidermis, dermis, or both. They may appear as an abrasion or blister.

Grade 3

Grade 3 ulcers show full-thickness skin loss, and subcutaneous fat may be visible. The depth of the ulcer will vary according to the location on the body, and in areas where there is little adipose tissue, such as on the heels, the ulcer is likely to be shallow. In areas where there is a lot of fatty tissue, grade 3 ulcers may be very deep, and the true depth of the ulcer may be obscured by slough in the wound bed.

Grade 4

Grade 4 pressure ulcers have full-thickness tissue loss, with exposed or directly palpable bone or tendon, and will often show tunnelling in the tissues. Grade 4 ulcers can extend into muscles, fascia, tendons, or joint capsules.

Skin care

Prevention and management of moisture-associated skin damage and pressure ulcers require nurses to ensure that all decision-making and practice is grounded in professional knowledge and practical skills and framed by professional values, teamwork, and respectful and empathic communication.

Local policies and procedures will guide appropriate nursing interventions and actions, but these are likely to include:
- Continence assessment and management.
- Regular skin assessment and inspection.
- Regular completion of a pressure ulcer risk assessment.
- Regular repositioning of people who are immobile.
- Using high-specification foam or alternating airwave mattresses.
- Using heel protectors.
- Nutritional assessment and/or dietetic referral.
- Maintaining and monitoring hydration.
- Reducing the risk of constipation.
- Pain management.

Effective preventative skin care is likely to include:
- Helping people with personal hygiene.
- Cleansing skin with a pH-balanced foam cleanser.
- Using moisturizers to restore epidermal function.
- Applying topical barrier creams.

If a person develops a pressure ulcer, then the management plan and reporting procedures will be determined by local policy. This is likely to include:
- Inspecting and documenting the surface area and depth of pressure ulcers.
- Liaising with tissue viability services for specialist advice.
- Using aseptic non-touch technique (ANTT) when cleaning and dressing pressure ulcers.
- Using appropriate dressing treatments, according to local drug formulary and local policy, to maintain a warm, moist, non-toxic environment for wound healing.

Management of musculoskeletal pain

People with MSK conditions may have chronic pain caused by long-term degenerative disorders, acute pain associated with traumatic injury, or post-operative pain following elective or emergency surgery.

Treatment priorities will differ, depending on whether the pain is chronic or acute. Typically, the management of chronic MSK pain focuses on controlling pain levels and achieving an acceptable quality of life and functionality in social and vocational contexts.

Acute MSK pain management focuses on reducing pain to acceptable levels to assist with recovery and prevent post-operative complications.

All healthcare organizations are likely to have local guidelines for pain management which are based on the WHO 'analgesic ladder'. Local policies and procedures for prescribing, administering, and recording analgesic regimes should always be followed.

In MSK pain, multimodal analgesia is often used, particularly in chronic pain conditions. Multimodal pain management will typically escalate a combination of analgesics and neuropathic and adjunct drugs until pain relief is achieved.

The multimodal approach aims to prevent and control pain, avoid unnecessarily high doses of one type of analgesic, and minimize side effects. Examples of typical drugs include:

- *NSAIDs*: such as ibuprofen, diclofenac, naproxen, and celecoxib.
- *Weak opioids*: such as codeine, dihydrocodeine, and tramadol.
- *Strong opioids*: such as morphine, fentanyl, buprenorphine, oxycodone, and pethidine.
- *Adjuncts*: such as antidepressants, anticonvulsants, steroids, and benzodiazepines.

(See also ➲ Chapter 23, Pain.)

Mobility and rehabilitation

Rehabilitation and restoration of function is important in minimizing the potential complications of short- or long-term immobility associated with MSK conditions.

Following emergency or elective MSK surgery, or for people who have long-term degenerative disorders, it is most likely that an MDT will be involved in planning and supporting rehabilitation, mobility, and restoration of function. MDTs are likely to include medical staff, physiotherapists, nurses, and occupational therapists.

Physiotherapists can give people support and advice on using crutches, walking frames, walking sticks, and other mobility aids correctly. They can also advise on appropriate exercises to restore movement and function. However, it is important to note that in long-term MSK conditions, or following trauma or elective surgery, resumption of full function is not always possible.

There will normally be local policies or procedures to guide rehabilitation and mobility planning, such as an expectation that the majority of people who have had a total knee replacement should be full weight-bearing post-operatively. However, some people will have instability in the joint, or may be very frail, or have post-operative pain or nausea which will limit their ability to mobilize as expected. Therefore, mobility, appropriate exercise, and rehabilitation plans will need to be specific to each individual.

Depending on the nature of any surgery or other treatments, there will be different types of mobility plans which support healing and resumption of function. In general terms, these can be described as:

- *Full weight-bearing*: placing full body weight on the affected leg as normal. This is usual for total hip and total knee replacements. Crutches or frames will be required initially, with the person able to work towards independent mobility at their own pace.
- *Weight-bearing as tolerated*: placing as much weight through the affected limb as feels comfortable, letting pain and discomfort be the guide. Crutches or frames will be required initially, with the person able to work towards independent mobility at their own pace.
- *Partial weight-bearing*: placing a reduced amount of weight through the affected leg. This is sometimes predetermined as a percentage proportionate to the person's body weight. Partial weight-bearing may be used for people who have had total hip and total knee replacements. Crutches or frames will be needed.
- *Toe-touch weight-bearing*: where the floor should only be touched for balance. No weight is borne through the leg, and crutches or frames are required to facilitate movement.
- *Heel weight-bearing*: body weight can be placed through the heel of the foot, but no weight must go through the toes. This is used where there has been surgery on the front of the foot. Crutches or walking sticks may be helpful.
- *Non-weight-bearing*: no weight can be placed on the affected leg, and mobility aids such as crutches or frames are necessary. Usually used after ankle surgery and some foot surgery.

Clinical investigations in musculoskeletal conditions

- *X-rays* are the primary method of investigation used to identify fractures, dislocations, and joint disease such as OA.
- *Ultrasound scan* can be used to detect soft tissue lesions such as a rotator cuff muscle tear in the shoulder. Abscesses, joint effusions, and haematomas can also be identified.
- *CT* scans give a three-dimensional image of a bone, joint, or fracture.
- *MRI* is often used to show details of the spinal column, joint and muscular abnormalities, bone tumours, and soft tissue masses.
- *Bone scans* involve IV injection of a radioisotope, before bone is scanned for the presence of metastatic disease, tumours, bone infections, and other inflammatory changes such as loosening of a hip or knee replacement.
- *Nerve conduction studies* are used to identify damage to peripheral nerves, both motor and sensory. Electrodes are placed on the skin over the muscles being tested, and a small electrical current is delivered to the skin.
- *EMG* involves inserting a small needle into a muscle to detect the electrical activity and any muscle or nerve damage. EMG is often used to diagnose conditions such as carpal tunnel syndrome.
- *Arthroscopy* is an investigative procedure where a small camera device is inserted into a joint. It enables diagnosis of the joint problem. Biopsy or therapeutic surgery can be performed at the same time.
- *ECG and/or echocardiogram* are commonly used as part of a falls assessment where there is actual or potential MSK trauma or fracture.

Laboratory tests

Where a person presents with an MSK disorder, this may be a result of another underlying condition or an associated complication which has not been diagnosed or treated. In these cases, useful laboratory tests include:

- Biochemical bone profile—serum calcium, phosphate, and alkaline phosphatase.
- Serum U&Es.
- FBC.
- Serum protein electrophoresis.
- ESR and CRP.
- Serum creatine kinase (CK).
- Urinalysis/MSU.
- Urine Bence–Jones protein (BJP).
- CXR.
- ABGs.
- Blood cultures.
- TFTs.
- LFTs.
- Blood glucose.
- Serum B12 and folate.

When an older person has suffered a fracture, they may experience an episode of acute confusion or delirium, which is common in cases of fractured neck of femur. Some laboratory services offer a 'confusion screen' which is a combination of blood tests used to identify biochemical, microbiological, or other causes of confusion.

Key nursing considerations

When working with people with MSK or rheumatologic disorders, their families, and significant others, all nursing practice and decision-making is framed by professional knowledge, values, and teamwork, and grounded in respectful, empathic communication.

For effective clinical decision-making, it is important to engage with both the person and their family, interpret any information they give within the framework of professional nursing knowledge, and be guided by local policies and procedures to determine appropriate courses of nursing action.

For all people with MSK and rheumatologic conditions, these are likely to include:

- Ongoing clinical assessment and observations.
- In MSK trauma, assess the risk of peripheral neurovascular deterioration and compartment syndrome.
- Timely and accurate record-keeping and reporting.
- Effective communication with the MDT.
- Timely and accurate reporting of any observations, clinical measurements, or changes in the person's condition.
- Liaison with specialist services such as physiotherapists, occupational therapists, pain specialists, and tissue viability specialists.
- In a hospital environment, calculate EWS and adjust care in accordance with local track and trigger escalation plans.
- Monitor blood pressure, heart rate, oxygen saturation, temperature, respiratory rate, and urine output.
- Complete a falls risk assessment.
- Assess VTE risk and apply preventative devices as indicated.
- Assess risk for moisture wounds and pressure ulcers.
- Assess and monitor nutritional status.
- Assess any restricted mobility, and note any mobility aids used or needed.
- Complete any clinical investigations ordered.
- Prepare for surgery in line with local policies and procedures.
- Pain and medicines management.
- Support resumption of mobility as appropriate.
- Inform the person of any procedures or investigations which are being carried out.
- Clearly explain all nursing actions and interventions.
- Support patients, families, and carers in understanding the MSK condition and its implications.
- Work with patients, families, and carers to address the functional, psychological, and social impact of the MSK condition.
- Seek to clearly and honestly allay any patient and family anxieties.
- Maintain a safe and calming environment for recovery.
- As far as possible, ensure physical comfort.

(For details of specific clinical procedures, see ➲ *Oxford Handbook of Clinical Skills in Adult Nursing*.)

Useful sources of further information

- Arthritis ℘ www.arthritisresearchuk.org, www.arthritiscare.org.uk
- Back Care ℘ www.backcare.org.uk
- British Pain Society ℘ www.britishpainsociety.org
- European Pressure Ulcer Advisory Panel ℘ www.epuap.org
- Fibromyalgia ℘ www.ukfibromyalgia.com
- Lupus UK ℘ www.lupusuk.org.uk
- NHS Choices ℘ www.nhs.uk/Conditions
- NICE ℘ www.nice.org.uk
- Osteoporosis ℘ www.nos.org.uk
- Prosthetic limbs ℘ www.limbless-association.org

Drugs frequently prescribed for musculoskeletal and rheumatologic conditions

Drugs frequently prescribed for MSK and rheumatologic conditions are listed in Table 20.1. *All drug doses listed in this table are adult doses.* This table is only to be used as a guide, and the current *BNF* should be consulted for further advice. Nurses should involve themselves only in the administration of medications which fall within their sphere of competence.

Table 20.1 Drugs frequently prescribed for musculoskeletal and rheumatologic conditions

Anti-inflammatory drugs	Dose	Common side effects
Non-selective NSAIDs (ibuprofen carries the lowest risk for adverse GI effects, with piroxicam, ketoprofen, and ketorolac associated with the highest risk and indometacin, naproxen, and diclofenac as intermediate risk)	Ibuprofen: initially 300–400mg 3–4 times daily, increased if necessary to maximum of 2400mg daily; maintenance dose of 600–1200mg daily may be adequate. See *BNF* for doses of other NSAIDs	GI discomfort, nausea, diarrhoea, and occasionally bleeding and ulceration occur, particularly in the elderly; a degree of worsening of asthma may occur; hypersensitivity reactions. Increased risk for thrombotic events (e.g. MI and stroke). See *BNF* for full range of side effects and degree of risk with different NSAIDs
Selective NSAIDs, i.e. cyclo-oxygenase 2 (COX-2) inhibitors (as effective as non-selective agents and should only be used instead of a standard NSAID in patients at high risk for developing serious GI problems)	Celecoxib: OA, 200mg daily in 1–2 divided doses, increased if necessary to maximum of 200mg twice daily	As above
Osteoporosis	**Dose**	**Common side effects**
Bisphosphonates, e.g. alendronic acid	Alendronic acid— treatment of post-menopausal osteoporosis: 10mg daily or 70mg once weekly. Treatment of osteoporosis in men: 10mg daily	Oesophageal reactions, abdominal pain and distension, dyspepsia, regurgitation, melaena, diarrhoea or constipation, flatulence, MSK pain, headache

(Continued)

Table 20.1 (Contd.)

Rheumatologic conditions		
Gout	**Dose**	**Common side effects**
Colchicine	For acute treatment of gout: 500 micrograms 2–4 times daily until pain relieved or vomiting/diarrhoea occurs; maximum of 6mg per course; course not to be repeated within 3 days Prevention of gout attacks when starting allopurinol: 500 micrograms twice daily	Nausea, vomiting, abdominal pain; excessive doses may cause profuse diarrhoea, GI haemorrhage, rashes, and renal and hepatic damage
Allopurinol	Prophylaxis of gout: initially 100mg daily, preferably after food, then adjusted according to plasma or urinary uric acid concentration; maintenance dose of 100–200mg daily in mild conditions, 300–600mg daily in moderate conditions, 700–900mg daily in severe conditions; doses over 300mg daily given in divided doses	Rashes (*withdraw* therapy, though if mild, re-introduce gradually—discontinue immediately if recurrence); hypersensitivity reactions occur rarely (see *BNF* for further details and more side effects)
Febuxostat	Treatment of chronic hyperuricaemia in gout: 80mg once daily, increasing to 120mg once daily if serum uric acid level is >6mg/ 100mL after 2–4 weeks' treatment	GI disturbances, abnormal LFTs, oedema, and headache. Rare, but serious, hypersensitivity reactions (see *BNF* for further details)
Rheumatoid arthritis	**Dose**	**Common side effects**
Methotrexate	7.5mg *once weekly* (as a single dose normally of 3 × 2.5mg tablets), adjusted according to response, maximum total weekly dose of 20mg	Mucositis, myelosuppression, anorexia, abdominal discomfort, intestinal ulceration and bleeding, diarrhoea, and many more (see *BNF*)

(Continued)

Table 20.1 (Contd.)

Hydroxychloroquine	Administered on expert advice; 200–400mg daily; maximum of 6.5mg/kg using ideal body weight	GI disturbances, headache, and skin reactions (rashes, pruritus); many more less common side effects (see *BNF*)
Sulfasalazine	Administered on expert advice and normally as enteric-coated tablets; initially 500mg daily, increased by 500mg at intervals of a week to a maximum of 2–3g daily in divided doses	Rashes, GI intolerance, and occasional leucopenia, neutropenia, and thrombocytopenia; hypersensitivity reactions For sulfasalazine, see ➋ Table 17.2, Drugs frequently prescribed for gastrointestinal conditions, p. 306
Leflunomide	Initially 100mg once daily for 3 days, then 10–20mg once daily	Diarrhoea, nausea, vomiting, anorexia, oral mucosal disorders, abdominal pain, increased blood pressure, headache, and many more (see *BNF*)

Conditions of the eyes, ears, nose, and throat

Introduction

Many disorders of vision and hearing are concomitant with the growing elderly demographic, and conditions of the eyes, and ears, nose, and throat (ENT) are often associated with other health states. Whilst ophthalmic and ENT interventions are largely the domain of distinct clinical specialisms, general adult nurses are likely to encounter people with eyes and ENT conditions across all care settings. This chapter outlines key facts about eyes and vision disorders and ENT conditions which are likely to be useful to the general nurse. Important nursing considerations for decision-making and practice are outlined, and an overview of frequently prescribed medications is presented in a summary table.

Eye conditions

Disorders of the eye and visual pathway can range from minor transient irritations or infections through to sight-threatening ophthalmic conditions. Eye conditions may also be indicative of other underlying pathology or disease processes.

People suffering from eye conditions may develop profound anxiety about the possibility of blindness or be concerned about the nature of any invasive clinical investigations or treatments needed. Eye conditions also have the potential to impact on all areas of a person's life and work. People who are visually impaired may become socially isolated as a result of difficulties in recognizing people, or have limited confidence in their ability to undertake everyday activities.

Styes (hordeolum)

Styes are an infection of lash follicles in the lid margin, and the infective response results in a cyst and the production of pus. Treatment of styes is with lid hygiene, warm compresses, and application of topical antibiotic drops or ointments.

Chalazion (meibomian cyst)

This is a hard lump in the meibomian gland that often follows a staphylococcal infection and which usually resolves spontaneously. Treatment includes lid hygiene and lid massage, and persistent cases may require incision and curettage under local anaesthesia.

Basal cell carcinoma

This is a common malignancy of the eyelid. It may start as a pearly nodule that becomes ulcerated with time. Treatment includes excision, curettage, cryotherapy, or radiotherapy.

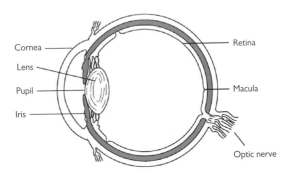

Figure 21.1 Structure of the eye.

Reproduced from George Castledine and Ann Close, *Oxford Handbook of Adult Nursing*, (2009) with permission from Oxford University Press.

Blepharitis

Is an extremely common chronic infection of the eyelid margins. It causes red, itchy, crusted, and scaly lids. It is sometimes associated with conjunctivitis. Treatment includes removing crusts and scales by frequent soaking with warm compresses. Antibiotics or steroid drops may be required if the condition persists.

Dacryocystitis

Dacryocystitis is inflammation of the lacrimal sac, causing redness, swelling, and watering of eyes due to a blocked tear duct. Pus may exude from the tear ducts, and inflammation may spread to surrounding tissues and lead to systemic infection. A diagnostic swab of discharge should be taken before antibiotics are prescribed.

Conjunctivitis

This may be due to allergy, bacterial infection, viruses, or *Chlamydia*. Eyes are often gritty, sticky, itchy, and sore, with discharge and mild photophobia, but no change in vision. Conjunctivitis is often bilateral.

Any discharge should be removed with scrupulous eye hygiene, and cosmetics and lotions should be avoided. Antibiotic eye drops, such as chloramphenicol, are often prescribed for bacterial and viral infections, and for allergic conjunctivitis, a range of anti-allergy drops are available. In severe or persistent cases, topical steroids or antihistamine drops may be prescribed by an ophthalmologist.

Ectropion

Ectropion is a turning-out of the lower eyelid. This condition can cause eye irritation and watering, and the condition may be unsightly. Surgery may be needed.

Entropion

Entropion is a turning-in of the lower eyelid. This condition can cause severe eye irritation and watering, and the eyelashes of the turned-in lid can irritate the cornea. Taping the lower eyelid to the cheek can give temporary relief, but in the longer term, corrective surgery may be required.

Photophobia

Is painful sensitivity to light and may be indicative of other underlying conditions or neurological disorders (see also ➜ Chapter 16, Neurological conditions).

Corneal abrasion or ulcer

Is a result of traumatic injury to the cornea of the eye by grit, dirt, or a foreign object scratching the surface, often experienced by contact lens wearers. Abrasion or ulcers cause intense pain and photophobia and, if not treated, can result in permanent damage to the eye. Treatment is usually by antibiotic and steroid drops. These are often administered hourly in the first instance, and with reducing frequency as the cornea improves.

Keratoplasty

This is the procedure of corneal grafting to replace a severely damaged cornea. It is performed under general anaesthesia, and the graft is generally from a donor.

Eye pain

Pain is often severe if it is due to corneal abrasions, foreign bodies, scleritis, or acute glaucoma. It tends to be less severe in conjunctivitis, keratoconjunctivitis, and optic neuritis. Eye pain may also be due to referred pain, trigeminal neuralgia, shingles, migraine, and tension headaches. It may also occur post-operatively or after laser treatment.

Dry eyes

Dryness causes irritation and redness and is due to reduced secretion or evaporation of tears, or mucin deficiency in tears. 'Artificial' tear drops can be inserted to provide relief.

Periorbital cellulitis

This is an inflammation to the area surrounding the eyeball, often affecting the eyelid and the skin surrounding the outer aspect of the eye, and can include the upper cheek.

Periorbital cellulitis may follow a period of sinusitis or periorbital injury. People present with fever, eyelid swelling, pain, general malaise, and discharge and congestion of the eye. Complications include retinal vein occlusion, optic nerve compression, blindness, and cavernous sinus thrombosis.

The condition is generally treated with IV antibiotics, followed by a course of oral antibiotic therapy. Blood cultures to determine appropriate antibiotic therapy are normally needed, and consultation with specialist ENT services should be sought.

Macular degeneration

This is the leading cause of blindness in people over 65 years of age. It affects both eyes with deterioration in central vision, including blurring, distortion, dark spots, problems in bright sunlight, and difficulty adapting between dark and light. It causes problems with reading, writing, and facial recognition.

Risk factors include age, family history, sunlight, smoking, and diet. Management strategies include use of magnifying devices, large-print publications, talking books, and clocks. People with macular degeneration should consider registering as 'sight-impaired' if partially sighted or 'severely sight-impaired' if blind (ℜ www.rnib.org.uk).

Acute macular degeneration (AMD) is normally treated by photocoagulation, and some specialist centres treat wet AMD with photodynamic therapy and ranibizumab injection.

Cataract

Cataract refers to opacity of the lens, which is a leading cause of blindness worldwide, and is a priority area for the WHO (ℜ www.who.int). The condition is usually progressive, and people experience reduced ability to focus or perceive colour. Blurring or loss of vision, halos around objects, and increased glare are also common.

Causes include congenital infection (rubella), family history, age, obesity, diabetes, trauma, radiation exposure, and drugs (long-term steroid use). People presenting with cataracts may have an undiagnosed diabetic condition, which should be excluded.

Treatment includes surgical extraction, followed by plastic lens implant, normally as day-case surgery, with local anaesthesia. Post-operatively, antibiotics and steroid eye drops are given for around 2–4 weeks.

Following cataract surgery, people should avoid lifting, bending, smoky atmospheres, make-up, hairspray, and swimming. An eye shield can be worn at night to prevent inadvertent rubbing.

Glaucoma

In glaucoma, raised intraocular pressure causes damage to the optic nerve, leading to loss of vision. Glaucoma is usually chronic and known as primary open-angle glaucoma (POAG).

In POAG, the intraocular pressure is not so high as to cause pain, but it can cause considerable damage to the optic nerve. However, because it affects peripheral vision first, the person may be unaware, and it is often first noticed by an optician at a routine eye test.

Risks include age, family history, African origin, diabetes, thyroid eye disease, and short-sightedness. Medical treatment involves lowering the intraocular pressure, normally with topical prostaglandin agonists and/or β-blockers. Surgery may be necessary in some cases.

Much less common is acute angle-closure glaucoma. This is an ophthalmic emergency, in which the intraocular pressure is extremely high, causing substantial pain. The eye is red and hard, the cornea cloudy, and the pupil unreactive. This condition requires urgent treatment with drops (including pilocarpine) and IV medication (commonly acetazolamide). Treatment is peripheral iridotomy by laser surgery, which normally prevents recurrence.

People aged over 40 or who have a family history of glaucoma should have an annual eye screening.

Retinal detachment

Retinal detachment is also a serious ophthalmic disorder, which may lead to blindness. Risks include middle age, short-sightedness, and previous detachment.

Initially, people will see a shadow across the vision of the affected eye, and they may also see bright flashes or floaters in the field of vision, but there is no pain.

At a very early stage, retinal detachment may be treated by laser or cryotherapy under local anaesthesia. Most cases, however, require surgery by vitrectomy. In vitrectomy, the vitreous is removed from the eyeball, and either gas or silicone oil is used to reinflate the eye, which pushes the retina back into place. This is normally performed under general anaesthesia but can be undertaken with local anaesthetic.

Following retinal surgery, people are advised to keep their heads in a fixed position for 5–10 days to enable the gas or silicone oil to push the retina back into place. Where a gas bubble has been injected, it will normally take around 6 weeks to be absorbed. During this time, the patient is advised to alert the anaesthetist if they are admitted to hospital for any other surgery, and people should not travel by air whilst the gas remains in their eye.

The extent to which people are able to see after surgery depends partly on whether the retinal detachment extended to affect the central vision. If so, the ability to see fine detail may not return.

Diabetic retinopathy

Retinopathy is a known complication of diabetes, and over time people with diabetes may become increasingly visually impaired. Diabetic retinopathy is classified as three different types:

- *Background diabetic retinopathy*—where blocked, dilated, or leaky retinal capillaries become fragile and haemorrhage. It is usually asymptomatic and not sight-threatening.
- *Proliferative diabetic retinopathy*—where damaged blood vessels reduce blood supply to the retina, leading to growth of new fragile blood vessels, retinal scarring, and retinal detachment.
- *Diabetic maculopathy*—is ischaemia and/or leakage of fluid which reduces the function of the macula and affects central vision.

Laser photocoagulation can be used to treat both maculopathy and proliferative retinopathy. Appropriate treatment of the underlying diabetes is necessary, and people living with diabetes are offered annual eye screening, with retinal photography to monitor for ocular degeneration.

Other ophthalmic terms and conditions

See Box 21.1.

Box 21.1 Other ophthalmic terms and conditions

- Diplopia: double vision.
- Enucleation: removal of the eye.
- Evisceration: removal of the globe contents whilst retaining sclera and extraocular muscles.
- Exophthalmos: protrusion of the eyeball.
- Hyphaema: bleeding into the anterior chamber of the eye.
- Hypopyon: collection of pus in the anterior chamber of the eye.
- Nystagmus: involuntary rhythmic movement of the eyeball.
- Papilloedema: unilateral or bilateral oedema of the optic disc due to raised ICP.
- Scleritis: inflammation of the white of the eye.

Eye tests and clinical investigations

Disorders of the eye, or visual disturbances, may be a symptom of another (diagnosed or undiagnosed) condition, so clinical investigations and eye examination seek to exclude these conditions or causes:

- Renal disease.
- Hypertension.
- Diabetes.
- RA.
- MS.
- Head injury, neurological disease, or nerve damage—which may result in abnormal pupil reactions.
- Drugs such as anticoagulants, anti-hypertensives, and recreational drugs which can cause visual disturbances.
- Family history of eye disease.

Visual acuity

Visual acuity evaluates central vision and is tested (with spectacles or contact lenses if worn) using either Snellen's test board or LogMAR visual acuity test. Near vision can be tested by reading a book or newspaper.

Ophthalmoscopy

This is mainly used to examine the retina. It may detect retinal haemorrhage or exudate, retinal detachment, cupped discs (an indication of glaucoma), abnormal vitreous and blood, loose floaters, or red reflex. In addition, it can be useful to identify cataracts or abnormal pupils.

Viewing the retina is carried out in a darkened room, using prescribed mydriatic drops to dilate the pupil. Before these drops are administered, people should be advised that their vision will be blurred and they should not drive or be exposed to bright light until this wears off; normally, this takes a few hours.

Examination with a slit-lamp

This provides a slit of light of variable thickness and angulation that is viewed through a binocular microscope to give a magnified view of the structures of the front of the eye. Additional hand-held lenses are required to view the retina and optic disc at the back of the eye.

Selected other eye tests

- *Tonometry*: tonometry is used to measure IOP after topical anesthetic has been administered.
- *Fundus fluorescein angiography*: dye is injected into veins to highlight retinal blood vessels and detect any leakage and dilation.
- *Fundus photography*: is used to record the retinal appearance.
- *Visual field test (perimetry)*: visual field tests assess peripheral vision, as well as central vision, and measurements are used to produce a 'map' of a person's visual field.
- *CT scan*: CT of the head can be used to identify tumours affecting the occipital lobe and optic nerve.

- *X-ray*: where a person has eye or vision symptoms which may be related to an underlying condition, X-rays can be useful to detect associated problems, or for head and face damage which is affecting the eyes or vision.
- *Ultrasound scan*: these scans are useful for viewing structures inside the eye.
- *Laboratory tests*: if underlying conditions are suspected, FBC, blood glucose, U&Es, and a lipid profile may be necessary to assist in diagnosis.

Eye surgery

Approximately 80% of eye surgery is performed under local anaesthesia as day-case surgery, and many people presenting for eye surgery belong to the older age group.

For eye surgery, local policies and procedures should always be followed, but special attention may need to be given to people's anxieties about temporary or permanent loss of sight. The ability of people to care for themselves post-operatively or learning to live with a degree of impaired vision should also be assessed as part of any longer-term care plan.

Visual impairment

Visually impaired people may lack confidence when they are outside their familiar environment and may have difficulty orienting to a new or different place. Nurses should aim to minimize any distress or discomfort through active listening and thoughtful responses to people's concerns.

It is important to provide verbal guidance to the physical geography of the care setting and perhaps orient the person by walking with them around the care environment. Always walk at the person's pace and describe what they are approaching.

If the visually impaired person has a working dog, these should never be distracted.

For drivers with visual impairment, the DVLA needs to be notified (% www.gov.uk/government/organisations/driver-and-vehicle-licensing-agency). Air travel may be restricted for a time in certain conditions such as following eye surgery.

Key nursing considerations

Irrespective of the nature of the eye condition, nursing practice and decision-making are grounded in effective and empathetic communication, alongside clinical knowledge and skills.

A lot of ophthalmic practice is now the domain of specialist nurses or advanced practitioners, but general nurses may have occasion to work with people experiencing visual impairments, in both hospital and community settings.

Nursing practices will be determined by the nature of the ophthalmic diagnosis and treatment plan, and all local policies and procedures should always be followed. In the hospital setting, additional nursing time may be needed to orient people with visual impairment to the place of care.

- Carry out all admissions procedures and assessments according to local policies and procedures.
- Accurately monitor and record all clinical and ophthalmic observations.
- Complete any clinical investigations ordered.
- Accurately administer and record any prescribed pain relief, symptom relief, and other medications.
- Accurately record and report any changes to the person's condition within the MDT.
- Liaison with specialist ophthalmic services.
- Orient the person to the care environment and ensure their physical comfort.
- Clearly explain all actions and interventions.
- Give accurate explanations of likely events and investigations such as installation of eye drops or preparation for surgery.
- Maintain a safe and calming environment for recovery.
- Seek to allay patient and family anxieties.

Examination of the eye and visual function

- Observe and compare the person's eyes for swelling, discharge, stickiness, bruising, redness, the conjunctiva, clarity or abrasions of the cornea, shape and size of the pupils, and reaction to light.
- Note and report any visual changes or disturbances, including blurred or distorted vision, dark spots in the visual field, flashing light, floaters, and rainbow colours or halos around bright lights.
- Record photophobia, headaches, and pain.
- Clarify normal use of prescription glasses, reading glasses, varifocals, bifocals, contact lenses, or prosthetic eyes.
- Ascertain whether the person is registered as visually impaired or severely visually impaired (℞ www.rnib.org.uk) and their usual coping strategies.
- Clarify their normal work, and domestic and social situation.
- Assess any anxieties about their current eye condition.

Installing eye drops

- Explain the procedure and gain the person's consent.
- Decontaminate hands according to local policies and procedures.
- Ask the person to look up, and gently evert the lower lid.
- Insert the required number of drops into the lower conjunctival fornix, without touching the eye.
- Apply gentle pressure over the lacrimal sac (just below the medial aspect of the eye) to improve absorption into the eye.
- Ask the person to close their eyes, and wipe away any excess, moving from the nose outwards.
- Wash and dry hands.
- Wait 5–10 minutes if installing further drugs in the same eye.

Ear conditions

Disorders of the ear and auditory pathway can range from minor and transient infections through to serious neurological conditions and profound deafness. Ear conditions may also be indicative of other underlying pathology or disease.

It is estimated that approximately 1 in 6 people in the UK have hearing loss (🕮 www.actiononhearingloss.org.uk). People who are suffering from ear conditions may become socially isolated as a result of difficulties in hearing and an inability to participate fully in everyday social communication or interaction.

Ear conditions can affect the outer, middle, or inner ear (see Figure 21.2) and may also be associated with cranial nerve disorders.

Foreign body

Foreign bodies in the outer ear can cause pain, discomfort, hearing loss, and infection. A superficial foreign body can be removed by a suitably experienced practitioner. If there is any risk of damage to the eardrum, removal under general anaesthesia may be needed. Antibiotics may be prescribed to prevent infection.

Impacted ear wax

Impacted ear wax develops due to difficulty in shedding debris and wax in people who have narrow ear canals, or wear earplugs or hearing aid moulds. It can also be caused by using cotton buds to clean the ear. Over time, it can lead to increased hearing impairment and deafness. Treatment includes irrigation and microsuction but may require the use of topical

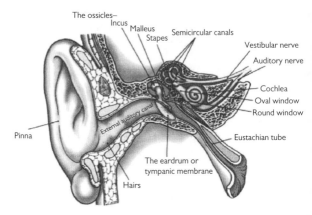

Figure 21.2 Simple diagram of the ear.

Reproduced from Rogan Corbridge and Nicholas Steventon, *Oxford Handbook of ENT and Head and Neck Surgery* 2e (2010), with permission from Oxford University Press.

drops such as olive oil or sodium bicarbonate to soften the wax before removal. *Removal of ear wax should only be attempted by clinical practitioners who have been appropriately trained.*

Otitis externa

Is a bacterial or fungal infection of the external ear and may be due to scratching (e.g. in eczema) or exposure to water ('swimmer's ear'). It results in pain, discharge, and swelling of the ear canal, sometimes involving the surrounding lymph nodes. Treatment includes aural toilet to remove debris, antibiotic and steroid drops, combination ointment, or antifungal drops. In some cases, an ear pack will be inserted to help keep the ear canal open. People with otitis externa will need pain relief, and referral to ENT specialist services may be required.

Furunculosis

Furunculosis is an infection of a hair follicle in the ear canal, which causes severe pain. Treatment includes pain relief, topical antibiotics, and steroid drops. If there is surrounding inflammation, oral antibiotics may be prescribed. It may be associated with an undiagnosed diabetic condition.

Ramsay–Hunt syndrome (herpes zoster)

Ramsay–Hunt syndrome is a rare condition, normally associated with a history of chickenpox or shingles. Vesicles appear in the external ear canal and around the ear. Pain, deafness, vertigo, and seventh cranial nerve palsy may occur. If facial palsy occurs, then measures to protect the eye, such as lubricant ointments, and taping the eye closed should be used. Pain relief is essential, and antiviral medications (e.g. aciclovir) and steroids may be helpful for treatment of palsy.

Post-auricular sebaceous cyst

This is an infection of a sebaceous gland behind the pinna and causes swelling, pain, and deformity. Mastoiditis, sore throats, and neck pain can be complications. Treatment for a cyst requires pain relief and may also involve excision and packing of the cyst under local anaesthesia. Cysts which have been packed will normally need daily dressing changes.

Acute otitis media

People with otitis media present with earache, conductive deafness, pyrexia, and general malaise, and the condition is common in children. Spontaneous perforation of the eardrum may occur, resulting in a cessation of pain and discharge of pus. Mastoiditis can be a complication. Otitis media is normally managed through pain relief and antibiotic therapy if the condition persists for >2–3 days. In the longer term or in cases of mastoiditis, surgical treatment by insertion of grommets may be indicated.

Glue ear

Otitis media with effusion may follow an acute episode of otitis media due to inadequate drainage via the Eustachian tube. It results in deafness and speech and language problems, and is common in children. Long-term antibiotics and mucolytics may be used, but the condition is often treated surgically by the insertion of grommets.

Cholesteatoma

A cholesteatoma is an uncommon condition, which is an abnormal collection of skin cells inside the ear, normally caused by damage, collapse, or trauma to the eardrum. A cholesteatoma normally affects one ear and is manifest as a persistent discharge and gradual hearing loss in the affected ear. If untreated, cholesteatoma can permanently damage the structures of the inner ear and lead to infection, vertigo, tinnitus, damage to facial nerves, or permanent hearing loss.

Ear bleeding or discharge

Bleeding or discharge from the ears is normally indicative of other conditions. Bleeding may occur as a result of trauma, infection, perforation of the eardrum, or basal skull fracture. With skull fracture, CSF may leak from the ears. Offensive discharge can occur in infections of the outer and middle ear.

Perforated eardrum

A perforated eardrum can result from direct trauma, fracture to the base of the skull, blast injury, or substantial changes in barometric pressure (e.g. in scuba diving). The person will experience pain, conductive deafness, and sometimes bleeding. Antibiotics are given to prevent infection, and attempts to clean or dry the ear should be avoided. People with a perforated eardrum are normally referred to specialist ENT services.

Mastoiditis

Caused by an infection in the middle ear extending to the mastoid cells and space. It results in pyrexia, tenderness and swelling, discharge, and hearing loss. Complications can include cranial nerve palsy, meningitis, and brain abscesses. Treatment is by IV antibiotics and analgesia.

Tinnitus

Tinnitus refers to any sound heard in the ear, which is not from an external source. People who experience tinnitus usually describe it as ringing, buzzing, or whistling sounds. The cause is often unknown but may be linked to exposure to loud noises, hearing loss, head injuries, Ménière's disease, raised blood pressure, stroke, vascular disorders, diabetes, and prescribed or recreational drugs.

Ear examination and audiogram investigations are needed, and unilateral tinnitus should be investigated by MRI to exclude damage to the cochlear–vestibular nerve. Tinnitus is very difficult to treat, and in severe cases, it can interfere with daily life and lead to depressive states. Tinnitus should always be investigated by ENT specialist services to exclude underlying conditions such as acoustic neuroma.

Ménière's disease

This is a relatively rare inner ear disorder which presents with episodes of vertigo, fluctuating hearing loss and tinnitus, and a sense of fullness in the ear. People may also experience nausea and vomiting. The cause is unknown but may be due to overproduction of endolymph fluid. Episodes can be triggered by factors such as stress, fatigue, alcohol, or flashing lights.

Treatment includes diuretics, a low-salt diet, avoiding triggers, and anti-emetics. The majority of cases are treated medically, but endolymphatic sac surgery and vestibular nerve section are surgical interventions which can also be used.

Acoustic neuroma

This is a rare benign neoplasm of the eighth cranial nerve that causes tin-nitus, asymmetrical sensorineural deafness, and vertigo. Treatment may be by conservative management of symptoms or through micro-surgery in specialist neurosurgical units.

Vertigo

Vertigo may be of central origin but is often caused by inner ear prob-lems and disturbance of the balance mechanisms in the ear. Vertigo may be accompanied by dizziness, and the person may experience falls or 'drop attacks' if the vertigo is sudden and intense. Attacks vary in severity and duration, and are often accompanied by nausea and/or vomiting. Treatment is by anti-emetic medicines and vestibular suppressant drugs.

Ear tests and clinical investigations

Disorders of the ear, or hearing impairment, may be a symptom of another (diagnosed or undiagnosed) condition, so ear examination and clinical investigations will seek to exclude:
- History of infectious diseases such as herpes, meningitis, and measles.
- Long-term use of prescribed medicines.
- Family history of ear problems.
- Trauma.
- Past surgery.

An auroscope is used to examine the external ear canal and eardrum. By gently pulling the pinna upwards and backwards (to straighten the ear canal), it will be possible to see wax, debris, foreign bodies, and the eardrum itself (unless wax is impacted against it).

Hearing tests
- *Voice tests*: these gauge a person's ability to hear speech. One ear is occluded, and words or numbers are whispered into the other ear which the person is then asked to repeat.
- *Tuning fork tests*: these are used to distinguish between conductive and sensorineural deafness.
- *Rinne's test*: compares a person's ability to hear a tone conducted by air and bone. People are asked whether a vibrating tuning fork is louder when placed on the mastoid process (bone conduction) or when placed in line with the external ear canal (air conduction).
  - In normal hearing, the tuning fork is heard more clearly when held in line with the external ear canal. In conductive hearing loss, the tuning fork is heard more clearly when placed on the mastoid process.
- *Weber's test*: compares bone conduction in both ears to determine whether unilateral hearing loss is conductive or sensorineural.
  A vibrating tuning fork is placed in the centre of the forehead.
  - People who perceive the sound in the midline have normal hearing.
  - People who perceive the sound better in the affected ear have conductive loss.
  - People who perceive the sound better in the unaffected ear have sensorineural loss.

Audiometry
Audiometry is the testing of a person's ability to hear various sound frequencies. Audiometry investigations can assess the differences between normal hearing, conductive hearing loss, and sensory hearing loss.
- *Pure tone audiometry* is used for general assessment of hearing and hearing loss by air and bone conduction. Pure tone signals are relayed either by a vibrator attached to the mastoid process (bone conduction) or via earphones (air conduction).
- *Speech audiometry* is used to assess a person's ability to understand speech. A tape of words at varying intensities is played, and the percentage of correct words repeated is plotted against a speech audiogram.

- *Tympanometry* (or impedance testing) tests for middle ear compliance. The pressure in the external ear canal is altered, and at each different pressure setting, sound is passed into the ear and the reflected sound energy is measured.
- *Audiometry electric response* is where surface-recording electrodes are placed on a person's head and used to study the response of different auditory pathways to sound.
- *Imaging*: CT scan, MRI scan, X-ray, or ultrasound scan may be used to assist in diagnosis or to exclude underlying conditions which are manifest as ear symptoms.
- *Laboratory tests*: in ear conditions, microbiological tests are most commonly used. If other conditions are suspected, then FBC, blood glucose, U&Es, and a lipid profile may be necessary to assist in diagnosis of an underlying condition.

Ear surgery

Myringotomy and insertion of grommets

These surgical procedures are undertaken for glue ear (mostly affecting children) or for malfunction of the Eustachian tube in other age groups.

A small incision is made in the tympanic membrane (eardrum), and a small tube (grommet) is inserted to facilitate drainage and prevent fluid and pressure accumulation in the ear.

Myringoplasty

This is a surgical procedure to repair a perforation in the tympanic membrane using a small graft. Post-operatively, people should be advised to avoid raising pressure in the middle ear by such things as vigorous nose blowing, flying, and extreme sports such as scuba diving and parachuting.

Mastoidectomy

This refers to the surgical removal of affected tissue from the mastoid cavity under general anaesthesia. Preoperatively, people will normally have an X-ray of the mastoid and hearing tests to determine baseline measurements against which the surgery can be evaluated.

Following mastoidectomy, there may be a pressure dressing in place for 1–2 days, and an ear pack for 10–14 days.

Pinnaplasty

This is an operation under general anaesthesia for people who have unilateral or bilateral protrusion of the pinna. It is designed to reduce the protrusion and involves a surgical cut behind the pinna and shaving or removal of excess cartilage.

Preoperative photographs of the ear(s) may be taken. The surgical wound is either sewn or glued, and a pressure dressing applied. This will remain in place for up to 2 weeks.

Stapedectomy

Surgery involves removal of the stapes ossicle in the middle ear and its replacement with a plastic prosthesis. It usually results in a dramatic improvement in hearing, but there is a risk of deafness and balance problems in approximately 2% of people.

Hearing loss and impairment

Deafness and hearing impairment can range from mild and transient to profound and permanent (see Box 21.2). Deafness and hearing impairment can be of gradual or sudden onset. It may be the result of a natural ageing process or the consequence of a disease. Deafness and hearing impairment can also be associated with speech, language, and general communication disorders in the longer term and can indirectly result in social isolation.

Box 21.2 Classification of hearing impairment and deafness

Classification	Softest sound level which can be heard without amplification
Mild hearing impairment	16–30dB
Moderate hearing impairment	31–70dB
Severe hearing impairment	71–90dB
Profound hearing impairment	Over 91dB
Deafness	Unable to hear at all. May be congenital or acquired deafnesc

---

Types of hearing loss

- *Sensorineural* hearing loss is caused by disorders of the inner ear, the cochlea, the acoustic nerve, or central auditory pathway.
- *Conductive* deafness is the result of disorders of the external or middle ear which prevent sound from reaching the cochlea. These include congenital deformities (such as atresia of the external ear), wax, perforation of the eardrum, ossicular chain disorders, Eustachian tube disorders, otitis media, and cholesteatoma (cystic growths in the middle ear).
- *Presbycusis* is the term for age-related hearing loss due to degeneration of the fine hair cells of the cochlea. High-frequency sounds are affected first.

Communication aids

Some people may have to communicate without sound and use a combination of lip reading, body language, and facial gestures. Others rely on sign language, and some may be helped by hearing aids or surgery.

Hearing aids

Are electronic battery-operated devices, worn externally, which amplify sound and transmit it to the ear through a speaker. All sounds, including background noises, are amplified.

Hearing aids are often worn behind the ear or in the ear canal itself. Modern hearing aids use digital technology which means that they are very discrete and can be programmed to individual hearing loss.

Cochlear implants

Cochlear implants are small electronic devices that are surgically implanted. The device lies underneath the skin behind the ear, and the wires are implanted in the cochlea. An external microphone device rests over the ear, and contact between the microphone and the device is via magnets. Cochlear implants then convert sound waves into electrical impulses that are processed by the auditory pathway.

Bone-anchored hearing aids (BAHAs)

These work by the conduction of sound waves reverberating in the mastoid, as distinct from the electronic signals used in cochlear implants. A metal plate is inserted beneath the skin behind the ear and anchored to the mastoid bone. There is a clip on the surface of the skin, to which a device that transfers sound waves into the mastoid bone is attached.

Listening equipment

Loop and infrared systems help the listener hear sounds more clearly by reducing background noise. They are often found in theatres, cinemas, banks, and shopping centres. Smaller systems can be set up in the home.

Neck loops, ear loops, loop amplifiers, or headphones can make listening to videos, TV, radios, and sound systems easier by clarifying and amplifying sounds. The majority of television equipment now incorporates a subtitle option for people with hearing impairments.

British Sign Language

British Sign Language (BSL) is the most widely used method of signed communication in the UK. It uses both manual and non-manual components, hand shapes and movements, facial expression, and shoulder movements. Some health services have access to BSL practitioners who can help health professionals communicate with deaf people who sign.

Finger spelling

Is often used in conjunction with BSL, and a range of words, often names of people and places, are spelt out on the fingers.

Other equipment

- Alarm clocks with flashing lights and vibrating pads.
- Fire alarms, smoke alarms, and door bells with flashing lights.
- Telephones with flashing lights, extra amplification, and induction loop to enable use of the 'T 'setting on the hearing aid.
- Text and video phones.
- Hearing dogs.

Enhancing communication with hearing-impaired people

Nurses may not always recognize when a person has a hearing impairment, particularly when they are not presenting with an ear complaint. People may seek to conceal what they perceive as a disability due to embarrassment. Hearing loss or impairment may be misinterpreted by nurses as communication or language differences.

When talking to people with hearing impairments, it is always important to create an environment conducive to talk, by reducing background noise and limiting distractions as far as is possible. Nurses should speak slowly and clearly to people and their families, and it is good practice to check regularly for understanding.

If hearing impairment is suspected, it may be appropriate to ask respectful questions about the person's hearing, and whether or not they use any hearing aids. It may be helpful to include translators or a sign language interpreter if these are available. It should also be recognized that it may take additional time to communicate with a person who has a hearing impairment, and it may be helpful for nurses to make sure their mouth is clearly visible and at the same level as the patient's face.

People with hearing impairments may benefit from referral to speech and language therapists, audiologists, and sign language or lip reading experts. They may also benefit from registering as hearing-impaired or deaf (see ℘ www.rnid.org.uk), where they can gain useful information about employment and other rights and access to local and national support services and networks.

Key nursing considerations

A lot of ENT practice is now the domain of specialist nurses or advanced practitioners, but general nurses may have many occasions to work with people with hearing impairments, in both hospital and community settings. It is important for general nurses to remember that hearing loss impacts on all aspects of daily life when working with people with hearing impairments.

Nursing practice and decision-making will be determined by the nature of the diagnosis and treatment plan, and all local policies and procedures should always be followed. In the hospital setting, additional nursing time may be needed to communicate with, and collect information from, a person with hearing impairment.

- Carry out all admissions procedures and assessments according to local policies and procedures.
- Accurately monitor and record all clinical observations.
- Complete any clinical investigations ordered.
- Accurately administer and record any prescribed pain relief, symptom relief, and other medications.
- Accurately record and report any changes to the person's condition within the MDT.
- Liaison with specialist audiology services or interpreters.
- Observe and compare the person's ears for swelling, redness, discharge, bleeding stickiness, pus, and pain.
- Note any signs of facial nerve palsy or evidence of recent surgery.
- Clarify any changes or disturbances to hearing or recent ear infections.
- Ascertain whether the person is registered as hearing-impaired (𝒥 www.rnid.org.uk) and their usual coping strategies and equipment used.
- Orient the person to the care environment and ensure their physical comfort.
- Provide pens, pads, and sign boards to facilitate communication.
- Assess any anxieties about their current condition.
- Assess their normal work, and domestic and social situation.
- Clearly explain all actions and interventions.
- Give accurate explanations of likely events and investigations such as preparation for surgery.
- Maintain a safe and calming environment for recovery.
- Seek to allay patient and family anxieties.

Nose and throat conditions

As part of the upper respiratory tract, the nose and throat may be prone to minor irritations and infections, which cause pain or discomfort but do not compromise respiratory function. However, more serious nose and throat conditions may result in life-threatening obstructions which require urgent treatment. The structures of the nose and throat are illustrated in Figure 21.3.

Foreign body

A foreign body in the nose usually occurs in young children, through the insertion of such things as beads, small toy parts, crayons, and sweets. It is usually unilateral and produces offensive or bloodstained discharge. If the foreign body is accessible, in the anterior part of the nose, it can be removed by a trained practitioner. The majority of foreign bodies get wedged in the middle meatus and rarely get inhaled. However, if there is a risk of dislodging and subsequent inhalation, removal under general anaesthesia may be necessary.

Foreign bodies in the throat are often fish and meat bones, other food, sharp objects, and small coins. These may lodge in the upper airway or be swallowed.

Foreign bodies which are swallowed often result in sharp local pain, retrosternal pain, dysphagia, and increased salivation. Swallowed foreign bodies should be investigated and can be identified on X-ray. Not all require clinical intervention; however, the risk of perforation or obstruction in the GI tract must be considered.

A foreign body which obstructs the upper airway is a clinical emergency. The Resuscitation Council UK (% www.resus.org.uk) recommends that severity of the obstruction should be assessed, by determining how well the person is able to cough. If the foreign body cannot be removed by coughing, then five back blows, followed by five abdominal thrusts (Heimlich manoeuvre), are advised. The foreign body may need to be surgically removed. (See also ➔ Chapter 26, Clinical emergencies.)

Nasal polyps

These are pedunculated sacs in the nose, which are usually bilateral. They are often related to allergies and are more common in men. Polyps cause nasal obstruction, watery or purulent discharge (if infected), post-nasal drip, and sneezing. Nasal polyps can also reduce smell and taste sensations. Treatment includes topical steroid drops or systemic steroids or surgical removal.

Sinusitis

This is an inflammation of the mucous membrane of the paranasal sinuses, due to obstruction, infection, or allergy. It may present as headache, facial pain, blocked nose, post-nasal drip, and changed voice resonance. Treatment is with antibiotics, analgesia, and decongestant sprays. In severe or persistent cases, the sinuses may be irrigated under anaesthesia.

Rhinitis

Rhinitis is an inflammation of the mucous membrane of the nose, which may be described as allergic or non-allergic. In allergic rhinitis, the condition is caused by an allergen, often pollen. There are several possible causes of

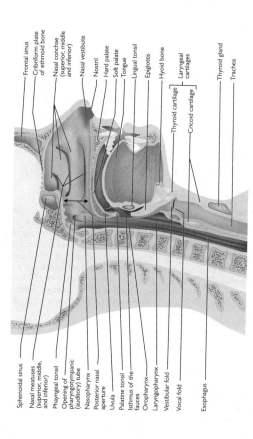

Figure 21.3 Structures of the nose and throat.

Reproduced from Marieb E N and Hoehn K, *Human Anatomy and Physiology (7e)* (2006), with permission from Pearson Education.

non-allergic rhinitis, which include viral infections, noxious fumes or smoke, and extreme temperatures. Rhinitis may also be caused by hormonal imbalances or hormonal contraception. Symptoms of rhinitis can include a blocked or runny nose, pain and discomfort, sneezing, and a reduced sense of smell, which may be treated with nasal drops and sprays and allergen testing. The condition can impact on a person's eating, drinking, breathing, speaking, and overall quality of life.

Epistaxis

Anterior nosebleeds are commonly seen in children where blood drips from one or both nostrils. It is usually due to nasal dryness, facial injury, violent sneezing, nose blowing or picking, foreign bodies, or common cold.

Posterior nosebleeds are more often seen in adults and may be related to underlying health conditions (e.g. hypertension, diabetes, tumours) or aggravated by drugs (warfarin, cocaine, aspirin). In the first instance, digital pressure should be used to stop the bleeding (see Box 21.3). If digital pressure is unsuccessful, invasive measures may be necessary.

- Nasal packing.
- Topical vasoconstrictor.
- Chemical cauterization (silver nitrate sticks).
- Intranasal balloon pack.
- Ligation under general anaesthesia (for arterial bleeds).

Nasal fractures

Direct trauma to the nose may result in fracture of nasal bones or the septum. Nasal fractures are often associated with a sports injury or road traffic accident. Fractures may be simple where the skin and mucosa are intact, or compound where nasal cartilage and bone are exposed. People may present with nasal deformity, swelling, obstruction, epistaxis, and soft tissue injury.

Treatment includes analgesia and control of bleeding, repair of soft tissue injury or abrasions, and in some cases reduction of the fracture. Fracture reduction can be done immediately or after 7–10 days when swelling subsides.

Nasal discharge

The characteristics of nasal discharge will be related to the underlying cause, and it may be clear, bloodstained, offensive, or infected and can be from one or both nostrils. Appropriate treatment will be determined by clinical examination and identification of the cause.

Box 21.3　Control of epistaxis by digital pressure

- Help the person sit in a position with their head forwards to prevent blood from entering the post-nasal space.
- Pinch the fleshy part of the nose, using the thumb and forefinger, for 10–30 minutes.
- Use an ice compress over the bridge of the nose, the back of the neck, or both, to promote vasoconstriction.
- Discourage the person from blowing their nose or sniffing (provide a receptacle for spitting).
- If available, wear PPE—gloves, mask, and eye protection.
- Note the duration and amount of bleeding.

Nasal tumours

The majority of tumours in the nose are benign, and these include nasal papillomas, which are wart-like growths, and nasal angiomas which cause severe epistaxis and require surgical excision.

Malignant lesions in the nose are not common and will often present very late. They may cause bloodstained discharge, nasal obstruction, and swelling of the lymph nodes and face.

Tonsillitis

This is a common throat condition, normally caused by streptococcal infection. People typically experience sore throat, dysphagia, fever, malaise, headache, swollen cervical lymph glands, and exudate on the tonsils. Treatment includes analgesia and local symptom relief, and antibiotics may or may not be prescribed. Tonsillitis may also be associated with glandular fever which manifests as additional back, groin, and axilla pain.

In severe cases, mostly in adults, tonsillitis can develop into peritonsillar abscess (quinsy). This condition results in worsening of symptoms, alongside earache, dysphagia, and difficulty opening the jaw. Treatment is by antibiotic therapy, and the abscess may need to be drained under general or local anaesthesia.

For people with recurrent tonsillitis, airway obstruction, sleep apnoea, quinsy, or suspected malignancy, a tonsillectomy may be necessary.

Laryngitis

Is an inflammation of the larynx, which is usually viral and is exacerbated by overuse of the voice, smoking, and drinking spirits.

Laryngitis causes hoarseness and laryngeal pain, and the condition can be treated by resting the voice, analgesia, and steam inhalation. Antibiotics are rarely needed.

Acute epiglottitis

This is a localized bacterial infection, which is more common in children. It causes swelling of the epiglottis, increasing dysphagia, stridor, and obstruction of the larynx. Treatment is by humidified oxygen therapy and IV steroids. Emergency intubation or tracheostomy may be required if the obstruction is compromising respiratory function.

Parotiditis

Parotiditis is an inflammation of the salivary glands, which is often caused by the saliva producing 'stones' or pus from infection. It is normally treated with antibiotics and analgesia, and people are also advised to eat sharp foods to stimulate saliva production and help clear the infected glands.

In some cases, the parotid glands may be removed under general anaesthesia. The procedure involves an external cut in the affected area and excision of the gland. This is usually performed after analysis by CT or ultrasound scan.

Laryngeal cancer

Is the most common head and neck tumour and is usually a squamous cell carcinoma. Smoking is the main risk factor, and people will present with hoarseness, pain, dysphagia, sore throat, and stridor. Diagnosis is by laryngoscopy and biopsy, and treatment is normally by surgery and radiotherapy. If the condition is detected early, the prognosis is often good.

Nose and throat tests and clinical investigations

Laryngoscopy

The larynx and nasopharynx can be examined by use of a laryngoscope. Indirect laryngoscopy, using mirrors or reflectors, is used to assess the mobility of the vocal cords or to locate a foreign body.

Fibre-optic laryngoscopy can also be used to visualize the entire nasopharynx and larynx. A flexible endoscope is introduced through the nose after topical anaesthesia has been applied. This is a useful approach for people who experience severe gagging.

Rigid endoscopy for examination and biopsy may be performed under general anaesthesia.

Laboratory tests

Any laboratory tests will vary, depending on local policies and procedures, and the person's known or suspected conditions. Routine laboratory testing may include FBC, group, cross-match and save (if surgery is scheduled), PT, and partial thromboplastin time (PTT).

- *Imaging plain X-rays* are useful for identifying bony structures of the head and neck and identifying foreign bodies.
- *CT and ultrasound scans* can be used for evaluating glandular and sinus disease and identifying the size and location of tumours.
- *MRI with or without contrast medium* can be used for investigation of the spaces, sinuses, tissues, and structures of the nose and throat.
- *Culture and sensitivity tests*—if a bacterial infection of the nose, throat, or glands of the head and neck is suspected, then samples of pathogens may be taken for microbiological culture and sensitivity testing.

Nose and throat surgery

Nasal polypectomy

Polyps are removed under local or general anaesthesia and normally sent for histology.

Nasal septoplasty

Where the nasal septum has become damaged after trauma, surgery involves lifting the mucosa, trimming the cartilage, and replacing the mucous membrane. Silastic nasal splints may be used to prevent adhesions and are removed after around 7 days.

Nasal septorhinoplasty

This surgical procedure is the same as septoplasty but also includes breaking and resetting of the nasal bones to give a visibly straighter nose.

Manipulation of nasal bones

This surgery is performed under general anaesthesia, usually after a traumatic nasal injury that has resulted in fracture. It normally has to be performed within 14 days of the injury to have effect and is predominantly a day-case procedure.

Functional endoscopic sinus surgery (FESS)

Chronic sinusitis results in abnormal mucus production and drainage, and FESS operates via an endoscope to restore normal sinus drainage by correcting anatomical abnormalities, removing diseased mucosa, removing polyps, and enlarging drainage channels.

Post-operatively, a rare complication of FESS is rapid eye swelling due to bleeding into the eye socket. This is a clinical emergency and must be treated promptly to prevent blindness.

Tonsillectomy

The removal of the tonsils under general anaesthesia and normally requires an inpatient stay in hospital.

Parotidectomy

Refers to the procedure to remove a parotid gland under general anaesthesia. Following surgery, the person will not be able to produce saliva in the same way and may need to use spray, gel, or lozenge saliva substitutes.

Thyroid lobectomy

This is the removal of either the left or right lobe of the thyroid gland, which may be necessary as a result of malignancy or overactive or underactive thyroid function. The surgery involves removal of the enlarged lobe through an incision to the front of the neck.

Total thyroidectomy

Total thyroidectomy is normally carried out in cases of malignancy. The procedure is similar to thyroid lobectomy, but the whole thyroid gland is removed. People will have to take thyroxine medication for life, as they will no longer naturally produce it. They also need long-term monitoring of serum calcium levels, and possibly short- or long-term calcium supplements, as the parathyroid glands regulate calcium.

Laryngectomy

Where the larynx is removed, it is normally because of malignancy. People who have a laryngectomy will no longer be able to speak using their vocal cords, so they will need to learn a new method of communication. People who are finding communication difficult may become very upset or frustrated, so it is important that nurses respect the person's dignity and communicate with them in an empathic and respectful manner.

In preparation for laryngectomy surgery, the person should have consultation with speech and language therapy services or meet someone who has previously had a laryngectomy.

Communicating with people following laryngectomy

It is important that people who are no longer able to communicate verbally do not become socially isolated. In both hospital and domestic environments, nurses may need to spend additional time with people to ensure that they are 'heard' and understood.

In the immediate post-operative period, a writing board and pens, signs, and picture boards may help people to communicate with staff and their families. It is also important that they are provided with a working bell or buzzer.

Although the person may no longer be able to speak themselves, it is important that nurses continue to speak *to them* in their normal voice, at a normal rate, and maintain appropriate eye contact.

Text or email messaging may provide a useful adjunct to new ways of communicating, but in the longer-term, people who have had a laryngectomy may opt to learn an alternative means of verbal communication.

- *Oesophageal speech*—where pockets of air are retained in the oesophagus and forced into the mouth to form words or syllables.
- *Electrolarynx*—is a hand-held, battery-operated device which produces electronic vibrations. It is placed on the throat and the person uses the vibrations to help form words.
- *Tracheoesophageal puncture*—is a voice prosthesis inserted into a surgically created fistula. The person speaks by forcing air through the prosthesis into the oesophagus and the mouth to form words.

Tracheostomy

A tracheostomy is an opening in the anterior wall of the trachea, which may be temporary or permanent, and is necessary to facilitate adequate ventilation.

In respiratory failure, a tracheostomy can be used to reduce the effort of breathing and may also be useful for people who require assisted ventilation over a protracted period or need regular removal of bronchial secretions.

Tracheostomy may also be an emergency treatment for an acute airway obstruction, or part of the strategy for living with a long-term neurological disorder which requires intermittent ventilatory support.

In the hospital environment, people who have a tracheostomy will often be nursed in a high-dependency area or ITU. If they are receiving ventilator support, it is important that inspired gases are humidified and that accidental extubation is avoided. In case of accidental extubation, spare tracheostomy tubes, dilators, and suction equipment should be readily available. If the tracheostomy tube is stitched into place, stitch cutters should also be available.

People with a tracheostomy will be unable to communicate verbally, so all the strategies and techniques outlined for communicating with people after laryngectomy also apply. Bronchial secretions can be aspirated through a tracheostomy tube, but this should only be carried out by healthcare staff who are appropriately trained in the technique.

(See also ➲ *Oxford Handbook of Clinical Skills in Adult Nursing*.)

Key nursing considerations

A lot of ENT practice is now the domain of specialist nurses or advanced practitioners, but general nurses may have occasion to work with people with nose and throat conditions in both hospital and community settings.

Nursing practice and decision-making will be determined by the nature of the diagnosis and treatment plan, and all local policies and procedures should always be followed. In the hospital setting, additional nursing time may be needed to communicate with, and collect information from, a person with a nose or throat condition.

- Carry out all admission procedures and assessments according to local policies and procedures.
- Accurately monitor and record all clinical observations
- Examine the person's nose and throat, and observe any airway problems, infections, tissue damage, stridor, cough, obstruction, discharge, pain, and bleeding.
- Complete any clinical investigations ordered.
- Accurately administer and record any prescribed pain relief, symptom relief, and other medications.
- Accurately record and report any changes to the person's condition within the MDT.
- Assess their ability to communicate verbally, and explore any alternative communication systems used.
- Provide pens, pads, and sign boards to facilitate communication.
- Liaise with speech and language therapy services, or local or national support networks if appropriate.
- Assess any anxieties about their current condition.
- Assess their normal work, domestic, and social situation.
- Clearly explain all actions and interventions.
- Give accurate explanations of likely events and investigations such as preparation for surgery.
- Maintain a safe and calming environment for recovery.
- Seek to allay patient and family anxieties.

Useful sources of further information

- Royal National Institute for the Blind (RNIB) ✆ www.rnib.org.uk
- International Glaucoma Association (IGA) ✆ www.iga.org.uk
- Macular Society ✆ www.macularsociety.org
- Driver and Vehicle Licensing Agency (DVLA) ✆ www.gov.uk/government/organisations/driver-and-vehicle-licensing-agency
- Action on Hearing Loss (formerly Royal National Institute for Deaf People) ✆ www.actiononhearingloss.org.uk
- Vestibular Disorders Association ✆ www.vestibular.org
- Ménière's Society ✆ www.menieres.org.uk
- National Institute on Deafness and Other Communication Disorders ✆ www.nidcd.nih.gov
- British Deaf Association ✆ www.bda.org.uk
- Hearing Links ✆ www.hearinglink.org
- National Association of Laryngectomee Clubs ✆ www.laryngectomy.org.uk
- British Thyroid Association ✆ www.british-thyroid-association.org

Drugs frequently prescribed for eye, ear, nose, and throat conditions

Drugs often used for eye, ear, nose, and throat conditions are listed in Tables 21.1 to 21.3. *All drug doses listed in this table are adult doses.* This table is only to be used as a guide, and the current *BNF* should be consulted for further advice. Nurses should involve themselves only in the administration of medications which fall within their sphere of competence.

Table 21.1 Drugs frequently prescribed for eye conditions

Antibiotics	Dose	Common side effects
Chloramphenicol 0.5% drops	Apply 1 drop every 2 hours; reduce frequency as infection is controlled, and continue for further 48 hours after healing	Transient stinging
Anti-inflammatory	**Dose**	**Common side effects**
Betamethasone	Apply one drop every 1–2 hours until inflammation is controlled, then reduce frequency	Potential 'steroid glaucoma' and/or 'steroid cataract' in susceptible patients; thinning of the cornea and sclera
Mydriatics/cycloplegics	**Dose**	**Common side effects**
Cyclopentolate drops 0.5% and 1% Tropicamide drops 0.5% and 1%	Single or normally short-term use	Transient stinging, raised IOP; on prolonged administration: local irritation, hyperaemia, oedema, and conjunctivitis may occur; toxic systemic reaction to cyclopentolate (and atropine eye drops) may occur in the very young and very old
Treatment of glaucoma	**Dose**	**Common side effects**
β-blocker drops, e.g. betaxolol and timolol	Apply twice daily	NB. systemic absorption may occur, therefore see side effect profile (for β-blocker drugs, see ➲ Table 15.2, Drugs frequently prescribed for cardiovascular conditions, p. 226); other side effects include ocular stinging, burning, pain, itching, dry eyes, erythema, and allergic reactions

(Continued)

Table 21.1 (Contd.)

Prostaglandin analogue drops, e.g. latanoprost	Apply once daily in the evening	Brown pigmentation, blepharitis, ocular irritation and pain, darkening/thickening/lengthening of eyelashes, conjunctival hyperaemia, transient punctate epithelial erosion, skin rash
Acetazolamide tablets/capsules	0.25–1g daily in divided doses	Nausea, vomiting, diarrhoea, loss of appetite, taste disturbance, paraesthesiae, flushing, headache, dizziness, fatigue, irritability, depression, thirst, reduced libido, metabolic acidosis and electrolyte disturbances on long-term therapy
Pilocarpine drops	Apply up to four times a day, depending on preparation used	Ciliary spasm leading to headache and brow ache, which may be more severe in initial 2–4 weeks of therapy; ocular side effects include burning, itching, blurred vision, conjunctival vascular congestion, vitreous haemorrhage, pupillary block, and lens changes with chronic use
Tear deficiency	Dose	Common side effectc
Hypromellose drops	Use hourly or as required	Few recorded

Table 21.2 Drugs frequently prescribed for ear conditions

	Dose	Common side effects
Betamethasone drops	2–3 drops every 2–3 hours, reduce frequency when relief obtained	Few recorded
Steroid drops combined with antibacterial, e.g. Gentisone HC®, Predsol N®, and Sofradex®	2–4 drops 3–four times daily (NB. Gentisone HC® is administered 3–4 times daily and at night)	Local sensitivity reactions
Cerumol® drops	Apply a generous amount (normally five drops) whilst patient lying down, with affected ear uppermost for 5–10 minutes	Possible irritation
Betahistine tablets	Initially 16mg three times daily, preferably with food; maintenance 24–48mg daily	GI disturbances, headache, rashes, and pruritus

Table 21.3 Drugs frequently prescribed for nose, throat, and mouth conditions

	Dose	Common side effects
Topical nasal decongestants	Ephedrine: 1–2 drops in each nostril, up to 3–4 times daily when required Xylometazoline: 2–3 drops into each nostril, 2–3 times daily when required; maximum duration of 7 days	Local irritation, nausea, headache; after excessive use—tolerance with diminished effect, rebound congestion, and possibly cardiac effects
Pseudoephedrine	60mg four times daily	Tachycardia, anxiety, restlessness, insomnia
Beclometasone	100 micrograms (two sprays) into each nostril twice a day; maximum of 400 micrograms (eight sprays) daily; when symptoms controlled, one spray into each nostril twice daily	Dryness, irritation of nose and throat, epistaxis; nasal septal perforation can occur, usually following nasal surgery
Mupirocin nasal ointment NB. reserve for eradication of nasal carriage of MRSA	Apply 2–3 times daily to inner surface of each nostril for 5 days	Few recorded

(Continued)

Table 21.3 (Contd.)

	Dose	Common side effects
Chlorhexidine and neomycin cream	Eradication of nasal staphylococci: apply to nostrils four times daily for 10 days Prevention of nasal carriage of staphylococci: apply to nostrils twice a day	Few recorded
Hexetidine, mouthwash/gargle	15mL undiluted 2–3 times daily	Occasional numbness or stinging
Nystatin suspension	100,000U held in mouth four times daily after food for 7 days (continue for 2 days after lesions resolved)	Oral irritation and sensitization; nausea also reported

Surgery

Introduction

When working with people who are having any type of surgery, the primary nursing responsibility is minimizing risk and maintaining patient safety. Nurses should always act within the limits of their knowledge, skills, and competence. All nursing decision-making in relation to surgery is framed by legal and ethical considerations, professional values, and teamwork, and grounded in respectful, appropriate communication skills. Anaesthetics, recovery, and operating departments are specialized areas of nursing practice, but general adult nurses will be involved in preparing people for surgery and in supporting them whilst they are recovering, until they are discharged from hospital. Community nurses may continue with post-operative care and rehabilitation once the person returns home. All organizations have policies and procedures for surgical safety, and it is incumbent on nurses to operate within local guidelines and legal requirements.

Types of surgical procedure

Surgical procedures encompass a wide range of different techniques, by means of which surgeons can examine and treat conditions and diseases in any of the body systems. Surgical interventions can be described in terms of whether they are a planned (elective) procedure or an emergency intervention.

- *Elective surgery* is normally the result of a process of clinical investigation and careful consideration of treatment options for any given health condition.
- *Emergency surgery* is normally a result of trauma or a clinical emergency and is usually performed for serious life-threatening conditions.

Minor surgical procedures under local anaesthesia can be performed in GP surgeries, health centres, outpatient clinics, or day-case units. More invasive surgical procedures which require general anaesthesia can also be performed in day-case units, but more commonly in operating theatres. Emergency lifesaving surgery may be performed in clinical environments, ICUs, or operating theatres.

- *Open surgery* is the most common type of surgery and is characterized by an incision, normally made into the thoracic or abdominal cavities or the limbs. Open surgery incisions are closed by staples or sutures.
- *Keyhole surgery* is carried out through a very small incision. Fibre-optic light sources, along with surgical instruments, are inserted through the incision. Keyhole surgery is used for an increasing number of conditions and is less traumatic than open surgery.
- The principles of *laparoscopic surgery* are similar to those of keyhole surgery, but laparoscopic surgery refers particularly to abdominal and peritoneal operations. Laparoscopy is commonly used in the diagnosis and treatment of abdominal or pelvic conditions.
- *Microsurgery* techniques use powerful magnifying devices and specialized instruments, such as micromanipulators or laser beams, to carry out the surgical procedure. Microsurgical techniques are used to operate on cells or minute body structures such as small arteries, the nervous system, the ear, or inside the eye.
- *Computer-assisted surgery (CAS)* uses computer technology for surgical planning and for guiding or performing surgical interventions. CAS is also known as computer-aided surgery, image-guided surgery, and surgical navigation (ℜ www.rcseng.ac.uk).
- CAS has been an important factor in the development of *robotic surgery*, which has the potential for some surgical procedures to be carried out remotely.

Surgery

Surgery is a treatment option in numerous health conditions, and in many cases, it can have dramatic effects on a person's health status. However, surgery can also cause significant harm to people.

The WHO (℀ www.who.int) reports surgical mortality rates of approximately 0.5–5% and that complications after inpatient operations occur in up to 25% of people. It is also estimated that around half of adverse events in hospitals are related to surgery and surgical care.

The WHO has undertaken a number of global and regional initiatives to address surgical safety and, through the work of international expert groups, has defined a set of core safety standards for member states. The standards address safe anaesthesia, safe site surgery, safe surgical teamwork, and prevention of surgical site infections.

The WHO 'checklist' for safe surgery describes procedures before anaesthesia, before skin incision, and before leaving the operating department, and they recommend that local users and specialist groups add to these checklists as necessary to address particular risk factors.

Before anaesthesia

- A patient has confirmed their identity, the site of the operation, and the procedure to which they have consented.
- The person's consent has been recorded.
- If applicable, the site for surgical incision has been marked.
- An assessment of the person's fitness for anaesthesia has been carried out, and a functioning pulse oximeter is in place.
- All the operating department team is aware of any allergies and whether there is any risk associated with the person's airway.
- Where there is a risk for blood loss in excess of 500mL, blood for transfusion is available.
- Good venous access has been established.

Before skin incision

- Confirm all team members have introduced themselves by name and role.
- Check and verify the identity of the patient.
- The operating surgeon to confirm the site, the anticipated procedure, the expected duration of the surgery, any anticipated critical events, or expected blood loss.
- The anaesthetic team to review any notable conditions and preparedness for incision.
- Nursing or operating department attendants to confirm the sterility of instruments, equipment checks and availability, and that relevant X-rays or other imaging are correctly displayed.
- To confirm whether antibiotic prophylaxis or other prescribed medicines have been administered.

Before leaving the operating theatre

- The procedure has been recorded in patient and theatre records.
- Instrument, swab, sponge, and needle counts are correct.
- Any specimens are correctly labelled.
- Whether there are any equipment problems to be addressed.
- Surgeon, anaesthetist, and nurse to have agreed key features for recovery and post-operative management.

The WHO surgical safety checklist has also been found to be feasible for use in emergency surgery (% www.who.int/patientsafety/safesurgery/ss_checklist/en/).

Adverse surgical incidents

An incident is defined as an event which could have, or did, result in unnecessary damage, loss, or harm to patients, staff, visitors, or members of the public. A serious incident involves unexpected or avoidable injury or death of one or more patient, staff, visitor, or member of the public.

Incidents which compromise patient safety and are largely preventable are referred to as 'never events' (⅍ www.gov.uk/government/publications/the-never-events-list-for-2011-12). In relation to surgical incidents and never events, these are normally related to wrong site surgery or retained swabs or instruments.

- A surgical intervention performed on the wrong site or organ.
- A surgical intervention performed on the wrong person.
- A surgical procedure which requires further urgent surgery.
- A procedure performed without consent.
- One or more instruments or swabs unintentionally retained following an operation.
- An operation or other invasive procedure to remove retained instruments or swabs.
- Complications arising from procedures to remove retained instruments or swabs.
- Complications arising from instruments or swabs which are not detected or removed.

Surgical incidents can also arise from miscalculations on the part of surgeons or anaesthetists which result in such things as excessive blood loss or acute airway obstruction, which should have been anticipated.

All surgical incidents and never events have to be reported. In the UK, these are reported to health care commissioners, and the information is made available to the public through NHS web pages. In the event of an adverse surgical incident of any sort, the quality of written records and the way the incident is reported are of central importance.

All healthcare organizations have local policies and internal processes for accident or incident reporting, and these should always be followed.

Surgical trigger tools and case note review are useful to identify perioperative adverse events and measure the overall level of harm within an organization. The surgical trigger tool developed by the NHS Institute for Improvement and Innovation describes how to undertake retrospective case note reviews (⅍ www.institute.nhs.uk/safer_care/safer_care/trigger__tool_portal.html).

Preoperative preparation

Preoperative preparation and assessment may begin several weeks prior to planned surgery to ensure that the patient is both as healthy as possible and properly informed. Preoperative assessment is essential for assessing risk and planning post-operative rehabilitation. It is often carried out in specialist clinics and in hospital or community settings. Many preoperative clinic services are led by advanced nurse practitioners or specialist nurses.

Prior to surgery, people will also need an assessment of their fitness for anaesthetic, which may or may not be part of the general preoperative assessment, depending on local policy and practice.

Preoperative assessment and preparation may include some of the following observations, measurements, or interventions:
- Baseline measurements of vital signs.
- X-rays or other imaging techniques.
- Blood or other samples.
- Respiratory function tests.
- Weight.
- Health history.
- Drug history.
- Allergy history.
- Nutritional history.
- Mental capacity assessment.
- Psychological assessment.
- Bowel preparation.
- Mobility assessment.
- Dental implants, crowns, false teeth.
- Communication difficulties or aids used.
- Domestic and social circumstances.

Venous thromboembolism (VTE)

VTE is a potential risk for people having surgery and NICE suggests that all patients should be assessed for VTE risk. Those at increased risk should be offered prophylactic interventions prior to surgery.

Indicators of increased risk include:
- People who have active cancer or are having cancer treatment.
- Those aged over 60 years.
- People admitted to critical care facilities.
- People who are dehydrated.
- People with known thrombophilias.
- Obesity with a BMI over $30kg/m^2$
- One or more significant medical co-morbidities such as heart disease, metabolic, endocrine, or respiratory disorders, acute infectious diseases, or inflammatory conditions.
- A personal history, or first-degree relative with a history of, VTE.
- People who use HRT.
- People using oestrogen-containing contraceptives.
- Varicose veins with phlebitis.
- Women who are pregnant or have given birth within the previous 6 weeks.
- People who have had or are expected to have significantly reduced mobility for 3 days or more, along with any of the known risk factors.

People admitted for surgical procedures, or following trauma, are also considered to be at increased risk of VTE in any of the following circumstances:

• Where the surgical procedure with a total anaesthesia and surgical time is going to be longer than 90 minutes.
• If the surgery involves the pelvis or lower limb and the total surgical time is expected to exceed 60 minutes.
• Where the surgery involves an acute inflammatory or intra-abdominal condition.

(See ℘ www.nice.org.uk/guidance/CG92.)

People who are considered at risk for VTE should also be assessed for their risk of bleeding, before pharmacological treatments to prevent clotting are used prophylactically.

Risk factors for bleeding include:
• Active bleeding.
• Acquired bleeding disorders (such as acute liver failure).
• Current use of anticoagulants known to increase the risk of bleeding.
• Lumbar puncture/epidural/spinal anaesthesia expected within the next 12 hours.
• Lumbar puncture/epidural/spinal anaesthesia within the previous 4 hours.
• Acute stroke.
• Thrombocytopenia.
• Uncontrolled systolic hypertension (230/120mmHg or higher).
• Untreated inherited bleeding disorders.

The risk for VTE can also be reduced by ensuring that people having surgery do not become dehydrated and are supported in mobilizing as soon as possible after surgery.

Mechanical VTE devices may be used for surgical patients, and the type of device will be based on the clinical condition, the nature of the surgery, and patient choice.
• Anti-embolism stockings (thigh or knee length).
• Foot impulse devices.
• Intermittent pneumatic compression devices (thigh or knee length).

(See also ➔ Chapter 12, Risk assessment.)

Preoperative fasting

The purpose of preoperative fasting is to minimize the risk of aspirating gastric contents during anaesthesia, surgery, or recovery, and the length of preoperative fasting will be determined by the type of surgery and local practice protocols.

Typically, preoperative fasting will be around 6 hours prior to surgery, and it is normally recommended that no alcohol is consumed within 12 hours of surgery. However, intake of water or clear fluid up to 2 hours before general anaesthesia is considered safe in healthy adults and may improve patient comfort and well-being.

Some prescription medicines may need to be stopped for hours or days before surgery, but this will be determined by the anaesthetist.

If the person is dehydrated, it may be necessary to commence an infusion of IV fluids prior to surgery.

Consent to surgical treatment

Consent is a person's agreement for a health professional to carry out any examination, intervention, or treatment, including surgery. In cases such as measuring blood pressure, the consent may be given verbally, but for surgical procedures, this is normally required as written informed consent. In the UK, the Mental Capacity Act established in law the conditions to safeguard people who may not be able to make decisions about their care and treatment, including consenting to surgical interventions.

• In order to be valid, consent must be given voluntarily, freely, and without pressure or undue influence by a person who is mentally competent.

• To give informed consent to surgery, the person must be appropriately informed and able to understand the nature and purpose of the procedure.

• People must also have the mental capacity to comprehend and retain information which can inform their decision-making. In addition, they need to be able to communicate their informed decision.

• Competent adults are entitled to refuse treatment, even when it would benefit their health.

Healthcare organizations will all have policies and procedures for securing informed consent from patients, and these should always be followed. Normally, it is the responsibility of the health professional carrying out the surgery for ensuring consent is secured before treatment begins. Consent can also be obtained by staff who have been trained and assessed in the practice and to whom the responsibility has been delegated.

In teaching or research centres, people may also be asked to consent to the possibility of tissue samples being retained and used for future research studies. They may also be asked permission for videos to be recorded or photographs taken for future teaching purposes.

People can selectively consent to surgical procedures and choose not to be involved in research or teaching, without prejudice. All surgical patients who may originally consent to contributing to teaching and research should always be informed that they may withdraw consent at any time, without detriment to their treatment.

Enhanced recovery after surgery (ERAS)

Enhanced recovery is an approach designed to help people recover more quickly after having major surgery. Although ERAS programmes are about recovery, they are always implemented preoperatively.

Many UK hospitals have enhanced recovery programmes in place, and there are different protocols and practices for different surgical procedures. However, the key principles of ERAS programmes are that:
- People are as healthy as possible before surgery.
- They receive the best possible care during their operation.
- They receive the best possible care whilst recovering.
- People are actively involved in their care.

The focus of most enhanced recovery programmes are pain management, nutrition, exercise, mobility, and relaxation, and wherever possible, minimally invasive surgical techniques.

Where enhanced recovery programmes are in place, it is often the case that GPs are involved in preparing people for their surgery and helping to stabilize any health conditions which may affect the operation.

Following surgery, nutritional and physiotherapy services are normally involved in rehabilitation and mobilization. People are discharged from hospital as soon as they can be reasonably expected to resume normal activities, with or without family or community health services support.

Safety in anaesthetic and recovery rooms

Risks in the operating theatre largely involve adverse incidents and never events related to procedures and process, and those arising from the necessary presence of medical gases and hazardous substances. A lot of nursing work in the anaesthetic room, operating theatre, and recovery room is therefore concerned with minimizing these risks, which include:

• Wrong patient.
• Wrong operation.
• No consent, or consent which does not adequately cover the procedure.
• Medication or transfusion errors.
• Patient injury as a result of positioning, moving and handling, gases, equipment, human error.
• Cardiorespiratory collapse.
• Surgical haemorrhage.
• Retained swabs or instruments.
• Failure of medical gas supply.
• Staff injury related to moving and handling, gases, hazardous substances, instruments, and equipment.
• Loss or damage to specimens.

Nursing in anaesthetic departments and recovery rooms is a specialist area of practice, and in the UK, this specialist area of nursing decision-making is framed by the standards of the British Anaesthetic and Recovery Nurses Association (⅏ www.barna.co.uk).

The association describes practice competencies in five key domains—ethics, scope of practice, education, clinical practice, and monitoring and assessment standards, all of which are informed by, and consistent with, the NMC standards (⅏ www.nmc.org.uk).

These anaesthetic and recovery standards recognize that people who have general anaesthesia are unable to maintain their own interests, dignity, or confidence from the point of induction until their return to full consciousness. Nurses who work in anaesthetic and recovery departments therefore have a central role in protecting and supporting patient interests whilst the patients are unconscious and vulnerable.

Nurses working in anaesthetic and recovery departments are members of MDTs who are responsible for the safety and care of all patients having treatment which needs general or local anaesthesia, sedation, or analgesia. The work may be in many clinical environments, including:

• Theatre suites or operating department complexes.
• Day-case surgery departments.
• Clinical investigation departments (such as cardiac catheter laboratories, endoscopy or radiology services).
• Delivery suites.
• Pain management services.
• Dental services.
• Psychiatric services.

The aim of nursing in the recovery room is to minimize the effects of the anaesthetic and promote recovery of consciousness and relative comfort, to a point where a patient may be returned safely to the ward or clinical area. Recovery from anaesthesia is normally signalled by a patient regaining airway and breathing control, cardiovascular stability, and the ability to respond to verbal instructions. An EWS system may be used. (For details of EWS, see also → Chapter 26, Clinical emergencies.)

Assisting recovery may involve a limited period of intensive oxygen therapy, extubation, administration of post-operative analgesia, suction of the upper airway, and administration of blood or IV fluids. Nurses working in recovery rooms focus on providing a safe environment, continuously monitoring the patient's condition, and preventing surgical complications in the immediate post-operative period.

The scope of anaesthetic and recovery nursing practice will normally be determined by local policies, procedures, and codes of practice, which must always be followed. These may include:

• Pre-surgical assessment clinics.
• Securing informed consent.
• Receiving patients from wards and clinical areas.
• Contributing to pre-incision checking.
• Checking of anaesthetic machines and equipment.
• Assisting in anaesthesia, sedation, or analgesia.
• Intubation and assisted ventilation.
• Management of IV lines and fluids.
• Moving and positioning of anaesthetized patients.
• Ongoing monitoring of the patient during surgery.
• Monitoring patients in the recovery area.
• Extubation.
• Pain relief and IV drug therapy.
• Handover of recovered patients to wards and clinical areas.
• Administration of local anaesthetic.
• Administration or management of regional anaesthetic blocks.

Maintaining safety for people in their progress from wards and clinical areas to the anaesthetic room, theatre, recovery room, and back to the ward is dependent on clear and effective communication between the numerous health professionals and ancillary staff involved.

For general nurses, it is important that they maintain clear and accurate patient records and effectively exchange patient information with their colleagues in the operating theatres. General nurses can also be an important source of information and comfort to people who are having surgery, both pre- and post-operatively.

Safety in the operating theatre

In the operating theatre itself, specialist theatre nurses are normally involved in patient management, assisting surgeons and circulating duties. Their working practices are framed by the WHO safe surgery 'before incision' and 'before leaving the operating theatre' conditions. In addition, theatre nurses may be involved in such tasks as:

- Positioning patients on the operating table.
- Ensuring good access to the operation site.
- Positioning theatre lighting.
- Adjusting operating tables.
- Ensuring surgical instruments are sterile and kept separate from non-sterile instruments.
- Sterile scrubbing, gowning, and gloving procedures.
- Preparing patient's skin.
- Positioning sterile drapes.
- Counting instruments, swabs, needles, tapes, blades, screws before, during, and after surgery.
- Recording batch numbers of any prostheses, implant, and inserts used.
- Tracking theatre trays and instruments after surgery.
- Collection and labelling of specimens.
- Cleaning instruments.

(See also ➲ Chapter 5, Record keeping and social media.)

Post-operative safety

When a patient has regained an acceptable LOC and is physiologically stable, they will normally be transferred back to the ward or clinical environment. Different specialties and departments will have their own protocols for post-operative care and management, and these should always be followed.

- Post-operative monitoring will normally involve a period of intensive observations and measurement of vital signs, the surgical wound, and wound drainage, and administration of IV fluids and prescribed pain relief.
- People who have had general anaesthesia and surgery may suffer from nausea and vomiting, which may or may not be related to their analgesic medication.
- Following surgery, patients are at risk for haemorrhage from the wound or the site of surgery, or from accidental damage to blood vessels during the surgical procedure.
- Signs of post-operative bleeding would be tachycardia with a weak thready pulse, low blood pressure, and cold, clammy skin. The wound dressing and any wound drains may also show excessive blood loss, so these should be regularly observed.
- People who have had surgery which involved a protracted length of time under anaesthesia and on the operating table, or those who have had considerable blood loss, may be at increased risk for developing hypothermia or pressure damage to the skin and bony prominences. Local procedures for the management of hypothermia or pressure ulcers should be followed.

(See also ➋ Chapter 26, Clinical emergencies and ➋ Chapter 20 Musculoskeletal conditions.)

In the post-operative period, general nurses should aim to ensure, as far as is possible, physical comfort and an environment that is conducive to healing and recovery.

People who are involved in an ERAS programme may be supported in mobilizing a few hours after surgery and be encouraged to eat and drink as soon as they are able to tolerate it. For other people, mobilization and resumption of eating and drinking may be determined by the nature of the surgery, local practice protocols, or the surgeon's preferences.

In the longer term, post-operative recovery is focused on the resumption of physical functions and, in some cases, adaptation to a new life situation or body image, which may be temporary or permanent. Recovery and adaptation will be influenced by a range of physical, psychological, or social factors:

- Persistent post-operative pain.
- The nature of the diagnosis and prognosis.
- Fear of complications.
- Expectation of further treatment.
- Disability.
- Fear of dying.
- Fear of hospitals and healthcare.

- Premature discharge.
- Availability of continuing care and support.
- Perceived ability to cope with normal life following discharge.
- Effect on self-identity and body image.
- Effect of surgery and its implications for family and significant others.
- Effects on work and social life.

Post-operative pain management

Most people will experience pain after surgery. Effective pain management can reduce morbidity, anxiety, and surgical complications and facilitate healing. A person's post-operative pain experience can be influenced by factors other than physical sensations:

- Individual expectations.
- Personal characteristics.
- Lack of understanding or information.
- Organizational factors.

Post-operative pain management will normally follow local protocols that have been developed by multi-professional teams of anaesthetists, surgeons, nurse specialists, therapists, and pharmacists. Some healthcare organizations will have a specialist pain team for helping in the management of post-operative pain.

Post-operative pain management strategies will normally employ pain assessment tools, prescribed medication (nurse-administered and patient-controlled), and non-pharmacological interventions. (See also Chapter 23, Pain.)

Blood transfusion

Some people who have surgery may need blood transfusion either before, during, or after surgery. Before surgery, blood transfusion may be necessary to treat an underlying anaemia and ensure the person is fit for general anaesthesia. During or after surgery, a common indication for blood transfusion is rapid or excessive blood loss.

The consequence of surgical blood loss is that blood pressure falls rapidly because of the reduced circulating volume, and cellular oxygen supply is significantly compromised by the loss of red blood cells.

All surgical procedures will have an estimated amount of blood loss, and where this is expected to be significant or the person has been assessed as at high risk of bleeding, blood will have been grouped and cross-matched for use during surgery.

All hospitals will have protocols for collecting blood for transfusion, checking before administration and recording the details of the transfusion in patient records and/or a central log. *Local protocols for safe blood transfusion should always be followed.* These will normally involve procedures for:

- Verifying the person's identity.
- Checking compatibility of the blood.
- Accurately recording details of the transfusion (as indicated by local practice policy).
- Measuring temperature, pulse, blood pressure, respiratory rate, and oxygen saturation levels 15 minutes after commencing the transfusion.
- Repeating these measurements at intervals specified by local policy to monitor adverse transfusion reactions.
- Observing the cannula for extravasation or inflammation.
- Reporting any observed or measured changes in the patient's condition as a matter of urgency.
- Observing any indications for stopping the transfusion.

In wards or clinical areas, it is not always necessary to use blood-warming equipment, but these may be necessary for patients who are anaesthetized in operating theatres.

Adverse transfusion reactions

Adverse reactions to blood transfusions can be due to infection or circulatory overload, but can also occur as a result of a serious immune response, such as an acute haemolytic reaction or anaphylaxis. These are clinical emergencies, and the transfusion should be stopped immediately and urgent medical help sought. Signs of blood transfusion reactions include:

- Pain.
- Fever.
- Chills.
- Rigor.
- Flushing.
- Urticaria.
- Tachycardia.
- Palpitations.
- Hypertension.

- Hypotension.
- Dyspnoea.
- Respiratory distress.
- Bone, muscle, or chest pain.
- Headache.
- Nausea and vomiting.
- Oliguria.

In the case of a person reacting to a blood transfusion, local incident reporting procedures should be followed, and an accurate and contemporaneous nursing report should be written.

Transfusion reactions need to be reported to the national service for serious blood reactions and events, and all equipment and blood containers need to be retained for inspection.

(See also *Oxford Handbook of Clinical Skills in Adult Nursing*.)

Surgical wounds

Management of surgical wounds is normally determined by local practice protocols, and some places will employ infection control and tissue viability specialists who can assist in the management of complex surgical wounds.

Wound healing is associated with the operative procedure and whether or not the surgical wound has been closed. In healing by primary intent, the edges of the skin are aligned and the wound closed by sutures, clips, staples, or tape.

In some cases, wound healing is by secondary intent where the wound is left open and heals by granulation, contraction, and epithelialization. This is normally used where there is considerable tissue loss, where an incision is shallow but has a large surface area, or for drainage of an abscess or pus.

There are four phases in wound healing:

- *Inflammatory phase*: the formation of a blood clot joins the wound edges loosely and stimulates an inflammatory response, swelling, heat, redness, and pain, which starts healing and repair. This requires energy and nutrition (0–4 days).
- *Regenerative phase*: granulation tissue starts the process of wound contraction. A new capillary network is formed. The length of this stage is variable but is approximately 24 days in wounds healing by primary intent.
- *Epithelialization*: the wound is covered by epithelial cells which migrate across the wound surface or along the suture line.
- *Maturation phase*: the wound becomes less vascularized, scar tissues become comparable to normal tissue, and tensile strength increases.

The wound healing process can be compromised by poor nutrition and dehydration. Obesity can also delay healing, and some health conditions, such as diabetes, can also delay wound healing.

Potential complications of surgical wounds

- *Haemorrhage* may occur during surgery or up to 10 days afterwards. Primary and intermediary haemorrhage can be a result of surgical technique, whereas secondary haemorrhage (around 7–10 days) is normally due to infection.
- *Infection*—the risk for wound infection can be increased by environmental factors such as surgical techniques and dressing changes. In older or obese people and those with diabetes or taking steroids or immunosuppressive medications, the risk for wound infection is increased. Signs of wound infection include inflammation, pyrexia, pain, and sometimes exudate, bleeding, or pus.
- *Dehiscence* is where a wound healing by primary intent breaks down or 'splits'. It may require surgical toilet or repair.
- *Scarring*—in some people, excessive collagen deposits can cause unsightly hypertrophic scars, which may eventually require surgical excision.

Principles of wound management

Local policies and procedures should always be followed, but key principles include:

- Dressing changes should always use ANTT.
- If there are signs of infection at dressing change, a wound swab should be taken.
- Offer analgesia before a dressing change.
- Use appropriate dressings to promote wound healing (check the local formulary).
- Wound dressings should:
  - Be absorbent.
  - Be comfortable.
  - Be non-adherent and non-toxic.
  - Minimize pain and trauma at dressing change.
  - Not require frequent or unnecessary changes.
- Seek advice from specialist tissue viability nurses (if available) for complex or challenging wound management.
- Removal of sutures or staples will be a matter of local procedure, but this is normally between 7 and 10 days post-operatively. People may have sutures removed in outpatient clinics, in GP surgeries, or by community nursing services.
- Involve the person and any family or carer in wound care, and explain the importance of asepsis and prevention of infection.

Recovery after surgery

With elective surgery, people will normally have an expected date of discharge, consistent with the nature of their surgery and local policies and procedures. It is often the case that people and families can make discharge arrangements at the time of admission.

Some hospitals employ staff members whose responsibility is coordinating discharge planning, and it is normal practice in UK hospitals for discharge summaries, and sometimes checklists, to be included in patient records.

People with complex health conditions or unexpected complications may need specific longer-term support after surgery, so plans for discharge may need to include arrangements for rehabilitation or convalescence or engagement with community or social services. Depending on the nature of the surgery, people may also be provided with written information outlining what it is normal to expect during recovery. These may include information about:

- Fatigue and tiredness for a period of time after general anaesthesia.
- Wound care, signs of wound infection, and arrangements for wound dressings.
- Resuming everyday activities.
- Exercise and any rehabilitative exercise specific to the surgery.
- Prescribed medication and pain relief.
- Contact information.
- Arrangements or appointments for review and follow-up.

Useful sources of further information

- *Oxford Handbook of Perioperative Practice*
- British Anaesthetic and Recovery Nurses Association ℳ www.barna. co.uk
- Royal College of Surgeons ℳ www.rcseng.ac.uk
- Informed consent ℳ www.health-ni.gov.uk/publications/ consent-guides-healthcare-professionals
- ERAS programmes ℳ www.nhs.choices
- National Patient Safety Agency ℳ www.npsa.nhs.uk
- NPSA Patient Safety Alert: WHO surgical safety checklist (adapted for England and Wales) and supporting information ℳ www.nrls.npsa.nhs. uk/alerts
- Never events ℳ www.nrls.npsa.nhs.uk/neverevents
- VTE guidelines ℳ www.nice.org.uk/guidance/CG92
- Mental Capacity Act 2005 ℳ www.mind.org.uk

Pain

Introduction

It is widely recognized that the experience of pain is unique to the individual, which makes caring for people in pain a challenge. Nurses have a humanitarian and professional duty to provide effective pain relief for people in their care, whether in a hospital or hospice environment or in the community setting. Many places now employ specialist pain nurses or teams to help manage acute, chronic, or end-of-life pain.

Definition of pain

Pain is described by the International Association for the Study of Pain as '*an unpleasant sensory and emotional experience, associated with actual or potential tissue damage, or described in terms of such damage*' (% www.iasp-pain. org/).

Most people will experience pain at some time, whether this is in response to an acute injury, after surgery, or as the result of a long-term health condition.

Some pain is protective and acts as an early warning sign to alert people that tissue damage has occurred or is about to occur. In these circumstances, painful stimuli activate specific pain receptors (nociceptors) to produce the sensation of pain. Pain can also be experienced when there is no evidence of tissue damage, as with some chronic pain conditions.

Pain is also an individual and an emotional experience. A person's perception and response to managing their pain can be influenced by a wide range of factors. These include:

- Previous experience of pain.
- Age.
- Gender.
- Personality.
- Expectations and associations.
- Emotional state and coping strategies.
- Information and understanding.
- A medical diagnosis.
- Cultural background.
- Socio-economic circumstances.

The individual nature of the pain experience means that a person's unique experience is a central consideration in nurses' decision-making and practice when helping people manage their pain.

Acute pain

Acute pain is that which has a recent onset, is most likely of limited duration and usually has an identifiable cause. Acute pain is associated with trauma, invasive procedures, surgery, some medical conditions, and some cancers.

- Post-operative pain is due to tissue trauma caused by the surgical incision and related tissue injury.
- Somatic pain is associated with the skin, muscle, bone, joints, and connective tissue.
- Visceral pain is related to the thoracic, pelvic, and abdominal viscera.

Characteristics of acute pain

- Sudden onset.
- Associated with trauma or disease.
- Ranges from mild to severe.
- Is relieved by treatment.
- Is of limited duration.
- Subsides as healing takes place.
- May develop into chronic pain.

Causes of acute pain

- Trauma.
- Inflammation/infection.
- Surgery.
- Diagnostic procedures (e.g. lumbar puncture).
- Invasive procedures (cannula insertion, injections).
- Wound dressing changes.
- MI.
- Obstetric pains (labour and childbirth).
- Headaches, migraine, earache, toothache.
- Exacerbation of chronic conditions (acute-on-chronic pain).

Untreated acute pain may eventually result in the development of a severe chronic pain condition, which can be both functionally devastating and difficult to treat. In addition to severe psychological and emotional consequences, untreated acute pain can also have damaging effects on the body systems.

- *Psychological effects*—the cognitive and emotional response to pain can give rise to:
  - Anxiety.
  - Fear.
  - Agitation.
  - Insomnia.
- *Respiratory effects*—an inability to take deep breaths or cough as a consequence of pain can result in:
  - Sputum retention.
  - Infection.
  - Atelectasis (lung collapse).
  - Hypoxia.
  - Respiratory failure.

- *Cardiovascular effects*—tachycardia and hypertension often associated with acute pain can lead to:
  - Increased oxygen requirements.
  - Increased cardiac effort.
  - Angina.
  - MI.
- *GI effects*—pain causing disturbance in gut activity may cause:
  - Nausea.
  - Vomiting.
  - Paralytic ileus.
- *Neuroendocrine effects*—metabolic changes and release of stress-related hormones related to pain may result in:
  - Electrolyte imbalance.
  - Retention of sodium and water.
  - Acute urinary retention.
  - Protein breakdown.
  - Poor wound healing.
- *Musculoskeletal effects*—immobility due to acute pain may lead to:
  - Muscle spasms.
  - Increased risk of DVT.
  - Increased risk of pressure ulcers.
  - Prolonged hospital stay for inpatients.

In hospital environments, poor pain management is a common cause of distress and a reason for complaints. Good pain management not only gives people physical comfort, but can also help prevent medical or surgical complications and accelerate recovery and rehabilitation.

In modern health services, many places now have protocols for 'fast-track' or 'accelerated' surgical care for suitable people. These protocols normally involve laparoscopic or keyhole surgery, enhanced nutritional regimes, early mobilization, and early discharge.

The success of these programmes is dependent on the effective management of post-operative pain. Pain management in 'enhanced recovery' programmes may include regional analgesia, low doses of local anaesthetic, and opioid drugs. (See also ⟱ Chapter 22, Surgery.)

Chronic pain

The Royal College of Anaesthetists describes chronic pain as ' . . . *that which persists beyond the expected time of healing following injury or disease*' (⌖ www.rcoa.ac.uk).

Chronic pain is normally recognized as having been continuous for >3 months, but complex pain problems may present earlier. Chronic pain may also have a damaging effect on a person's ability to function normally and eventually develop into a debilitating condition.

Characteristics of chronic pain
- An unclear history.
- Persistent beyond the expected time of healing.
- Muscular wasting, loss of core strength, weight loss.
- Fatigue.
- Persistent insomnia.
- May impact on normal daily functioning.
- May impact on mobility.
- May have profound lifestyle effects.
- Often has emotional and psychological effects.
- Rarely resolves.
- Complex and difficult to manage.

Causes of chronic pain
- MSK sources.
- Fibromyalgia.
- Abdominal pains.
- Headache (migraines).
- Angina.
- Peripheral neuropathy.
- Peripheral vascular disease.
- Stroke.
- Diseases of the CNS (e.g. MS).
- Cancer.
- Related to life events such as loneliness, relationship problems, and bereavement.
- Complex regional pain syndrome (CRPS).

The incidence of chronic pain is increasing, and in some people, there is no clear identifiable cause. Where chronic pain has a known cause, this may be described as nociceptive pain or neuropathic pain.
- Nociceptive pain is related to the stimulation of pain receptors. It may be associated with non-malignant MSK factors and malignant cancer pains.
- Neuropathic pain may be caused by a disturbance in sensory processing in nerves, in the central or peripheral nervous system.
- Damage can be due to trauma, surgery, infection, diabetes, ischaemia, malignancy, chemotherapy, or radiotherapy.
- Neuropathic pain has some different features to nociceptive pain and is often described by people as burning, stabbing, shooting, or 'like an electric shock'.

- People with neuropathic pain may also describe altered sensory experiences, e.g. allodynia (a response to a stimulus that does not usually cause pain) or hyper-analgesia (an excessive response to a painful stimulus).
- Neuropathic pain can be very difficult to treat, and antidepressant and anticonvulsant drugs are sometimes used.

Complex regional pain syndrome (CRPS)

- CRPS is a chronic condition which normally affects the limbs and results in motor, autonomic, and sensory changes. CRPS is often associated with a primary injury but persists long after healing has occurred.
- CRPS is characterized by periods of intense pain, swelling, and hypersensitivity to touch or temperature. People with CRPS may also experience unusual sensations in the limb, discoloration of the skin, changes in hair and nails, oedema, joint stiffness, and tremors.
- During periods of intense pain and associated symptoms, people with CRPS may not be able to work and may need support in everyday activities.
- CRPS is very difficult to treat, and strategies for managing the condition include analgesia, relaxation techniques, physiotherapy, and occupational therapy interventions. One of the ways to manage CRPS pain is through spinal cord stimulation (SCS). This is an implantable device which positions an electrode in the epidural space in the spinal cord. The person with CRPS has control over the device, and when stimulated, the SCS device relieves pain through causing paraesthesiae over the painful limb. SCS is not suitable for all people with chronic pain (⅍ www.nhs. uk/Conditions/Complex-Regional-Pain-Syndrome/).

Management of chronic pain

The management of chronic pain is focused on restoring or maintaining function, providing physical relief, or facilitating a comfortable end of life.

Strategies normally involve a combination of physical therapies, cognitive behavioural coping strategies, drugs, and adjuvant therapies such as TENS, acupuncture, and relaxation.

People with chronic pain are normally supported in living with their condition by a multi-professional specialist pain team. These may be in community clinics or hospital-based specialist centres. The specialist pain team may include anaesthetists or other medical practitioners, clinical psychologists, specialist nurses, physiotherapists, and occupational therapists. Pain teams also work in partnership with palliative care services.

Assessing pain

As pain is a unique experience, people with similar medical conditions, or having the same surgical procedures, may respond very differently to pain.

An accurate assessment of an individual's pain is essential to ensure effective pain management, and nurses need to listen carefully and respectfully to people's accounts of their pain.

There are a number of tools which have been developed to help nurses and other health professional assess people's pain, and the acronym 'SOCRATES' can be a useful aid to nurse decision-making in many clinical conditions:

- *Site*: where is the pain?
- *Onset*: when and how did the pain start?
- *Character*: is the pain sharp, dull, aching, or stabbing?
- *Radiation*: does the pain go anywhere?
- *Associated features*: nausea, vomiting, diarrhoea, or sweating?
- *Time*: is the pain constant or intermittent?
- *Exacerbating features*: what makes pain better or worse?
- *Severity*: how bad is the pain on a scale of 0–10?

Pain assessment tools

Self-report pain assessment tools are widely used in nursing and healthcare, and they are based on a person being able to allocate a 'score' to the intensity of their pain.

Behavioural observation tools are also available for people who may not be able to do this, such as very young children, young people, and adults who are unable to communicate in some way or people with dementia.

Visual analogue scales (VAS)

A VAS is a horizontal or vertical line drawn on paper, anchored by 'no pain' at one end and 'unbearable pain' at the other. People place a mark on the line to indicate the severity of their pain (see Figure 23.1).

Whilst the concept of VAS is straightforward, some people may find them difficult to understand, and it is debatable whether they are able to quantify any meaningful change to assist nursing practice and decision-making.

Numerical rating scales

Numerical rating scales are similar to VAS but use numbers to rate the intensity of pain. The scale ranges from 0 = no pain to 10 = unbearable pain (see Figure 23.2).

Visual analogue scale (VAS)

No pain -- unbearable pain

Figure 23.1 Visual analogue scale.

Numerical scale

No pain 0---1---2---3---4---5---6---7---8---9---10 unbearable pain

Figure 23.2 Numerical rating scale.

Verbal rating scale (VRS)

A VRS consists of a range of descriptors on a continuum. People select the description that best describes their pain (see Box 23.1).

Box 23.1 Verbal rating scale (VRS)

0 = no pain

1 = mild pain

2 = moderate pain

3 = severe pain

The PAINAD behavioural scale

The PAINAD (Pain Assessment in Advanced Dementia) scale was developed to assess pain in individuals with advanced dementia. The assessment scores a person's facial expression, body posture, changes in behaviour, and vocalizations (see Table 23.1).

There are other behavioural pain scales available, and these types of assessment tools may be useful when working with any adults who are unable to communicate effectively.

Multi-dimensional pain assessment tools

The McGill pain questionnaire is an example of a multi-dimensional pain assessment tool, which is widely used in clinics for people with chronic pain. It scores the person's pain experience across a range of different categories.[1]

1 Melzack R (1975). The McGill Pain Questionnaire: major properties and scoring methods. *Pain*, 1, 277–99.

Table 23.1 The PAINAD behavioural tool

Instructions: Observe the patient for five minutes before scoring his or her behaviours. Score the behaviours according to the following chart. The patient can be observed under different conditions (e.g. at rest, during a pleasant activity, during care giving, after the administration of pain medication).

Behaviour	0	1	2	Score
Breathing independent of vocalization	Normal	Occasional Laboured breathing Short period of hyperventilation	Noisy laboured breathing Long period of hyperventilation Cheyne–Stokes respirations	
Negative vocalization	None	Occasional moan or groan Low-level speech with a negative or disapproving quality	Repeated trouble calling out Loud moaning or groaning Crying	
Facial expression	Smiling or inexpressive	Sad Frightened Frown	Facial grimacing	
Body language	Relaxed	Tense Distressed pacing Fidgeting	Rigid Fists clenched Knees pulled up Pulling or pushing away Striking out	
Consolability	No need to console	Distracted or reassured by voice or touch	Unable to console, distract, or reassure	

Total score:Scoring: the total score ranges from 0 to 10 points. A possible interpretation of the scores is: 1–3 = mild pain; 4–6 = moderate pain; 7–10 = severe pain

Reprinted from *Journal of the American Medical Directors Association* 4(1), Warden V et al, Development and Psychometric Evaluation of the Pain Assessment in Advanced Dementia (PAINAD) Scale: 9–15., Copyright.

Pharmacological pain management

Good pain management is dependent on an accurate assessment of a person's pain and a consideration of appropriate analgesic treatments or non-pharmacological management options.

Pain management is designed to enable people to resume a normal lifestyle or function, or to help them manage comfortably within the limitations of their clinical condition. Good pain management plans will involve:

- Identifying safe and effective treatments.
- Using a stepwise approach to titrating analgesia.
- Using multi-modal combinations of analgesia.
- Aiming to minimize the side effects of medicines.

The WHO analgesic ladder

The WHO analgesic ladder was designed originally for use in the management of pain associated with cancer, but it is frequently used as a guide to a stepwise approach to titrating analgesia in general pain management (see Figure 23.3).

- *Step 1*—non-opioid drugs: preparations such as oral paracetamol is used for mild to moderate pain, and IV for moderate to severe pain. Paracetamol can be used in combination with strong opioids, such as morphine, to improve analgesic effects, especially after surgery.
- *Step 2*—weak opioid drugs: codeine and tramadol work on opioid receptors, producing analgesic effects. Codeine can be used in combination with paracetamol, metabolizing to morphine.

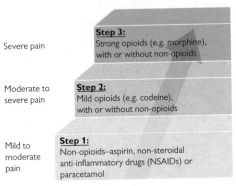

WHO ANALGESIC (PAIN RELIEF) LADDER

Severe pain	**Step 3:** Strong opioids (e.g. morphine), with or without non-opioids
Moderate to severe pain	**Step 2:** Mild opioids (e.g. codeine), with or without non-opioids
Mild to moderate pain	**Step 1:** Non-opioids—aspirin, non-steroidal anti-inflammatory drugs (NSAIDs) or paracetamol

Figure 23.3 The World Health Organization analgesic ladder.

Adapted from WHO's cancer pain ladder for adults, Copyright (2016) ℗ http://www.who.int/cancer/palliative/painladder/en/ Accessed June 2017.

• *Step 3*—strong opioid drugs: strong opioid drugs, such as morphine, oxycodone, fentanyl, and diamorphine, are used for severe pain and have demonstrated efficacy in a variety of visceral pain conditions. The dose and frequency should be titrated for people who are terminally ill.

Although morphine is a powerful analgesic, people with persistent non-malignant pain, who need >180mg a day, will need specialist consultations and advice. It may be that a reduced dose of morphine, with or without other interventions, is needed to help manage their pain.

Adjuvant agents

Adjuvant agents are drugs or therapies given in addition to the main treatment to maximize the effectiveness of pain management strategies. These may include the following.

Non-steroidal anti-inflammatory drugs (NSAIDs)

NSAIDs, such as ibuprofen and naproxen, are effective in pain associated with inflammation. However, their use is contraindicated in people with GI disorders, asthma, and cardiac or renal conditions.

Anti-epileptic and antidepressant drugs

Anti-epileptic and antidepressant medicines can be useful in neuropathic pain, as they inhibit the release of neurotransmitters. Drugs such as gabapentin, pregabalin, and amitriptyline may be used.

Other drugs

Muscle relaxants, such as baclofen and diazepam, are useful to control pain associated with muscle spasm, and corticosteroids can be useful for inflammation in painful joints. Inhaled Entonox® can be used for wound dressing changes, labour, and childbirth.

Local analgesia

The use of local anaesthetic techniques in pain relief is particularly useful in day-case surgery:

• Topical applications to the skin for insertion of cannulae.
• Wound infiltration for minor or intermediate surgery (e.g. hernia repair).
• Nerve blockade (e.g. intercostal block for fractured ribs).
• Plexus blockade (blocking a group of nerves).
• Transversus abdominis plane (TAP) blockade on either side of the abdominal wall for pain relief following surgery.
• Intrathecal (spinal) injection used in laparoscopic or orthopaedic surgery.
• Epidural analgesia through continuous infusion or patient-controlled epidural analgesia (PCEA), via an in-dwelling catheter.

Patient-controlled analgesia (PCA)

This is where a patient self-administers small intermittent IV bolus doses (usually 1mg) of an opioid, usually morphine, by means of a 'demand' button when they feel pain. A safety 'lock-out' system (normally 5 minutes) enables the opioid to take effect before another dose can be delivered.

Where patients are using a PCA device, there must be regular and routine observations of their vital signs, pain scores, and any side effects. Local policies and procedures for the management of PCA must always be followed.

Patient-controlled epidural analgesia (PCEA)

Epidural analgesia is administered by injection or through an indwelling catheter in the epidural space. It is widely used in obstetrics and in the management of post-operative pain relief, including 'enhanced recovery' programmes.

Patient safety is the most important aspect of PCEA, and there must be regular and routine observations of vital signs, pain scores, and side effects. Local policies and procedures for the management of PCEA must always be followed.

Non-pharmacological pain management

Non-pharmacological therapies are a useful adjunct to medicines in pain management and also have considerable utility in their own right. Use of non-pharmacological measures should always be considered, as they can provide considerable comfort to people in pain.

However, nurses should not administer alternative or complementary therapies, unless they have been trained and are competent in their use (℞ www.nmc.org.uk). Alternative and complementary therapies include the following.

Acupuncture

Chinese acupuncture involves the placement of fine needles in the skin at specific points on the body, based on observation of the tongue, eyes, and pulse. Western medical acupuncture is based on Chinese principles but works from a medical diagnosis.

Acupressure

Is similar to acupuncture but uses finger pressure on the acupuncture points, rather than needles.

Physiotherapy

Exercise can be an effective therapy for people with acute and chronic pain. These may include respiratory or MSK exercises. Exercises are particularly relevant for people with chronic pain to prevent muscle deconditioning and joint stiffness and improve core muscle strength.

Hydrotherapy

This is supervised exercise in water. The weightlessness experienced in warm water reduces stress on joints, muscles, and other connective tissues.

Thermotherapy

This is where heat, normally through heat pads, is applied directly to relieve pain, stiff joints, and muscle aches and spasms.

Transcutaneous electrical nerve stimulation (TENS)

TENS devices use electrodes placed around peripheral nerves to transmit electrical impulses and block pain pathways. The intensity of the impulses is controlled by the person using the machine, and TENS are useful for people who want to be active partners in the management of their own condition.

Cognitive behavioural therapy (CBT)

CBT works through the person's own thoughts and behaviour patterns which may be influencing their experience of pain. CBT uses a range of techniques, including distraction, guided imagery, deep breathing. and relaxation.

In CBT, people are taught to explore the meaning of pain and develop strategies to deal with negative thoughts and feelings. CBT techniques are often combined with exercise in multidisciplinary pain management programmes.

Aromatherapy

Involves the use of essential oils to treat a medical condition or induce relaxation. Aromatherapy may or may not include massage. It is important to determine whether there are particular aromas or oils to which people may be allergic.

Massage

Massage is the therapeutic manipulation of soft tissues of the body and is usually carried out over and around the site of the pain. It is contraindicated in areas that are actively inflamed or where there are open wounds, damaged skin, lumps, or tumours.

Reflexology

This is based on a belief that the body's natural healing mechanisms can be enhanced by the application of pressure to specific areas of the feet and hands.

Therapeutic relaxation

Guided imagery aims to help the person with pain to concentrate on a peaceful, pleasant image. They are then asked to describe sensory details of the image, whilst breathing slowly and deeply.

Muscle relaxation

Involves a focus on a particular muscle group. People use their hands to gradually work their way around their body, tense the muscles for 5–7 seconds, and then relax and concentrate on the sensations that relaxation brings.

Meditation and mindfulness

Are other methods used to counteract stress associated with pain and anxiety by producing a relaxation response.

Hypnotherapy

Hypnotherapy uses hypnotic techniques to help a person achieve a trance-like state, which allows them to become more relaxed and open to suggestion. Hypnotherapy is contraindicated in patients with severe psychological health problems such as depression or psychosis.

Key nursing considerations

General nurses will often deal with people in acute pain, whilst people with chronic pain conditions will most often be in the care of specialist pain teams or community nurses. In all cases, professional values, knowledge, and teamwork are essential to effective pain management. Respectful and empathic communication skills are essential.

In an emergency situation, the priority is always to deal with any life-threatening situation, and then treat the acute pain. Any local practice policies or protocols for pain management should always be followed.

All local practice guidelines relative to the person's clinical condition should be adhered to and, in addition, nursing practice and decision-making in pain management will encompass some or all of the following:

- Assess the person's pain by looking and listening.
- Use the SOCRATES (or other) acronym to guide observations and questions.
- Use an appropriate pain assessment tool, as specified by local practice protocols.
- Allow the person to express their pain experience in their own words.
- Accurately administer and record any prescribed pain relief, within the required standards of practice for safe medicines management ℳ www. nmc.org.uk).
- Ensure analgesia is titrated as appropriate for the level of pain.
- Administer drugs on time and as prescribed, and never keep a patient waiting for pain relief.
- Safely administer and record any adjuvant or other therapies.
- Evaluate the efficacy of previously administered pain medication or therapies.
- Record and document pain assessment scores on a regular basis, in accordance with local policies and clinical guidelines.
- Accurately measure and record vital signs, including temperature, pulse, blood pressure, respiratory rate, oxygen saturation, EWS, pain scores, sedation levels, and nausea, in accordance with local policies and guidelines.
- Observe posture for signs of guarding or protecting the painful area.
- Observe body language for signs of agitation.
- Observe any crying, moaning, and facial distortions.
- Accurately record the person's condition in the nursing records.
- Accurately report the person's condition in the MDT.
- Seek guidance from a specialist pain, or palliative care, team if necessary.
- Clearly explain all actions and interventions in the pain management plan to the patient and any family or carers.
- Seek to clearly allay patient and family anxieties.
- As far as possible, ensure physical comfort.

People living with chronic pain

People with chronic pain and their families may have misconceptions or misunderstandings about the nature of pain and its treatment. They may also find the lived experience of chronic pain is very frightening.

Effective management of chronic pain is dependent on people having an adequate understanding of their pain, so that they can manage it appropriately. This may require nurses to share their knowledge of prescribed drugs, and their effects and side effects to reach a concordance about the medicines regime with the person and their family.

People may also need to be supported in developing coping strategies, which may involve referral to specialist pain services, alternative or complementary therapies, or local support groups.

People with learning disabilities, those with mental health problems, and elderly people are at particular risk of poor pain management, so special attention should be paid to their particular needs. (See also ➔ Chapter 4, Medicines management.)

Useful sources of further information

- Fibromyalgia Network ℘ www.fmnetnews.com
- International Association for the Study of Pain ℘ www.iasp-pain.org
- Low back pain ℘ www.nice.org.uk
- National Patient Safety Agency ℘ www.npsa.nhs.uk
- Neuropathic pain (quick reference guide) ℘ www.nice.org.uk
- Royal College of Anaesthetists ℘ www.rcoa.ac.uk

Drugs frequently prescribed for pain management

Drugs which are frequently used for pain management are listed in Table 23.2. *All drug doses listed in this table are adult doses.* This table should only be used as a guide, and the current *BNF* should be consulted for further advice. Nurses should involve themselves only in the administration of medications which fall within their sphere of competence.

Table 23.2 Drugs frequently prescribed for pain management

Non-opioid analgesics	Dose	Common side effects
Paracetamol	500–1000mg every 4–6 hours to a maximum of 4g daily	Rare, but rashes and blood disorders reported. *Important*—liver damage (and less frequently renal damage) following overdose
NSAIDs	**Dose**	**Common side effects**
Non-selective NSAIDs (ibuprofen carries lowest risk for adverse GI effects, with piroxicam, ketoprofen, and ketorolac associated with highest risk, and indometacin, naproxen, and diclofenac as intermediate risk)	Ibuprofen: initially 300–400mg 3–4 times daily, increased if necessary to maximum of 2400mg daily; maintenance dose of 600–1200mg daily may be adequate (See *BNF* for doses of other NSAIDs)	GI discomfort, nausea, diarrhoea, and occasionally bleeding and ulceration occur, particularly in the elderly; a degree of worsening of asthma may occur; hypersensitivity reactions. Increased risk of thrombotic events (e.g. MI and stroke) See *BNF* for full range of side effects and degree of risk with different NSAIDs
Compound analgesic preparations	**Dose**	**Common side effects**
Co-codamol 30/500 (paracetamol 500mg and codeine phosphate 30mg)	1–2 capsules/tablets every 4–6 hours when necessary; maximum of eight capsules/tablets daily	As above for paracetamol, plus constipation, drowsiness, nausea, and vomiting
Co-dydramol 10/500 (paracetamol 500mg and dihydrocodeine 10mg)	1–2 tablets every 4–6 hours; maximum of eight tablets daily	As above
Opioid analgesics	**Dose**	**Common side effects**
Codeine	30–60mg every 4–6 hours when necessary See *BNF* for doses of other weak opioids	Nausea and vomiting, constipation, drowsiness, dry mouth; side effects as for morphine (see below) may be seen with larger doses

(Continued)

Table 23.2 (Contd.)

Morphine	Dose and frequency dependent on condition being treated and formulation used See BNF for details	As above; larger doses may cause respiratory depression, hypotension, and muscle rigidity See BNF for full range of side effects
Diamorphine	Dose and frequency dependent on condition being treated and formulation used See BNF for details	As above; larger doses may cause respiratory depression, hypotension, and muscle rigidity See BNF for full range of side effects
Oxycodone	Dose and frequency dependent on condition being treated and formulation used See BNF for details	As above; larger doses may cause respiratory depression, hypotension, and muscle rigidity See BNF for full range of side effects
Fentanyl	Dose and frequency dependent on condition being treated and formulation used See BNF for details	As above; larger doses may cause respiratory depression, hypotension, and muscle rigidity See BNF for full range of side effects
Buprenorphine	Dose and frequency dependent on condition being treated and formulation used See BNF for details	As above; larger doses may cause respiratory depression, hypotension, and muscle rigidity See BNF for full range of side effects
Tramadol	50–100mg, up to a maximum of every 4 hours; total of >400mg not usually required	As above; larger doses may cause respiratory depression, hypotension, and muscle rigidity See BNF for full range of side effects
Neuropathic and functional pain	**Dose**	**Common side effects**
Amitriptyline (NB. Unlicensed indication)	Initially 10mg at night, increased gradually to 75mg at night; higher doses under specialist supervision	Dry mouth, blurred vision, constipation, nausea, difficulty with micturition; cardiovascular side effects (ECG changes, arrhythmias, postural hypotension, syncope, tachycardia); many more side effects (see BNF)

(Continued)

Table 23.2 (*Contd.*)

Gabapentin	300mg once daily on day 1, 300mg twice daily on day 2, then 300mg three times daily on day 3, increasing by 300mg according to response every 2–3 days to maximum of 3.6g daily (some patients, including the elderly, may benefit from a lower starting dose and slower titration)	Nausea, vomiting, dry mouth, weight gain, confusion, drowsiness, and dizziness; many more side effects (see *BNF*)
Pregabalin	150mg daily in 2–3 divided doses, increased if necessary after 3–7 days to 300mg daily in 2–3 divided doses, increased further if necessary after 7 days to a maximum of 600mg daily in 2–3 divided doses (some patients, including the elderly, may benefit from a lower starting dose and slower titration)	Dry mouth, constipation, vomiting, dizziness, drowsiness, irritability, impaired attention; many more side effects (see *BNF*)
Ketamine	An anaesthetic drug, which may be used at sub-anaesthetic doses for control of neuropathic pain in palliative care Available for oral, buccal, and SC administration and dose titrated to patient need 100–400mg/day orally	Raised ICP, tachycardia, hypertension, hallucinationc

Palliative care

Introduction

Palliative care is a specialized area of nursing practice, but also one which embraces all people who are living with a life-limiting or life-threatening illness. The purpose of palliative care is to enable a person and their family or significant others to live as full a life as possible within the constraints of their health condition. Palliative interventions often begin at an early stage of a long-term or life-limiting illness, and may be concurrent with active treatment interventions. Palliative care continues until death, and although many palliative care services are delivered by specialist teams, general nurses will also be involved with people in a range of clinical or domestic environments.

Principles of palliative care

Palliative care is defined by the WHO (⌖ www.who.int) as a holistic approach to helping people, and their families, who are living with life-limiting and life-threatening illnesses, to achieve the best possible quality of life.

Palliative care is a specialist area of healthcare practice which involves an MDT perspective to identify, assess, and help address and manage a person's physical, psychological, spiritual, and social needs. Members of a palliative care MDT will include some or all of the following:

- Consultant in palliative medicine.
- Specialist medical registrar/trainee.
- Palliative care nurse specialist.
- Registered nurse.
- Healthcare assistant.
- Social worker.
- Physiotherapist/occupational therapist.
- Complementary therapist.
- Pastoral worker.
- Religious representative.
- Counsellor.
- Clinical psychologist.
- Mental health/psychological therapist.
- Pharmacist.
- Dietician.
- Volunteer.

Palliative interventions may begin early in a person's illness and be provided alongside other treatments and interventions. It also extends to helping people who are thought to be in the last 12 months of their life, and those who are dying (see also ➲ Chapter 25, Death and dying).

The key characteristics of palliative care described by the WHO are that the approach:

- Provides relief from pain and other distressing symptoms.
- Affirms life and regards dying as a normal process.
- Intends neither to hasten nor to postpone death.
- Integrates the psychological and spiritual aspects of care.
- Offers a support system to help people live as actively as possible until death.
- Offers a support system to help the family and friends cope during a person's illness and in their bereavement.
- Uses a team approach to address the needs of people and families, including bereavement counselling if indicated.
- Will enhance quality of life and may also positively influence the course of illness.
- Is applicable early in the course of illness in conjunction with other therapies that are intended to prolong life, including those investigations needed to better understand and manage distressing clinical outcomes.

History and development of palliative care

The origins of palliative care date back to fourth-century Europe and the role of religious communities in caring for pilgrims, the sick, and the dying. The modern hospice movement was pioneered in the UK by Dame Cicely Saunders, with the opening of St Christopher's Hospice over 50 years ago. The original philosophy of holistic care for dying people now extends to those facing life-threatening or life-limiting illness, within any setting. This has led to the recognition of palliative care as a medical specialty.

Historically, many palliative care services have been funded through the voluntary sector, with a focus on care for people with end-stage cancer. However, there is now widespread recognition of the importance of palliative care not only for people with malignant disease, but also for those with long-term health conditions such as heart and respiratory failure, neurological diseases, and dementia.

Palliative care services are becoming more integrated into general healthcare provision, although access to good-quality care at the end of life is not yet universal.

Contemporary palliative care

Hospices still play an important role in the provision of palliative care services, but they are no longer seen purely as places for people who are dying. Modern hospices also focus on providing specialist palliative support for people and families with complex issues relating to illness.

Palliative care is increasingly provided within hospital, community, and care home settings and as outpatient and day therapy services.

Holistic and MDT working is central to the palliative care approach, and contemporary palliative care is now more clearly defined (ℛ www.ncpc. org.uk).

- *Palliative care generalist*: those providing day-to-day care for people, families, and carers in their homes and in hospitals.
- *Palliative care specialist*: those who specialize in palliative care such as consultants in palliative medicine and clinical nurse specialists or advanced practitioners.

Many people will receive good generalist palliative care support without the need for involvement of specialist services. However, a referral for specialist advice and support should be made when the knowledge and skills necessary to meet a person's needs extend beyond the limits of the generalist practitioner. These may include:

- Advice on the management of complex pain.
- Symptom management.
- Psychosocial and spiritual issues.
- Hospice at home.
- Inpatient and outpatient hospice services.
- Specialist GP services.

Specialist palliative care teams will normally have defined referral criteria, and they are often able to provide additional support to people, families, and general nurses through education and training.

The combination of generalist and specialist palliative care services should enable appropriate support to be provided in any environment. This is particularly important when a person is approaching the end of their life.

It is recognized that whilst most people indicate a preference to die within their own home, the majority of people within the UK die in an acute hospital setting. The availability and access to effective, well-coordinated palliative services are essential in enabling a person to die in the place of their choice.

The impact of life-limiting or life-threatening illness

All people have a spiritual dimension, whether this is expressed overtly as a religious belief or is understood as that which gives the person and their life meaning. Life-limiting or life-threatening illness can impact on this core of a person's being, causing a profound sense of loss or spiritual distress, which can result in emotional and psychological pain. This may be experienced and manifest in various ways:

• Fear of dying.
• Loss of self-efficacy or control.
• Loss of independence.
• Reduced physical functioning and increased dependence.
• Changed body image and embarrassment.
• A perceived diminished role within the family.
• Changed relationships.
• Isolation from family, friends, and social networks.
• Changes to a person's role within society.
• Existential questions relating to the sense of self, reason, and being.
• Anger towards self, family, medical professionals, and religion.
• Sadness, hopelessness, anxiety, and/or depression.

The effects of life-limiting or advanced illness on mental health can often go unrecognized, leading to lack of treatment and support.

The ability to identify when a person may be in emotional or psychological pain is an important nursing responsibility. It is central to securing appropriate and effective support. Whilst nurses need to be aware of their individual capabilities and limitations, the ability to communicate with empathy and compassion is everyone's responsibility (see also ➡ Chapter 6, Communication in a healthcare context, ➡ Chapter 7, Dignity and respect, ➡ Chapter 8, Culturally sensitive communication, ➡ Chapter 9, Communicating concerns in healthcare, ➡ Chapter 10, Conflict resolution, and ➡ Chapter 11, Breaking 'bad news').

Effective support is likely to require discussion within the MDT and referral to specialist palliative care professionals. Psychological services may be needed.

This team approach is very important, as anxiety and depression can be disguised and may only be manifest through physical symptoms.

• *Anxiety*—physical symptoms may include palpitations, chest pains, sweating, dizziness, headaches, irritability, restlessness, stomach pain, excessive flatulence, diarrhoea, and sleep disorders.
• *Depression*—physical symptoms associated with depression include such things as lethargy, appetite loss, GI tract disturbances, sleep disorders, excessive tiredness, and poor concentration. A person with severe depression may also have suicidal thoughts, feelings of worthlessness, hallucinations, and/or delusions.

Advance care planning

Advance care planning (ACP) refers to the discussions and planning for the future between a person and the people providing care. In order to engage with ACP discussions, a person must be assessed as having mental capacity (www.legislation.gov.uk). If it is expected that the ill person may lose mental capacity or become unable to communicate at some point in the future, then this planning should take place at an early stage of the illness trajectory.

However, it is recognized that having ACP discussions may be very difficult for all involved, so it is important to identify the most appropriate health professional to participate in this discussion. Any health professionals involved must be able to use effective, sensitive, and compassionate communication skills, and have a comprehensive understanding of ACP and the Mental Capacity Act.

- ACP is founded on an understanding of the wishes, values, and personal goals that may be important to a person.
- It is a voluntary process, and no one should be coerced into having ACP discussions.
- ACP provides an opportunity for a person to state their preferences and wishes for future care and to discuss any potential treatment options.
- ACP should be an ongoing process, and plans regularly reviewed in partnership.

Once agreement on an ACP has been reached, this should be documented and communicated to key persons involved in care provision. Family members should only be informed if this is what the person wishes. Outcomes of ACP may include:

- *An advanced statement*: indicating a person's wishes and preferences. This will help medical and nursing teams consider what is important to the person when making decisions regarding care and treatment if they lose mental capacity.
- *An advanced decision to refuse treatment (ADRT)*: specifying a person's formal decision to refuse treatment in specific circumstances. An ADRT may be legally binding, dependent on whether it is assessed as valid at the time indicated.
- *The appointment of lasting power of attorney*: someone is nominated by the ill person to make decisions on their behalf if they lose mental capacity. This is a formal decision which must be made whilst the person has mental capacity and must be registered with the Office of the Public Guardian.

Symptom management

Uncontrolled physical symptoms in advanced illness can cause substantial distress and significantly impact on quality of life. Symptoms can stem from multiple causes:

- Symptoms directly related to the disease process.
- Symptoms secondary to the effects of treatments such as radiotherapy or chemotherapy.
- Symptoms related to the limitations of the disease such as immobility and constipation.
- Other co-morbidities which may be present, in addition to the primary disease such as arthritis.

The assessment and management of symptoms in palliative care are an important nursing role within the MDT. In advanced illness, symptoms such as pain, fatigue, anorexia, cachexia, nausea and vomiting, and dyspnoea are common.

Pain

Although pain can be understood as a physiological process, it also involves complex emotional and cognitive components, resulting in an individual and subjective experience.

Whilst not all people will experience pain, it is one of the most prevalent symptoms of advanced disease and can be a source of considerable distress. Pain can result in profound physical and emotional suffering which impacts on quality of life.

Different concepts are used to describe and understand pain associated with life-limiting or life-threatening conditions.

- *Nociceptive pain*—relates to neurotransmission of messages indicating actual or potential tissue damage. Examples of how this type of pain may be described include dull, aching, or throbbing.
- *Neuropathic pain*—refers to 'nerve' pain which is transmitted by a damaged or malfunctioning nervous system. This type of pain may be described as sharp, shooting, or burning.
- *Acute pain*—usually has a recent onset and is of limited duration. It is often associated with autonomic responses such as raised pulse and sweating. Acute pain may be protective against further injury.
- *Chronic pain*—is persistent and present for a longer period. It may be related to a chronic disease, but the cause is not always easily identifiable.
- *Incident pain*—is pain which occurs on movement.
- *Pain threshold*—the subjective minimum level at which a person perceives something as painful.
- *Pain tolerance*—the subjective maximum level of painful stimulus that a person is able to accept.

Supporting people in pain

Effective management of pain should be an ongoing process, which includes regular review and re-assessment, and monitoring the effects of any interventions to alleviate pain.

Pain tools can be a valuable aid to the assessment and management of pain. It is important to understand which assessment tools are in use within local practice and ensure that they are used appropriately.

Once the nature and source of pain have been identified, appropriate interventions can be delivered, which may involve pharmacological and non-pharmacological approaches.

A detailed summary of pain assessment tools and pharmacological and non-pharmacological management of pain is included in ⊃ Chapter 23, Pain.

Fatigue

Fatigue is an intense, subjective feeling of weakness, tiredness, and loss of energy, which affects many people with advanced disease. Fatigue has the potential to affect a person's ability to function and may result in emotional and psychological distress.

Effective and empathic communication skills are essential in understanding an individual's experience of fatigue and the impact it has on quality of life and everyday activities.

There may be a point where intervention for fatigue is no longer appropriate due to the potential distress the intervention itself may cause. It is therefore important that fatigue is assessed and reviewed regularly:

• Acknowledge the symptom, and express willingness to support the person.
• Explore potential causes such as emotional concerns, pain, sleep disturbance, depression, dehydration, and medications.
• Communicate with the MDT regarding the potential use of drug therapy to alleviate fatigue.
• Liaise with the MDT to treat other secondary causes (e.g. anaemia, infection).
• Help to establish a person's priorities and identify goals.
• Work with the MDT and the person to develop a management plan for engaging in appropriate activities, exercise, and rest periods throughout the day.
• Consider the use of a fatigue diary if appropriate.
• Monitor, review, and document the impact of any interventions.

Anorexia

Appetite is a mechanism associated with food intake, but there are also complex social and cultural meanings attached to appetite and eating. Whilst food has an essential physiological role, it can also be a very important component of psychosocial and cultural behaviours.

Loss of appetite (anorexia) during advanced illness can be extremely distressing for both the person experiencing it and their family. The ill person may be unable to engage in the social interaction that is linked to eating or be unable to tolerate the food which has been prepared for them. Anorexia has the potential to trigger distressing behaviours and complex emotions, including frustration, anxiety, worry, anger, and guilt in others.

In some disease conditions, anorexia may be associated with the loss of lean body mass (cachexia), irrespective of the level of nutritional input. This can be particularly distressing for both the ill person and their family and friends.

To provide support to people who have anorexia or cachexia associated with advanced disease, nurses should aim to help alleviate the social distress. Talking about the impact the particular illness has on appetite, and the nature of weight loss and cachexia, can be useful to help understanding.

- Identify which foods the person prefers to eat and is able to tolerate.
- Encourage the preparation of food that is presentable and appealing, and can be eaten in a place where the person feels comfortable.
- Assess and monitor food and fluid intake, and liaise with other appropriate professionals such as dieticians, dentists, and doctors if necessary.
- Establish whether there are any contributing factors or reversible causes affecting appetite such as the illness itself, body image, medicines, treatments, strong smells, nausea, constipation, anxiety, and taste changes.
- Observe the physical appearance of the mouth and tongue for signs of oral infection, inflammation, sores, dentures which no longer fit, and anything mechanical which makes eating difficult.
- Encourage regular oral hygiene if it can be tolerated.
- Allow opportunities for discussion of feelings and social and cultural beliefs around food and eating.

If the ill person is unable to tolerate oral nutrition and fluids, the use of enteral feeding and artificial hydration can be considered. It is important that any discussions relating to artificial hydration and nutrition are undertaken by appropriately qualified health professionals and include, wherever possible, people, their families, and significant others.

Nausea and vomiting

Nausea and vomiting (emesis) are often discussed together; however, it is important to recognize that they are distinct symptoms. Although a person with advanced disease may have both symptoms, and nausea will often precede vomiting, one symptom can be present without the other.

Nausea and vomiting are triggered by the stimulation of receptors and neurotransmitters, via the GI tract, chemoreceptors, the vestibular centre, and the cerebral cortex and limbic system.

Accurate assessment will help identify possible causes of nausea or vomiting, and the potential treatments or anti-emetic medications which can be prescribed.

Gastrointestinal causes
- Oral infection and stomatitis.
- Enlarged abdomen due to enlarged liver, tumours, or ascites.
- Constipation or faecal impaction.
- Intestinal obstruction.
- Inflammation (e.g. peritonitis).
- Gastric stasis (e.g. due to medications, anticholinergics).
- Gastric irritation (e.g. ulcer, NSAIDs).

Chemical causes
- Medications such as morphine.
- Chemotherapy.
- Radiotherapy.
- Hypercalcaemia.
- Uraemia.

Neurological causes
- Raised ICP, brain tumour.

Infection
- Local or systemic.

Psychological causes
- Fear and anxiety.

Assessment and management of nausea and vomiting

As with all other aspects of palliative care, thorough assessment and effective communication are central to nursing practice and decision-making in helping people with nausea and vomiting.

- Assess the onset and pattern of the symptoms, precipitating factors, and any related symptoms.
- Observe the timing of symptoms and factors which make it worse or better.
- In vomiting, establish the volume and frequency.
- Determine whether there are any other related symptoms such as pain, drowsiness, and confusion (which may indicate biochemical disturbances).
- Assess whether medications may be contributing to the nausea and vomiting (e.g. morphine, anticholinergics, NSAIDs).
- Consider whether nausea or vomiting may be related to constipation or immobility.
- Assess mouth health, and look for any signs of systemic infection.
- Give physical support to people who are vomiting, and maintain their safety, wearing PPE if available.
- Maintain privacy and dignity, especially in a clinical environment.
- Offer mouthwashes and mouth care.
- Ensure any anti-emetic medications are appropriately prescribed and administered; monitor, review, and report their effect.
- Monitor fluid intake and output, in accordance with organizational policy.
- Liaise with the MDT for review of symptoms and management.
- Consider complementary therapies.

The oral absorption of medications may be affected by nausea and vomiting, so prescribed medicines may have to be administered by an alternative route.

Dyspnoea

Breathing difficulties have a high prevalence in advanced illness and can be attributed to a number of physical, psychological, or emotional causes. Dyspnoea may be directly related to a respiratory condition such as COPD or lung cancer, or to other conditions such as heart failure, pleural effusion, anaemia, or respiratory tract infection.

As with pain, dyspnoea has multiple dimensions and can be a very frightening experience for people. As with all aspects of palliative care, effective and compassionate communication is essential to providing support.

Assessment and management of dyspnoea

- Establish the ill person's perspective of their breathing difficulties and the impact it is having on their daily activities and quality of life.
- Liaise with the MDT to address potential reversible causes, and decide upon the most appropriate management plan.
- Asses the onset and pattern of symptoms and any precipitating factors, related physical signs or symptoms, or changes in the underlying condition.
- If oxygen is prescribed, consider the most appropriate method of administration.
- Ensure prescribed medications are administered; monitor, evaluate, document, and communicate their effects to the MDT.
- A referral for dyspnoea management may be helpful.
- If possible, ventilate the environment through opening windows or using fans to allow a flow of cool air. It is important to establish whether this is helpful and can be tolerated.
- Consider complementary techniques such as relaxation, aromatherapy, or massage.

(See also ⊃ Chapter 14, Respiratory conditions.)

The family and significant others

Supporting a person's family and those important to them is an integral part of palliative care. Family members can be an invaluable support and help to provide physical and emotional care, which can be beneficial for all concerned. However, advanced illness will affect different family members in very different ways and will invariably impact on interpersonal dynamics.

Sensitive, compassionate, and effective communication will help to gain an understanding of the relationships and roles within the family and can help in assessing the impact of the illness. It may also help to establish the appropriate type and level of support the family want or need.

Providing support

Some people may want to include their family in all discussions and decisions about their care, whilst others, for various reasons, will ask to exclude them. A person's wishes should always be respected, and their permission sought to discuss their care with family members.

- Be pro-active in opening discussion with significant others about their feelings, and actively listen to what they say.
- Help them discuss any concerns, worries, or fears they may have.
- Address the family's understanding and information needs, without compromising the patient's wishes.
- Support and coordinate discussions relating to care planning, and ensure that appropriate MDT professionals are involved.
- If appropriate, enable the family and others to be involved in providing nursing support, ensuring all risks have been assessed and addressed.
- Be alert to family members' needs and whether those who have been caring for the patient are experiencing carer fatigue, and how they can best be supported.

(For further information on family support, grief, and bereavement, see also ➔ Chapter 25, Death and dying.)

Other nursing considerations

The philosophy underpinning nursing practice and decision-making in palliative care is holistic and person-centred. It respects the person and their family, with a focus on supporting and maintaining quality of life as defined by the person.

Person-centred nursing practice and decision-making include partnership care planning and a process of shared decision-making relating to all appropriate interventions, choices, and goals. The holistic approach is founded on effective, compassionate, and empathic communication.

Whilst some nursing activities will be concerned with delivering clinical interventions and assisting with physical functions, a lot of palliative nursing is about providing a sense of 'being there' for the person and their family. This includes actively listening and allowing them time and space to talk about themselves, their feelings, and the impact of their illness.

Not all people will want to talk about their illness, and people should never feel pressured into discussions of this nature; however, the opportunity should be available if this is important to them. There may not often be an answer to existential questions such as 'why did this happen to me?' But a genuine, humane response can be a useful intervention in itself.

Useful sources of further information

- Care Quality Commission (2016) *A different ending: end of life care review* ℘ www.cqc.org.uk/content/different-ending-end-life-care-review
- Gold Standards Framework ℘ www.goldstandardsframework.org.uk/
- Mental Capacity Act (2005) ℘ www.legislation.gov.uk/ukpga/2005/9/contents
- National Council for Palliative Care ℘ www.ncpc.org.uk/palliative-care-explained
- National Council for Palliative Care (2011) *Capacity, care planning and advance care planning in life-limiting illness: a guide for health and social care staff* ℘ www.ncpc.org.uk/freedownloads
- National Institute for Health and Care Excellence (2011, updated 2017) *End of life care for adults.* Quality standard [QS13] ℘ https://www.nice.org.uk/guidance/qs13
- Scottish Palliative Care Guidelines. *Weakness/fatigue* ℘ www.palliativecareguidelines.scot.nhs.uk/guidelines/symptom-control/weakness-fatigue.aspx
- World Health Organization ℘ www.who.int/cancer/palliative/definition/en/

Chapter 25

Death and dying

Introduction

An important aspect of nursing practice is caring for people in the last days and hours of their life, whether in a hospice, a clinical environment, or their own homes. Whilst death may be sudden and unexpected, or the anticipated result of an intractable health condition, effective support of dying people and their families is an important aspect of nursing and care. The UK Leadership Alliance for the Care of Dying People (⌗ www.england.nhs.uk) describes five key principles to guide nurses who are working with people and families at the end of life.

The last days and hours of life

The Leadership Alliance approach stresses the importance of care which focuses on the needs, wishes, and preferences of the dying person, their family, and those identified as important to them.

It is also important to note that the five key priorities are relevant to care provided for a person who it is thought may die within days or hours. However, this in itself may be difficult to predict and, whilst nurses have a crucial role, a multi disciplinary team (MDT) approach to clinical decision-making is important.

The five priorities

- Recognizing the possibility that a person may be in the last days and hours of life, communicating this clearly, and making decisions and taking actions in accordance with the person's needs and wishes, ensuring that these are regularly reviewed and decisions revised accordingly.
- Maintaining sensitive communication between healthcare staff and the dying person and those identified as important to them.
- Involving the dying person and those identified as important to them in decisions about treatment and care to the extent that the dying person wishes.
- Actively exploring, respecting, and meeting (as far as possible) the needs of families and others identified as important to the dying person.
- Wherever possible, agreeing an individual plan of care (which includes food and drink, symptom control, and psychological, social, and spiritual support) and delivering it with compassion.

Clinical decision-making

Whether in a clinical environment or a person's home, the last days and hours of a person's life can be very distressing for the dying person, their families, the nurses, and other health professionals involved with them. It is likely that assessment and clinical decision-making in relation to dying people will be led by an experienced healthcare professional, and nurses should have a clear understanding of their role within the relevant MDT. They also need an understanding of local organizational policies for care in the final days of life.

An important first stage in clinical decision-making is the recognition that a person is, or is becoming, clinically unstable and may not recover despite treatment interventions and is therefore likely to be dying.

- This recognition may be arrived at after a comprehensive assessment of the potentially reversible causes of symptoms or through observed changes in the person's condition.
- All decision-making should be underpinned by an assessment, which includes the physical, spiritual, emotional, psychological, social, and communication needs, wishes, and preferences of the dying person, their family, and those important to them.
- Assessment should also include a sensitive appraisal of the person's understanding of the situation and their information needs.
- For family and significant others, a pro-active assessment of their needs is also important, as is offering them the opportunity to ask questions and discuss any concerns, worries, or fears they may have.
- Assessment of the dying person's mental capacity is important to confirm the ability and wishes of the person to engage and participate in decision-making.
- Nurses should be aware of the dying person's status as regards resuscitation or organ donation.
- Similarly, any related decisions, such as ADRT, and deprivation of liberty safeguards (DOLS).

It is also important for nurses to recognize and respect difference. In order to maintain dignity and compassion, it is necessary to actively listen to what the dying person and their families are saying and to respect their expressed views and wishes, even when these are different to the nurse's own.

Physical changes in dying people

A number of physical changes may occur in the last days and hours of life, so regular physical observation and ongoing assessment are necessary.

A dying person's condition may also stabilize or even appear to improve before death, but this does not necessarily indicate that the person will recover. It may therefore be necessary to help the person, and family, deal with false hopes or unrealistic expectations.

Whilst not all of the known physical changes will be observed in every dying person, it is important to document observations and assessments. Changes in the person's physical condition should be discussed with the MDT, the dying person (where appropriate), and the family. Physical changes may include:

- Reduced appetite and oral intake.
- Difficulty swallowing.
- Nausea and/or vomiting.
- Increased drowsiness.
- Dry, sore mouth.
- Reduced LOC, although the dying person may still respond and appear to be aware of the presence of others.
- Restlessness and/or agitation.
- Unconsciousness.
- Changes to the face and skin such as pallor, cyanosis, or mottled appearance, especially in the extremities.
- Changes to breathing pattern—shallow, fast, rapid, or slow and irregular (Cheyne–Stokes).
- Excessive respiratory tract secretions, causing 'noisy' breathing.
- Breathlessness.
- Muscle twitching (myoclonus).
- Retention of urine.
- Pain.

Key nursing considerations

The principal nursing responsibility towards dying people, irrespective of location or expectation of death, is to maintain the person's comfort and dignity.

Wherever it is feasible, an individual end-of-life care plan can be developed with the MDT, but it is recognized that, in emergency situations, this may not always be possible. Nonetheless, nurses should always respect the person's dignity and communicate appropriately and sensitively with the dying person and their families.

Nursing practice and decision-making are exercised through attention to physical care, spiritual support, and communication.

Physical care

Physical interventions should be focused on maintaining physical comfort and dignity at all times and, as far as is possible, respecting the wishes of the dying person and their family. It may also be helpful to involve the family or significant others in giving physical care to the dying person.

- Adjust the physical environment, general setting, and lighting and noise level to provide maximum comfort.
- Ensure privacy, but avoid isolation.
- Assess the person's level of functional ability, and assist them if necessary and appropriate.
- Help the person to eat and drink safely.
- Regularly review the person's ability to tolerate oral food and fluids.
- Consider whether clinically assisted nutrition and hydration are necessary, and refer to the MPT.
- Assess the condition of the person's mouth regularly, and help with mouth care as required.
- Regularly assess any physical symptoms.
- Regularly assess for pain.
- Observe for any non-verbal signs of pain, particularly if the person is no longer able to talk.
- Administer the most appropriate non-pharmacological relief for pain or other symptoms.
- Administer and accurately record any prescribed medications, and monitor and report their effects.
- Assess for difficulty in taking oral medications and, where necessary, ensure that an alternative administration route is prescribed.
- Support or fully attend to personal hygiene and toileting needs.
- Assess the skin for changes, and keep clean, dry, and comfortable.
- Assist or change the person's position, as necessary, to ensure physical comfort.
- Apply appropriate pressure-relieving aids where indicated.

Spiritual support

People who are dying may be a committed member of a religious faith and have specific needs associated with their religion. Similarly, those who do not have a religious belief may have a spiritual dimension to their lives, which is equally important to them. Nurses should also be aware that some people may not have any spiritual feelings at all, and these too should be respected. Nurses should therefore seek to identify what, if anything, is spiritually important and meaningful to the dying person and their family:

- Identify specific religious or spiritual needs.
- Contact an appropriate religious representative if the dying person or family asks you to.
- Assist with religious observances if acceptable to the person and their family.
- Acknowledge, respect, and support the spiritual needs of the family or people important to the dying person.

Communication

Therapeutically, the ability to communicate with empathy and compassion is important, for both the dying person and those important to them. The communication and information needs of both the person and the family must be identified and addressed sensitively.

Procedurally, inter-professional communication is also essential at this time, and the ability to liaise with nursing colleagues and medical and other healthcare staff is a crucial aspect of good nursing practice. It is also important that nurses maintain accurate records to ensure seamless nursing hand-over and continuation of care for the dying person and their family.

- Actively listen.
- Consider and assess the person's ability to communicate and engage in decision-making (mental capacity, cognitive status, or language).
- Ensure that explanations are provided before undertaking any clinical procedures or other interventions.
- Avoid 'talking over' the dying person.
- Seek to involve the dying person in dialogue with, or about, them.
- Maintain physical contact through the use of appropriate touch.
- Actively assess the understanding and information needs of the family.
- Allow the family to express concerns, worries, or fears.
- Provide explanations using a sensitive and compassionate approach.
- Keep the family informed about physical or other changes which are occurring.
- Liaise with, and involve, other members of the MDT when necessary and appropriate.
- Ensure that all nursing records are comprehensive and accurate.

Caring for a dying person and supporting their family can often be emotionally demanding and very stressful for health professional staff. Nurses should be aware of their own feelings and make use of any support available within the care team and the local organization.

After death

It is important to recognize that the approach to care and communication in the last days of a person's life can have a lasting impact on the family's experience of death and bereavement.

If the dead person or their family has particular religious beliefs, there may be customs and rituals associated with death and dying which need to be observed and respected.

In circumstances where a death is sudden or unexpected, the family or significant others may seek to express their distress, or anger, through formal complaints. Nursing records of care and interventions for the dying person will need to be reviewed as part of any inquiry into the circumstances of their death.

There are many practical actions which need to be undertaken following any death, and the central element of care provision is an ability to maintain dignity and respect for the deceased person and to provide compassionate care and support to the family.

In a hospital or other clinical environment, it is important that local organizational policy is always followed, including procedures for respectful removal of the body from the clinical area. Practical nursing duties after death may include:

- Informing the medical professional responsible for the person.
- Facilitating verification of death by a medical professional, or a senior nurse who has completed relevant training and is authorized to do so.
- Recording details of the death in accordance with local policy, which may include the time, persons present, the nature of death, and any medical or other devices in use.
- Specific immediate actions, such as referral to the coroner, may be necessary, so appropriate service managers need to be informed.
- If the deceased or their family had consented to organ donation, then the local organizational policy and procedure must be followed.
- If appropriate, carrying out procedures for honouring any cultural and religious beliefs, with involvement of religious representatives if relevant.
- In clinical environments, local policies and procedures should be followed to prepare the deceased person's body for safe transfer to the mortuary or funeral home.
- Following organizational policy, document and return any personal possessions to the deceased person's family.
- Involve the family in preparing for the removal of the body if this is something they wish to do.
- Allow the family sufficient time with the deceased, and avoid intruding.
- Listen to the family, and address any immediate questions or concerns, ensuring that these discussions are documented.
- Keep an accurate record of all nursing actions taken after death.
- If the person is in a clinical environment, ensure there is appropriate support for other patients who may be distressed, anxious, or frightened.
- Ensure the safety and well-being of all staff in contact with the deceased person.

A medical certificate stating the cause of death will normally be completed by a medical professional and provided to either the next of kin or a designated funeral director acting on the family's behalf.

Supporting the family at the time of death

Where a death is anticipated, the family or other people important to the deceased may be present at the death, so nurses need to be able to respond sensitively and appropriately to their reactions, which may be expressed in various ways:

- Open distress—crying, wailing.
- Emotional catharsis—anger, shouting, violent actions.
- Incongruous mood and behaviour—laughing.
- Subdued distress—sadness, resignation, or disbelief.
- Physiological reactions—fainting or hyperventilation.

Where a person's death is unexpected and families are not present at the time, nurses will need to deal with their reactions and address questions about the cause and manner of death. Additional consideration will need to be given to:

- How the family or named next of kin will be informed.
- Who the most appropriate person is to inform the family.
- How the family will be supported if they choose to see the deceased person in the clinical environment.

It is also important to be aware that even in cases where death is expected, not all families will choose to be present at the time of death. Some may not wish to attend the deceased person at all, and the decision of these people should always be respected.

Providing information

After a person has died, it is often part of local procedures and policy to provide practical information to a family, which may be in the form of information leaflets.

Written information should not replace compassionate verbal communication. Any information, whether written or verbal, should be provided in a manner which is respectful and sensitive to the particular needs of the family.

- Assess the specific information needs of the family.
- Address any questions openly and honestly.
- Ensure that any explanations are tailored to family needs.
- Include information about any necessary administrative and legal procedures.
- In line with local policy, provide practical written information such as how to register a death, bereavement support information, and how to begin funeral arrangements.
- Advise about when and where they, or the nominated funeral directors, can obtain the death certificate.

Referral to the coroner

If a person's death needs to be referred to the coroner, this may cause considerable additional distress to a family and may delay the disposal of the body. In these circumstances, nursing records may also need to be reviewed by the coroner's office.

Where a doctor is able to provide a medical cause of death, the death can be registered and the body disposed. In order to provide this certificate, the doctor must know what caused the death and must have seen and treated the person for that condition within the 14 days before they died.

Where there is no doctor available who can issue this certificate, the death must be reported to the coroner, but this does not necessarily mean that there will be an inquest.

There are several types of death that must always be reported to the coroner:

- All children and young people under 18 (even if due to natural causes).
- Deaths within 24 hours of admission to hospital.
- Deaths that may be linked to medical treatment, surgery, or anaesthetic.
- Deaths that may be linked to an accident, however long ago.
- Suicide or suspicion of suicide.
- Any other suspicious circumstances.
- Where there is a history of violence.
- Deaths that may be linked to the person's occupation (e.g. asbestos exposure).
- All people in custody (even if due to natural causes).
- All people detained under the Mental Health Act (even if due to natural causes).
- Some illnesses such as hepatitis and TB.

It might be very important to assure a family that not all referrals to the coroner necessitate a post-mortem examination or result in a public inquest (% www.gov.uk/after-a-death). It is often the case that the coroner only needs to review the medical and nursing case notes. Once the coroner has authorized the disposal of a body, the funeral arrangements can proceed.

Very often there is no need for the family to be involved with the coroner's office. The collection of a certificate to dispose of a body can be done by the designated funeral directors.

Loss, grief, and bereavement

Whilst loss takes many forms, bereavement generally refers to the loss of a person through death. Grief is the response to that loss, which may be a serious threat to health and well-being.

The challenge for people who have been bereaved is for them to find ways to cope physically, psychologically, emotionally, and socially and learn to live with their loss.

The classic twentieth-century work by the psychologist Kübler-Ross gave a new focus to ways of thinking about death and grief and originally described five stages in the grieving process. Since then, considerable effort has been dedicated to understanding grief and the grieving process.

There are many theories of bereavement, all of which have contributed significantly to the understanding of people's experiences and responses following a death. The critique of the more traditional theories is that they provide only a limited appreciation of the complexities of grieving.

Contemporary theories of loss, grief, and bereavement focus on individual expressions of grief and include how the bereaved person creates a sense of meaning, integrates the memory of the deceased person, and adjusts to the future. Responses to bereavement may also relate to a wider social or cultural context and the secondary losses which result from the death.

It is important to recognize that there is no 'right' or 'wrong' way to grieve, and each person will react in their own unique way and time.

Whilst it is recognized that grief is an individual experience, Box 25.1 outlines some examples of the physical, psychological, emotional, and social reactions which may occur following bereavement.

Supporting the bereaved

For nurses working in the acute clinical sector, their role in supporting the bereaved may be very limited. However, for those based in community or hospice environments, there may be a longer-term commitment to supporting people who are bereaved.

The grieving process may begin prior to a person's death in the form of anticipatory grief or mourning. This can relate to abstract losses such as the loss of an expected future, or the anticipation of everyday life without the dying person.

It is important to be aware of how different families experience grief and to work within professional role boundaries to provide appropriate support before the death and following bereavement. The care provided to a dying person and their family before and after a death is likely be an enduring memory for the bereaved.

Many people will access bereavement support through social networks, family, and friends. However, this may become difficult in circumstances where support networks are lacking or the family are geographically distant. Nurses can help people by directing them to more formal support organizations such as Cruse Bereavement Care (ᐦ www.cruse.org.uk).

Box 25.1 Grief reactions

Anger

Fear

Guilt

Sadness

Anxiety

Worry

Lack of concentration

Feelings of disconnection

Isolation

Confusion

Forgetfulness

Hopelessness

Yearning

Search for meaning

Loss of faith

Crying

Sleep disturbance

Loss of appetite

Chest tightness

Palpitations

Dry mouth

Numbness

Social withdrawal

It is important that nurses are able to recognize when specialist bereavement services may be necessary such as where a person continues to be overwhelmed by the physical, psychological, emotional, and social effects of grief.

Effective communication is an essential component for supporting bereaved people and in helping nurses assess where more formal bereavement support may be needed.

- Acknowledge the bereavement.
- Acknowledge your own feelings.
- Acknowledge any feelings of helplessness.
- Actively listen to what people are saying.
- Try to understand and acknowledge the person's perspective.
- Allow the bereaved person to express their feelings, emotions, and grief in their own way.
- Let them know their feelings are OK.

- Never assume to know how someone is feeling.
- Enable them to tell their story and to talk about the person who has died.
- Be aware of cultural variations in response to bereavement.
- Use both verbal and non-verbal communication skills, including touch if appropriate.
- Find out what is helping the person to cope with their grief.
- Be aware of any signs that the bereaved person is having difficulty coping with their grief.
- Encourage, and assist with, referral to GPs or specialist support if required.

(See also ➜ Chapter 6, Communication in a healthcare context, ➜ Chapter 7, Dignity and respect, ➜ Chapter 8, Culturally sensitive communication, ➜ Chapter 9, Communicating concerns in healthcare, ➜ Chapter 10, Conflict resolution, and ➜ Chapter 11, Breaking 'bad news'.)

Useful sources of further information

- The Leadership Alliance for the Care of Dying People ✍ www.england. nhs.uk/ourwork/qual-clin-lead/lac
- National Institute for Health and Care Excellence (2015) *Care of dying adults in the last days of life.* NICE guideline [NG31] ✍ www.nice.org.uk
- NHS Improving Quality Sustainable Improvement Team ✍ www. nhsiq.nhs.uk/improvement-programmes/long-term-conditions-and-integrated-care/end-of-life-care/care-in-the-last-days-of-life.aspx
- The functions of the coroner ✍ www.gov.uk/after-a-death
- Mental Capacity Act (2005) ✍ www.legislation.gov.uk/ukpga/2005/9/contents
- Cruse Bereavement Care ✍ www.cruse.org.uk
- Dying Matters ✍ www.dyingmatters.org/page/coping-bereavement
- NHS Choices (2017) *Coping with bereavement* ✍ www.nhs.uk/Livewell/bereavement/Pages/coping-with-bereavement.aspx

Chapter 26

Clinical emergencies

Clinical emergencies

A clinical emergency is a critical situation, which may be life-threatening. It is usually a sudden and unexpected event, happening anywhere, anytime, to anybody.

Emergency healthcare in the UK is increasingly provided by an integrated network made up of first responders, paramedics, air ambulance, major trauma centres, trauma centres, emergency departments, GPs, walk-in clinics, and minor injury units. However, an important part of nurse decision-making is prompt and appropriate response to clinical emergencies, wherever these occur.

Nurses may encounter a clinical emergency both within their work environment and outside it, and so should be aware of how to deal with emergencies in their own clinical setting, but should also have an understanding of the principles of basic first aid.

Whether providing emergency assistance in a work-based context or outside the remit of employment, nurses are always bound by the NMC Code, their terms of employment, and the laws of the country of practice (% www.nmc.org.uk/standards/code/).

- Prevention of injury and understanding the principles of how to deal with clinical emergencies are important for nurses working with people in all sectors of health services.
- Clinical emergencies often occur in hospital, when deterioration in a person's condition goes unrecognized or untreated. An understanding of local policies and procedures in the case of an emergency is essential.
- Nurses who are called to deal with a clinical emergency, in any setting, must maintain the highest level of professionalism and should be particularly mindful of their own feelings, comments, and reactions in an emergency situation.
- In clinical emergencies, nursing decision-making and practices are framed by professional knowledge, values, and teamwork, grounded in respectful, empathetic communication skills, which maintains confidentiality and people's dignity at all times.

Managing clinical emergencies

In any clinical emergency situation, nurse decision-making is focused on the nurse's knowledge and ability to recognize and respond appropriately to a potential or actual life-threatening circumstance.

Technical competencies, effective communication skills, and partnership working with the MDT are essential for an effective response to clinical emergencies. The key principles of managing clinical emergencies are the same, regardless of the context in which they occur:

- Rapidly assess the situation.
- Avoid any risk to yourself.
- Think before acting.
- Prevent further harm to the ill or injured person.

Emergencies outside hospital

For all clinical emergencies, outside of a hospital environment, the *SAFE* approach is recommended.

- *S*—Shout for help.
- *A*—Assess for dangers to the person and the rescuer.
- *F*—Free from danger.
- *E*—Evaluate the person.
- If the person is unresponsive and not breathing normally, then emergency services should be called (999 or 112), and basic life support (BLS) initiated.
- Commence cardiopulmonary resuscitation (CPR) at a rate of 120 chest compressions per minute, until help arrives.
- At the nurse's discretion, rescue breaths may also be given. If so, this should be at the rate of 30 chest compressions to two rescue breaths, repeated until help arrives (℠ www.resus.org.uk).
- The airway should be opened using the chin lift or jaw thrust technique, taking care to minimize movement of the neck (see Box 26.1).
- Where a person is alert and appears to be breathing normally, the clinical emergency can be further evaluated by questioning or talking to the person.

Box 26.1 Opening the airway

Head tilt–chin lift manoeuvre
- Place one hand on the person's forehead.
- Apply firm, but gentle, backward pressure using the palm of the hand.
- Place the fingers of the other hand under the chin.
- Lift the chin forward, supporting the jaw, and tilt the head back.

Jaw thrust manoeuvre
- Kneel near the top of the person's head.
- With both hands, grasp the angles of the lower jaw.
- Lift the jawbone up, and tilt the head back.

- If the person is able to respond to questions appropriately, then a patent airway, adequate breathing, and cerebral perfusion can be assumed.
- It is useful to maintain brief conversations with the person at short intervals to ascertain the LOC and comfort the person.
- A rapid respiratory rate or the person only being able to speak in short sentences normally indicates respiratory distress, which may lead to a rapid deterioration in their condition.
- An ambulance should always be called immediately for anyone complaining of chest pain.
- If trauma is the actual or suspected cause of the clinical emergency, then the cervical spine should be immobilized until clinical investigations can exclude any damage.
- If the person has suffered a traumatic injury, they should be immobilized and, if possible, the mechanism of the injury identified.
- Pressure should be applied to any external bleeding and, if feasible, the bleeding part should be raised above the level of the heart.
- The person should be kept safe and warm until help arrives.
- In clinical emergency circumstances, outside of a hospital or other clinical environment, it is important that the nurse projects an air of calm.
- It is also important to accurately report any observations or information about the person and the clinical situation to the emergency clinicians (normally a paramedic) who provide assistance.

(See also ➤ Table 26.2, Glasgow coma scale, p. 537.)

Emergencies in hospitals and other clinical environments

All healthcare organizations will have their own policies and procedures for responding to clinical emergencies, and these should always be followed.

Most local protocols and procedures will incorporate the UK Resuscitation Council's recommended *ABCDE* approach, and their guidelines for basic and advanced life support (🖰 www.resus.org.uk/resuscitation-guidelines/abcde-approach/).

The principles of the ABCDE approach to the critically unwell or injured person allow for systematic assessment of both the person and the situation. Each element is assessed and any life-threatening problem corrected, prior to moving on to the next step in the assessment.

The ABCDE approach facilitates early recognition of the need for help, promotes a team approach to emergency interventions and care, and supports ongoing re-assessment and evaluation of the person and the situation. In the community or outside a clinical environment, it may not be possible to correct all the immediate clinical problems, but nonetheless the ABCDE(F) approach should be used to guide assessment and facilitate an accurate 'handover' to the emergency services.

ABCDE(F) assessment

- *A—Airway*: assess airway patency, which should be established prior to moving on to the next part of the assessment. In people who have suffered a trauma, it is important to be aware of the risk of a potential injury to the cervical spine with some airway manoeuvres.
- *B—Breathing*: assess the efficacy of breathing. Any life-threatening conditions, such as asthma, tension pneumothorax, or pulmonary oedema, should be treated immediately.
- *C—Circulation*: assess circulation and, if impaired, treat the cause. Ensure that IV access has been established, in case emergency drug administration or fluid replacement is needed.
- *D—Disability*: assess the LOC through noting alertness, voice, pain, and unresponsiveness (AVPU). Aim to establish the cause of any loss of consciousness, as this may require re-assessment and urgent treatment of ABC.
- *E—Exposure*: assess the patient's overall condition and any injury by exposing the body for inspection, whilst maintaining the patient's dignity at all times.

It is worth noting that the '*F*', for *family*, is also an important nursing responsibility when dealing with people in clinical emergency situations. Whether in hospital or outside, it may well be that the nurse is the person who assumes, or is given, the task of informing or comforting the family or significant others.

The outcome of the ABCDE(F) assessment will determine the next steps to be taken.

Cardiopulmonary resuscitation (CPR)

If the person is unresponsive or not breathing normally, or cardiac arrest is evident, then the local emergency procedure should be followed immediately and life support commenced.

Cardiac arrest procedures in hospitals will incorporate the UK Resuscitation Council's ABCDE approach to assessment, and their guidelines for basic and advanced life support (℞ www.resus.org.uk/resuscitation-guidelines/abcde-approach/). In the first instance, nurses should:

- Call for help, the resuscitation equipment, and defibrillator.
- Lay the person flat.
- Open the airway using the chin lift or jaw thrust technique.
- Commence CPR at a rate of 120 chest compressions per minute, until help arrives.
- At the nurse's discretion, rescue breaths may also be given. If so, this should be at the rate of 30 chest compressions to two rescue breaths. This should be repeated until help arrives.
- If an automatic electrical defibrillator (AED) is available, attach to the patient and follow the instructions.
- Once help arrives, it is the nurse's responsibility to clearly and accurately communicate relevant information about the ABCDE assessment, the person, and the arrest situation to other members of the emergency team.
- A designated member of the emergency team, normally a person with advanced life support skills and training, will then manage the cardiac arrest and make clinical judgements about defibrillation, drugs, and any other relevant interventions.
- In clinical emergency situations, it is normal practice to exchange information between different healthcare professions using acronyms to ensure that key features of the emergency are noted and exchanged. Examples of these are SBAR and RSVP (see Table 26.1).
- If the person is conscious, it is important that nurses communicate timely and appropriate information to them about their situation and offer comfort wherever possible.

Table 26.1 Examples of acronyms used in clinical emergency situations

SBAR	RSVP
S—situation	R—reason
B—background	S—story
A—assessment	V—vital signs
R—recognition	P—plan

Key nursing considerations in clinical emergencies

In clinical emergency situations, nursing decision-making and practices are framed by professional knowledge, values, and teamwork and grounded in respectful, empathic communication skills.

Key nursing considerations listed here will apply to any clinical emergency situation, with the addition of other specific interventions directly related to the nature of the emergency.

Healthcare organizations will also have local policies, protocols, or guidelines for dealing with different clinical emergencies, and these should always be followed.

In all emergency situations

- Assess the person, using the ABCDE(F) approach.
- Call for assistance.
- Commence BLS, if indicated.
- Observe and accurately note the person's condition.
- Accurately time and report any observations, clinical measurements, or changes to the person's condition.
- If the person is conscious, obtain an account of the onset of the emergency and any associated medical conditions.
- Maintain a safe and calm environment.
- As far as possible, ensure physical comfort.

In emergency situations in hospitals or other clinical environments

- Establish IV access.
- Take blood samples for laboratory testing.
- Monitor blood pressure, heart rate, oxygen saturation, temperature, respiratory rate, LOC, and urine output.
- Re-assess and record vital signs as the clinical condition dictates.
- Calculate EWS, and adjust care in accordance with local track and trigger escalation plans.
- Manage any additional investigations ordered as part of local care protocol (e.g. ECG, radiological imaging).
- Safely and accurately administer any prescribed IV fluids, and accurately record fluid balance.
- Safely and accurately administer and record any prescribed medicines (including oxygen therapy).
- Clearly explain all actions and interventions to the patient and any family or carers present.
- Give accurate explanations of other likely events and investigations.

(For details of specific clinical procedures, see ➲ *Oxford Handbook of Clinical Skills in Adult Nursing*.)

Sepsis

An infection is the body's local response to invasion by, and multiplication of, bacteria, viruses, fungi, and parasites. Infections can often occur without symptoms, and these are known as subclinical infections. Some infections may provoke a body-wide systemic inflammatory response, and this severe and life-threatening condition is known as sepsis. In the UK, it is estimated that sepsis is responsible for >100,000 hospital admissions and around 37,000 deaths per year (℞ www.nhs.uk/Conditions/Blood-poisoning/Pages/introduction.aspx).

The criteria used to identify sepsis are contained within the systemic inflammatory response syndrome (SIRS). Whilst the SIRS criteria are not specific to sepsis, the presence of two or more SIRS criteria in the presence of an infection is assumed to be sepsis.

SIRS criteria

- Temperature >38°C or <36°C.
- Heart rate >90bpm.
- Respiratory rate >20 breaths per minute
- White cell count <4 or >12g/L.
- Altered mental state.
- Blood glucose >7.7mmol/L in those who are not diabetic.

Categories of sepsis

- *Sepsis*: the presence of two or more SIRS criteria with a known infection.
- *Severe sepsis*: sepsis with evidence of organ dysfunction, hypotension, or hypoperfusion. This may be demonstrated by reduced LOC, hypoxia, oliguria, and serum lactate measurement of >2mmol/L.
- *Septic shock*: shows the same symptoms as severe sepsis, with refractory hypotension (continued hypotension despite adequate fluid resuscitation) and a serum lactate measurement of >4mmol/L.

Whilst any person suffering from infection is at risk for sepsis, severe sepsis, or septic shock, people who are very young, frail, and elderly, those with multiple co-morbidities, and people who are immunocompromised are at greatest risk.

Investigation and treatment of sepsis

All people with sepsis require immediate intervention to determine the severity, identify the pathogen, initiate appropriate treatment, and prevent further deterioration. Healthcare organizations will normally have a clinical pathway or recognized 'care bundle' for the treatment of sepsis, and local procedures should always be followed. A widely used care bundle is the 'Sepsis Six'.

The 'Sepsis Six'
- Blood cultures (usually two sets from two different sites).
- Administration of antibiotics within 1 hour.
- High-flow oxygen.
- Serum lactate and FBC.
- IV fluid.
- Accurate measurement of fluid balance.

The severity of sepsis is classified by physiological and biochemical measures and the person's response to treatment. All those with severe sepsis or septic shock should be reviewed by the critical care team and may need a period of intensive care.

The central aspect of sepsis treatment is urgently commencing IV antibiotic therapy. Clinical research has suggested that for people with septic shock, there is a 7.6% increase in mortality for every hour delay in commencing antibiotic treatment. Treatments also include antipyretic drugs and inotropic or vasopressor medicines.

Key nursing considerations in sepsis

In addition to the key nursing considerations outlined on ➲ p. 524 of this chapter, particular attention should be paid to calculating EWS and adjusting nursing care in accordance with local track and trigger escalation plans.
- Establish and maintain IV access.
- Blood for culture and other laboratory tests.
- Timely administration of IV antibiotic therapy, antipyretics, and other prescribed medications.
- IV fluid replacement therapies.
- Prescribed oxygen therapy.
- Maintain a safe and calming environment for recovery.
- As far as possible, ensure physical comfort.

Useful sources of further information
- Surviving Sepsis Campaign ℘ www.survivingsepsis.org
- The UK Sepsis Trust ℘ www.sepsistrust.org

Shock

Shock is a life-threatening emergency, which occurs when oxygen supply is inadequate to meet the body's metabolic demand at the cellular level. In a hypoxic state, metabolic acidosis develops, and organ damage and death may result. Shock is normally due to a failure within the cardiovascular system. Shock requires prompt recognition and immediate treatment to ensure the best possible patient outcomes.

Types of shock

Hypovolaemic shock
- Normally occurs due to haemorrhage, as a result of trauma, fracture, GI bleeding, ruptured aortic aneurysm, or ruptured ectopic pregnancy.
- May also be due to severe fluid loss associated with burns, GI problems such as severe vomiting and diarrhoea, and intestinal obstruction.

Cardiogenic shock
- Occurs as a result of a failure in the pumping mechanism of the heart and significantly reduced cardiac output.
- Causes include MI, myocarditis, cardiac contusion, cardiac arrhythmias, and valvular rupture.

Obstructive shock
- This occurs when there is obstruction to the outflow of blood from the heart caused by blockage of the great vessels.
- Causes include massive PE, tension pneumothorax, and cardiac tamponade.

Distributive shock
- This occurs when there is impaired distribution of blood flow throughout the body, usually as a result of vasodilation.
- Causes include vasodilation due to sepsis or medication, altered distribution of flow due to anaphylaxis, sepsis, and arteriovenous shunting.

Neurogenic shock
- Is also a type of distributive shock, resulting from brain or spinal cord injury.

Physical signs of shock
- Tachypnoea with increased respiratory rate, and rapid and shallow breathing pattern.
- Tachycardia with a heart rate >90 is common but may not be present in patients with cardiogenic or neurogenic shock.
- Hypotension with systolic blood pressure <90mmHg in adults. Values may be higher in young, fit, or previously hypertensive patients.
- Poor peripheral perfusion, cool peripheries, clammy/sweaty skin, pallor.
- Low urinary output (oliguria), <50mL/hour in adults.

- Altered consciousness, dizziness, fainting, or weakness, especially on standing or sitting up.
- Distress and agitation.
- Neurogenic shock presents differently to other types of shock, with people having warm dry skin, due to loss of sympathetic nervous tone. This results in inability to redirect blood flow from the peripheries to the central circulation. This can lead to rapid heat loss and hypothermia.

Treatments

Treatments for shock will be dictated by the precipitating cause and may include:

- Emergency surgery.
- IV fluid replacement.
- Infusion of blood or blood products.
- IM adrenaline.
- Tranexamic acid.
- IV antibiotics.
- IV inotropic or vasoactive therapy.
- IV antihistamines.
- IV corticosteroids.

Key nursing considerations in shock

In addition to the key nursing considerations outlined on ➋ p. 524 of this chapter, particular attention should be paid to restoring haemodynamic status and, if possible, identifying the cause of the shock state. Shock can be exacerbated by fear and pain, so calm, empathic communication with people is important.

Anaphylactic shock

Anaphylactic shock is not due to blood loss or other failures of the cardiovascular system but is *a severe, potentially life-threatening, allergic reaction*.

Anaphylaxis should always be dealt with as a clinical emergency and treated with IM adrenaline as soon as possible. People who have a known and serious allergy most often carry their own dose of injectable adrenaline, of which friends and families may be aware. In these cases, first-line treatment is often managed by the person with the allergy. In other people, the first-line treatment is normally given by paramedics, pre-hospital services, or in accident and emergency departments. The most common allergens known to trigger reactions are:

- Insect stings.[1]
- Peanuts and tree nuts.
- Identified food groups (such as milk, eggs, seafood, strawberries).
- Some prescription medicines.

Exposure to a trigger allergen will normally cause an immediate allergic response, but in some cases, the reaction to the trigger may be delayed by several hours.

---

1 NHS Choices. *Insect bites and stings.* ✍ www.nhs.uk/conditions/Stings-insect/Pages/Introduction.aspx.

Signs of anaphylaxis
- Itching, or a raised, red skin rash.
- Swelling in the eyes, lips, hands, and feet.
- Swelling of the mouth, throat, or tongue.
- Breathing, wheezing, difficulties.
- Swallowing difficulties.
- Feeling light-headed or faint.
- Abdominal pain, nausea, and vomiting.
- Collapse.
- Unconsciousness.

Nursing considerations in anaphylaxis

In addition to the key nursing considerations for decision-making and practice in clinical emergencies (see p. 524), in anaphylaxis, it is important to ascertain whether the adrenaline auto-injector has been administered if the person carries one.

Haemorrhage and wounds

Haemorrhage

Haemorrhage can occur both externally and internally. External bleeding usually results from wounds caused by trauma or surgery, but may also be caused by an underlying medical condition such as hypertension which can result in severe epistaxis.

Internal bleeding occurs within body cavities and may also be caused by injury, surgery, or underlying health conditions. Bleeding into the brain may manifest as seizures or stroke, whilst bleeding into the abdominal cavity from such things as an aortic aneurysm or an ectopic pregnancy can present as severe abdominal pain.

Internal bleeding may occur spontaneously from underlying conditions such as a peptic ulcer, oesophageal varices, and some cancers. Haematological conditions such as haemophilia and clotting disorders are also a cause of haemorrhage.

Haemorrhage is usually classified by its source:

- *Arterial*: damage causes bright red, oxygen-rich blood to spurt out of the body in time with the heart rhythm.
- *Venous*: damage causes dark red blood to gush out profusely, depending upon the extent of the damage.
- *Capillary*: red and brisk at times or oozing, depending on damage.

Treatment of haemorrhage

Irrespective of its source, bleeding must be controlled. This may be achieved through application of external pressure and medication, or surgery may be necessary.

- Direct pressure is initially the effective way to manage external haemorrhage, but if an object is embedded in a wound, then pressure should be applied on each side of the embedded object or fragment.
- If possible, the bleeding area should be elevated to help control bleeding.
- IV fluid replacement may need to be administered, to restore circulating blood volume.
- Blood products and tranexamic acid may be prescribed
- It may be necessary to treat uncontrolled haemorrhage through emergency surgery.
- The first indication of internal bleeding will often be subtle, with only an increase in respiratory rate and subsequent elevation in heart rate evident.
- If unrecognized or untreated, internal bleeding can ultimately lead to hypovolaemic shock and/or death.

Key nursing considerations in haemorrhage

In addition to the nursing considerations outlined on ➲ p. 524 of this chapter, nurse decision-making and practice should focus on identifying the source and cause of bleeding and restoring haemodynamic status.

- Observe for signs of external haemorrhage, particularly following surgery or trauma or in people with a known underlying condition.

- Observe for signs of internal haemorrhage, especially in people at high risk such as those with a history of excessive alcohol consumption, abdominal aortic aneurysm, or peptic ulcer disease.
- Ensure that PPE is worn.
- Apply direct pressure to any obvious external bleeding points or to either side of any foreign body which remains *in situ*. If penetrating trauma is evident, do not be tempted to remove any retained foreign body.
- People with epistaxis should be sat forward to decrease the blood flow to the nasopharynx. The soft part of the nose should be held for 10–15 minutes with constant pressure. The person should be encouraged to spit out any blood which collects in the pharynx. (See also ➜ Chapter 21, Conditions of the eye, ears, nose, and throat.)
- If a person's condition deteriorates, summon help and commence BLS if necessary.

(For details of specific clinical procedures, see ➜ *Oxford Handbook of Clinical Skills in Adult Nursing*.)

Wounds

- *Laceration*—occurs when blunt forces cause the skin tissue to break open, often over a bony prominence. The extent of the laceration varies in length and depth and results in torn skin and irregular wound edges. Repair is usually by surgical closure.
- *Incision*—results from a cut in the skin made by a sharp object such as a knife or broken glass. Stab and slash wounds are classified as incisions. The extent of the incision varies in length and depth and is characterized by clean-cut edges. Repair is usually by surgical closure.
- *Contusion*—or bruises are a collection of blood under the tissue, which discolours the skin. Contusions are caused by blunt forces, and localized bleeding occurs and forms a haematoma, but no skin breakage occurs. Usual treatments include applying cold packs to the area and administering mild analgesic medications.
- *Abrasions*—are 'grazes' which result from blunt injury. Broken skin may contain dirt, which increases the risk of infection. Treatment involves cleaning all dirt and debris that is embedded in the skin to prevent a permanent skin tattooing effect. Abraded areas may be dressed with non-adherent material or left open to heal.
- *Avulsion*—refers to full-thickness tissue loss in which the wound edges cannot be approximated. Small avulsions heal by secondary intention. Larger avulsions may require skin grafting. A severe type of avulsion injury is a degloving injury in which the skin is peeled away from the underlying structures.
- *Puncture wounds*—are commonly caused by a sharp or, in some cases, a blunt object, which has sufficient force to penetrate the skin. Underlying structures should be checked for further damage. Treatment involves cleansing the wound, removing any foreign objects, and careful surgical repair and closure.

- *Subungual haematomas*—or nail injuries result from a blunt force injury to a fingernail or toenail. Increasing pressure from blood accumulation under the nail causes a throbbing pain. Treatment involves relieving the pressure by making a small puncture in the nail with a sterile needle or surgical pin.
- *Surgical wounds*—see ➲ Chapter 22, Surgery.

All but the most superficial of wounds should be assessed by a nurse or other clinician experienced in wound care. To promote optimal healing, and return to normal function, it is essential to exclude injury to any deep underlying structures, ensure thorough decontamination of the wound, and close it properly.

Wounds which have the potential to become infected may also be treated with tetanus vaccination, tetanus immunoglobulin, or antibiotics.

Neurological emergencies

Level of consciousness

Level of consciousness (LOC) is a term used to describe people's awareness of self and sensory stimuli in their immediate environment.

In nursing and healthcare, LOC is understood as a continuum ranging from people who are fully aware and awake, through those with mild loss of awareness, to those with a complete lack of response to sensory stimuli.

There are several known causes of deteriorating consciousness or unconsciousness, all of which require urgent intervention and ongoing treatment and monitoring.

• Hypoglycaemia.
• Hyperglycaemia.
• Drug overdose.
• Head injury.
• Stroke.
• SAH.
• Convulsions.
• Alcohol intoxication.
• Cardiac failure.
• Respiratory failure.
• Cardiac arrhythmias and arrest.
• Hypovolaemic shock.
• Anaphylaxis.
• Sepsis.
• Hepatic failure.
• Renal failure.
• Hypothermia.
• Hyperthermia.
• Meningitis.
• Encephalitis.
• Malaria and other tropical diseases.

Various measurement tools have been designed to assess LOC. For a rapid assessment, the *AVPU* scale can be used (see Box 26.2).

Box 26.2 AVPU scale for rapid assessment of level of consciousness

A—alert
V—responds to voice
P—responds to pain
U—unresponsive

An assessment tool in widespread use for a more detailed and ongoing assessment of LOC is the Glasgow coma scale. This gives a total score for baseline and subsequent measurements of LOC and is useful for monitoring changes in a person's condition (see Table 26.2).

Treatment of an unconscious state will be determined by whether or not the cause of unconsciousness is known. In some cases, unconsciousness can be treated by medical or surgical decompression.

Medical decompression normally involves IV administration of medications such as dexamethasone or mannitol, and surgical decompression through drilling burr holes in the skull to reduce the ICP.

Table 26.2 Glasgow coma scale

Test	Patient's response	Score
Eye opening		
	Spontaneously	4
	To speech	3
	To pain	2
	None	1
Motor response		
	Obeys verbal command	6
	Reacts to verbal command	5
	Identifies localized painful stimulus	4
	Flexes and withdraws from painful stimulus Abnormal flexion (decorticate position)	3
	Flexes and withdraws from painful stimulus Abnormal extension (decerebrate position)	2
	No response	1
Verbal response		
	Oriented and able to converse	5
	Confused or disoriented	4
	Random reply, inappropriate words	3
	Incomprehensible, moans, or screams	2
	None	c
Total score		

Reprinted from *The Lancet*, 2(7872), Teasdale G and Jennett B., Assessment of coma and impaired consciousness. A practical scale, Pages 81–4, Copyright (1974), with permission from Elsevier.

All altered LOCs will require regular measurement and recording of the LOC, together with observation of vital signs, according to local protocols. Treatments administered may include:

- IV fluids.
- Oral or IV glucose.
- Antidotes (e.g. naloxone).
- Anticonvulsants (e.g. phenytoin).
- Antibiotics.
- Adrenaline.
- IV vitamins (e.g. Pabrinex®).

Key nursing considerations in neurological emergencies

In addition to the key nursing considerations outlined on p. 524 of this chapter, in the care and management of a person who is unconscious, particular attention should be paid to regular assessment of LOC and regular monitoring of physiological and physical signs that may indicate clinical deterioration.

If the person is at risk of developing pressure ulcers, then careful and regular repositioning will also be required. People who are in an unconscious state for a long period of time may need physiotherapy interventions, in an attempt to maintain some muscle tone.

It is also important to continue speaking to the unconscious person and to ensure that no nursing actions or interventions are carried out without an explanation.

(For details of specific clinical procedures, see ➔ *Oxford Handbook of Clinical Skills in Adult Nursing*.)

Stroke and transient ischaemic attack

A stroke is defined as the rapid onset of a focal neurological deficit of vascular origin, lasting >24 hours and which may result in death within 24 hours. There are two main types of stroke:

- *Ischaemic stroke*, which is caused by atherosclerosis and/or thrombosis, and subsequent tissue damage associated with compromised perfusion of the brain. Ischaemic stroke is the most common type.
- *Haemorrhagic stroke* is less common and is sometimes referred to as intracranial haemorrhage. This is where brain injury is caused by blood vessels bleeding into the brain and surrounding structures.

Depending on the area of damage, a person with stroke may present with any of these symptoms:

- Numbness, weakness, or paralysis in the face, limbs, or other part of the body.
- Slurred speech.
- Blurred vision.
- Confusion or disorientation.
- Severe headache.
- Altered LOC.

Prompt diagnosis and initiation of treatment of stroke can have a significant impact on a person's eventual recovery and rehabilitation. In recognition of this, several screening tools have been developed and validated to aid rapid initiation of treatment where stroke is suspected. These tools are most often used by pre-hospital services and in emergency departments.

- *FAST* (Face, Arms, Speech, Test) checks the face and arms for weakness and asymmetry, whilst assessing the speech for slurring.
- *ROSIER* (Recognition Of Stroke In the Emergency Room) is a screening tool designed primarily for emergency department use. It builds on the FAST test through the addition of assessment of leg weakness and searching for any deficits in the visual field.

The first-line treatment for an ischaemic stroke is thrombolysis, but this is only effective within a 4.5-hour window from the onset of symptoms. Thrombolysis is contraindicated in haemorrhagic stroke.

Prompt assessment of people with stroke symptoms will include urgent CT imaging of the brain, to expedite the selection of appropriate treatments and ultimately improve patient outcomes. NICE guidelines identify indications for immediate brain imaging in acute stroke:

- People known to be taking anticoagulation therapy.
- People with a known underlying bleeding tendency.
- Glasgow coma scale score below 13.
- Unexplained, progressive, or fluctuating symptoms.
- Papilloedema, neck stiffness, or fever.
- Severe headache at onset of symptoms (ℛ www.nice.org.uk/guidance/cg68).

Transient ischaemic attack (TIA)

A TIA is an episode of focal neurological deficit, which resolves within 24 hours. Symptoms of TIA are similar to those of stroke but normally resolve without treatment. TIA symptoms often subside within a few minutes but can last a few hours.

- People with focal neurological symptoms should be treated as though they have had a stroke, until a stroke diagnosis has been excluded by clinical investigation.
- Those who have been diagnosed with TIA should have their ongoing risk for a subsequent stroke calculated using a validated risk assessment tool such as the ABCD2 score.
- The ABCD2 tool is validated to predict the short-term risk of stroke after a TIA using five criteria: age, blood pressure, clinical features of TIA, duration of symptoms, and diabetic status.
- People with an ABCD2 score >4 have a high risk of stroke and should be admitted to hospital for further investigations and possible surgery.

(See also ➔ Chapter 16, Neurological conditions.)

Key nursing considerations in stroke and TIA

In addition to the key nursing considerations outlined on ➔ p. 524 of this chapter, where a person has had a stroke, particular attention should be paid to regular assessment of LOC and regular monitoring of physiological and physical signs that may indicate clinical deterioration.

If the person is at risk of developing pressure ulcers, then a skin assessment and careful and regular repositioning will also be required. Local policies and procedures for acute stroke management should be followed, and in addition:

- Assess stroke symptoms with a validated tool (as in local protocol).
- Measure and record LOC.
- Do not allow the person to eat or drink anything until a swallowing assessment has been carried out (normally by speech and language therapists).
- Assist with any urgent investigation such as CT brain imaging.
- Accurately administer and record any prescribed thrombolytic therapy.
- In the hospital environment, calculate EWS and adjust care in accordance with local track and trigger escalation plans.
- Ensure timely and accurate reporting of any observations, clinical measurements, or changes to the patient's condition.
- Clearly explain all actions and interventions to the patient and any family or carers present.
- Seek to clearly and honestly allay patient and family anxieties.
- Maintain a safe and calm environment for recovery.
- As far as possible, ensure physical comfort.

Outside of the clinical emergency situation, longer-term care and treatment of people who have had a stroke are focused on rehabilitation and the restoration of optimum cognitive and physical functions.

Some places have specialist stroke services where intensive multidisciplinary rehabilitation is offered to suitable people. Stroke rehabilitation, in both hospitals and the community, is likely to involve physiotherapy, occupational therapy, speech and language therapy, dietetics, psychology, and mental health and medical services.

Rehabilitation of people who have had a stroke is often a long-term health project which is challenging for the affected person, their significant others, and the health professionals working with them.

Seizures

A seizure is a sudden, excessive, disorderly discharge of electrical impulses in the brain, which causes temporary alteration in the function of the CNS. Seizures may or may not result in unconsciousness. Also referred to as convulsions or fits, the causes of seizures include:

- Trauma to the brain.
- Tumours.
- Poisons.
- Drugs.
- High temperature.
- Hypoxia.
- Epilepsy.

Types of seizure

Relative to how much of the brain is involved, seizures are either focal or generalized. Focal seizures affect a specific, localized part of one of the lobes of the brain, whilst general seizures affect all lobes.

Seizures can start in any of the cerebral lobes. What happens during a seizure will vary, depending on which lobe, and in which part of the lobe, the seizure originates. People's symptoms will also be different.

The disordered electrical activity that causes a focal seizure can sometimes spread through the brain and develop into a generalized seizure. In this case, the focal seizure acts as a 'warning' which may be called an aura.

Auras are usually brief, lasting a few seconds, although some can last for much longer. An aura may manifest as an odd smell or taste or a visual or perceptual disturbance.

Once the epileptic activity spreads to both hemispheres of the brain, it rapidly becomes a generalized seizure, which is normally manifest as a tonic–clonic, tonic, or atonic seizure.

- *Tonic–clonic* seizures are those most commonly associated with epilepsy.
  - During the tonic phase, the person will lose consciousness and their body will go stiff.
  - During the clonic phase, the limbs will jerk and there may be urinary or faecal incontinence and clenching of the teeth or jaw. During the clonic phase, a person may stop breathing or have difficulty breathing and show cyanosis around the mouth.
- In *tonic* seizures, the person will lose consciousness and their body will go stiff, but this will not be followed by the twitching of the clonic phase.
- In *atonic* seizures, a person loses all muscle tone and drops heavily to the floor. These seizures are normally very brief and the person will often be able to get up again straightaway. However, people having atonic seizures are at risk for injury associated with the collapse.
- *Status epilepticus* occurs when a person has a seizure lasting longer than 30 minutes. This is a medical emergency requiring immediate treatment.

The recovery period following a seizure (known as the post-ictal phase) may be rapid or prolonged. During this period, a person may sleep or appear disoriented. They may also display odd or aggressive behaviour.

In the absence of any obvious underlying pathology, the causes of many seizures are unknown, but some triggers are:
- Not taking prescribed epilepsy medicine.
- Excessive tiredness.
- Stress.
- Alcohol.
- Drugs.
- Flashing, flickering, or stroboscopic lights.
- Menstruation.
- Hypoglycaemia.

(For more information on triggers, see ℘ www.epilepsy.org.uk/info/triggers).

Key nursing considerations in seizures
- Protect the person by clearing the immediate environment of hazardous objects which may cause injury.
- Protect their head with hands or soft padding.
- Do not move the person unless they are in immediate danger.
- Do not restrain the person or put anything in their mouth.
- Stay with the person to maintain their safety.
- Observe and accurately note the person's general condition.
- Measure and record the LOC according to local protocols.
- When possible, measure blood pressure, heart rate, oxygen saturation, temperature, respiratory rate, and LOC.
- Manage any investigations ordered as part of the local care protocol.
- Safely and accurately administer any prescribed IV fluids, and accurately record fluid balance.
- Safely and accurately administer and record any prescribed medications (including anti-epileptic drugs or oxygen therapy).
- Reassess and record vital signs as the clinical condition dictates.
- Accurately record all observations of the patient's condition.
- Ensure timely and accurate reporting of any observations, clinical measurements, or changes to the patient's condition.
- Clearly explain all actions and interventions to the person and any family or carers present.
- Seek to clearly and honestly allay patient and family anxieties.
- Maintain a safe and calming environment for recovery.
- Ensure physical comfort as far as is possible.

(See also ➲ Chapter 16, Neurological conditions.).

Respiratory emergencies

Respiratory diseases, or acute problems in other body systems, often result in a lack of oxygen reaching the tissues, which causes hypoxia. The body's first response to low oxygen levels is to increase the rate of respiration.

This means that a rapid respiratory rate (tachypnoea), shortness of breath, or other breathing difficulties are often the first clinical sign in a person whose condition is deteriorating.

Hyperventilation or tachypnoea is not always associated with respiratory disorders but may be a sign of respiratory compensation for a metabolic acidosis due to diabetes, sepsis, hepatic failure, or uraemia.

Causes of respiratory emergencies

- Asthma.
- COPD.
- Emphysema.
- PE.
- Hyperventilation.
- Hypoventilation.
- Status epilepticus.
- Allergic reaction.
- Obstruction by a foreign body (such as food, mucus, or dentures).
- Congestive cardiac failure.
- Anaemia.
- Anaemic heart failure.
- Pneumonia.
- Bronchitis.
- Epiglottitis.
- Rib fractures.
- Pneumothorax.
- Haemothorax.
- Contusion.
- Penetrating chest wall injury.
- Tetanus.

Symptoms associated with respiratory emergencies

- Tachypnoea.
- Breathlessness.
- Inability to speak in complete sentences.
- Dry or productive cough.
- Hoarse voice or noisy breathing (wheeze or stridor).
- Chest pain which is worse on inspiration.
- Temperature.
- Haemoptysis.
- Dizziness or fainting.
- Use of accessory muscles of respiration.
- Cyanosis, particularly around the skin and lips.
- Altered LOC.

Key nursing considerations in respiratory emergencies

In people with breathing difficulties, the physiological problems they are experiencing are likely to be compounded by a rising level of anxiety or panic at feeling they are unable to breathe. An important part of the care of these people is ensuring a safe and calming environment in which treatments can be carried out.

In addition to the nursing considerations outlined on ➲ p. 524 of this chapter, identifying the underlying cause of the respiratory emergency is central to effective nursing decision-making and practice.

- In the hospital environment, commence oxygen therapy for people with oxygen saturation level of <92% on room air.
- Ensure accurate and timely administration of any prescribed medications such as bronchodilators, adrenaline, antibiotics, steroids, diuretics, and analgesia.
- Calculate EWS and adjust care in accordance with local track and trigger escalation plans.
- Ensure timely and accurate reporting of any observations, clinical measurements, or changes to the patient's condition.

(See also ➲ Chapter 14, Respiratory conditions.)

Choking

Choking is an acute obstruction of the upper airways and can be a very frightening situation, both for the choking person and any observers. The universal sign of choking is when a person clutches their neck with one or both hands. The Resuscitation Council UK (℗ www.resus.org.uk) recommends that severity should first be assessed by determining how well the choking person is able to cough.

- With a mild obstruction, where the person still has an effective cough, they should be encouraged to cough to relieve the obstruction.
- With a more severe obstruction, where the person has an ineffective cough and is conscious, then five back blows, followed by five abdominal thrusts (Heimlich manoeuvre), are advised (see Figure 26.1).
- Where the obstruction is more severe, and the person is unconscious, then CPR should be commenced and urgent help sought.

(For details of specific clinical procedures, see ➲ *Oxford Handbook of Clinical Skills in Adult Nursing*.)

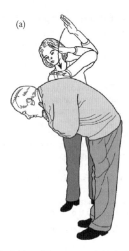

(a)

• If the back blows fail, carry out abdominal thrusts:

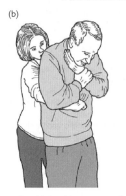

(b)

• Stand behind the patient and put both your arms around the upper part of the abdomen.

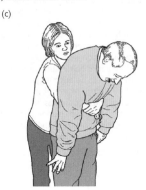

(c)

• Clench your fist and grasp it with your other hand.
• Pull sharply inwards and upwards with the aim of producing sudden expulsion of air, together with the foreign body, from the airway.

Figure 26.1 Back blow and abdominal thrusts.

Reproduced with kind permission from *Basic Adult Life Support Manual*, Chapter 10: Choking copyright (2015) Resuscitation Council UK.

Chest pain

Chest pain has multiple causes, which range from simple MSK pain to life-threatening MI and dissecting aortic aneurysm. Any person complaining of chest pain must be carefully assessed to establish the underlying cause.

With such a wide range of possible diagnoses, an accurate history is essential. This should include details of pain characteristics and the site, duration, and any known triggers of the pain. Some common causes of chest pain are:

Cardiac pain

- ACS is the umbrella term used to describe a range of conditions associated with disruption to the blood supply in the coronary arteries.
- Cardiac chest pain may be a result of STEMI, NSTEMI, angina, and UA.
- The pain associated with coronary conditions is typically described as a vice-like central chest pain which may radiate into the jaw and down one or both arms. It is usually associated with nausea and/or vomiting, shortness of breath, sweating, and pallor.

(See also ➜ Chapter 15, Cardiovascular conditions.)

Musculoskeletal chest pain

- Possible causes of MSK chest pain are muscle ligament strains, rib fracture, costochondritis, and local injury.
- MSK chest pain is typically described as a sharp, localized pain that is worsened by movement, coughing, and deep breathing.

Pleuritic pain

- Pleuritic pain may be caused by pleurisy, pneumothorax, and PE, and often has a sudden onset.
- The pain is normally located on the lateral aspect of the chest and may radiate to the shoulder or abdomen.
- Pleuritic pain is described as a sharp, localized 'stabbing' pain and is aggravated by movement, coughing, and deep breathing.

Gastrointestinal pain

- Chest pain associated with GI disorders is normally located in the lower substernal area where pain in the epigastric region spreads to the chest.
- It is typically described as a dull, aching pain and is often associated with meals. Causes include gastro-oesophageal reflux and gastritis.

Chest pain may also be associated with much rarer conditions such as:
- *Pericarditis*—where the inflammation of the pericardium causes a sharp, stabbing pain aggravated by deep breathing and lying flat.
- *Dissecting aortic aneurysm*—where internal bleeding causes a tearing pain in the anterior chest wall, radiating to the back and abdomen.
- *Skin conditions*—such as herpes zoster.
- *Sickle-cell disease*.
- *Pancreatitis*.

Key nursing considerations in chest pain

For people complaining of chest pain, the priority is that a rapid diagnosis is made, so that appropriate, and possibly lifesaving, treatment can be commenced. This may be medication, thrombolytic therapy, angioplasty, or emergency surgery (🕮 www.nice.org.uk).

Where healthcare organizations have local policies, protocols, or guidelines for dealing with people with chest pain, these should always be followed.

(For details of specific clinical procedures, see ➲ *Oxford Handbook of Clinical Skills in Adult Nursing*.)

Syncope

Syncope, or fainting, is a sudden temporary loss of consciousness, which is the result of a reduction of blood flow to the brain. Fainting is often preceded by a feeling of dizziness, nausea, light-headedness, and feeling hot, and there is usually a rapid recovery.

The person falls suddenly and appears very pale, cold, and clammy, with a slow pulse. Recovery is normally rapid. The lack of jerking movements, incontinence, or tongue biting differentiates syncope from a seizure.

Fainting is common in people who have been standing for long periods of time, which can result in pooling of blood and fluid in the legs, reduction of circulating blood volume, and decreased perfusion of the brain. Sudden collapse without any warning signs may also be the result of a cardiac arrhythmia. Common causes of collapse in adults include:

- Syncope due to a vasovagal episode.
- Cardiac arrhythmia.
- Epilepsy.
- Postural hypotension.
- Hypoglycaemia.
- Trauma.
- Witnessing or hearing an adverse event.
- Severe anxiety or phobia.
- Adverse drug reactions.

Key nursing considerations in syncope

In addition to the key nursing considerations outlined on ➔ p. 524 of this chapter, identifying the underlying cause of syncope is central to effective nursing decision-making and practice.

- Assess the person, using the ABCDE(F) approach.
- Call for help if cardiac collapse or seizure is suspected.
- Observe and accurately note the person's condition.
- Observe for signs of injury as a result of the collapse.
- Manage any investigations ordered as part of local care protocol.
- Ensure timely and accurate reporting of any observations, clinical measurements, or changes to the patient's condition.

(For details of specific clinical procedures, see ➔ *Oxford Handbook of Clinical Skills in Adult Nursing*.)

Poisoning

Poisoning may be accidental or the result of deliberate self-harm. Unintentional overdoses are common, particularly in elderly people with multiple co-morbidities and associated polypharmacy.

IV drug users are also at risk for accidental overdose, especially if they are unaware of the purity of the drugs they are using. Some people working with industrial chemicals may be at risk of poisoning if accidental exposure occurs.

Whether the act of poisoning is intentional or accidental, the initial treatment is the same. People who have deliberately harmed themselves may not always provide a clear and accurate history, and it may be necessary to gather information about the poisoning from family and friends.

Types of poisoning

- *Ingestion*—accidental or deliberate swallowing of poisons such as overdose of prescription medicines, recreational drugs, or noxious substances.
- *Injection*—accidental or deliberate injection of an overdose of prescription medicines or recreational drugs.
- *Inhalation*—accidental or deliberate inhalation of noxious gases, such as carbon monoxide, or recreational drug use.
- *Transdermal*—absorption of chemicals through the skin.

The National Poisons Information Service

All UK NHS organizations have online access to the National Poisons Information Service database (TOXBASE), and where a person is admitted to hospital with known or suspected poisoning, the database should be accessed.

Substance-specific monitoring and treatment advice will be provided by the poisons information service, and this may include:

- Giving activated charcoal for some ingested poisons, if within an hour of poisoning.
- Continuous monitoring of the patient, including cardiac monitoring and pulse oximetry.
- 12-lead ECG.
- ABG analysis.
- Blood glucose measurement
- IV access and blood tests, including FBC, U&Es, creatinine kinase, and specific serum drug levels such as paracetamol, digoxin, or theophylline.
- Administration of recommended antidote treatments such as acetylcysteine in the case of paracetamol overdose.

Key nursing considerations in poisoning

In addition to the key nursing considerations outlined on ➲ p. 524 of this chapter, all people with known or suspected poisoning should be assessed using the ABCDE(F) approach.

- Attempt to get a full history, particularly the name of the drugs or poisons ingested or exposed to, and the time of the poisoning.
- Access TOXBASE® for guidance on appropriate interventions.
- Overdose and poisoning is a time of high anxiety for most people, and for those who have intentionally harmed themselves, this is often at a crisis point. Special attention should be paid to allaying patient and family anxieties.
- All people who have taken an intentional overdose, or attempted deliberate self-harm with another type of poison, should be offered a referral to mental health services.

(For details of specific clinical procedures, see ➲ *Oxford Handbook of Clinical Skills in Adult Nursing*.)

Musculoskeletal injuries

Common injuries which present as clinical emergencies are those involving the muscle, tendon, ligament, bone, and surrounding soft tissues.

Trauma associated with MSK injuries often occurs in road traffic accidents, sports, and falls. As a clinical emergency, MSK injuries are most often given first-line treatment and care in the emergency department, which may be followed by surgical repair. MSK injuries are described according to the structures damaged:

- Fractures are breaks in the cortex of a bone.
- Dislocations are disruption to the integrity of a joint.
- Sprains are injuries to ligaments.
- Strains are injuries to muscles and tendons.
- Contusions and bruises are injuries to muscles and surrounding soft tissues.

Outside of the hospital environment, a person with a MSK injury should not be moved until the nature and extent of their injury has been assessed by a competent practitioner. (See also ➋ Chapter 20, Musculoskeletal conditions.)

Key nursing considerations in musculoskeletal emergencies

Outside the hospital environment

- Assess the person, using the ABCDE(F) approach.
- Call for assistance and emergency services.
- Observe and accurately note the person's condition.
- If the person is conscious, obtain an account of their accident.
- Seek information from any witnesses.
- Establish the site and intensity of any pain.
- Observe for deformity and discoloration, and assess the rate of capillary refill (this should be <2 seconds, and prolonged capillary refill suggests impaired circulation).
- Check for wounds and determine if the injury is open or closed.
- Apply a dressing to any wounds (if available), and attempt to apply direct pressure in order to control bleeding.
- Observe and palpate the area for abnormal movement.
- Check pulses distal to the injury, skin temperature, and sensation.
- Immobilize the painful area to prevent further damage to surrounding soft tissue and reduce pain.
- Apply ice, if available, to assist in the control of swelling.
- Elevate the injured area if appropriate.
- Clearly and accurately report all observations, and actions taken, to paramedics or other emergency services.
- On rare occasions, MSK injuries involve amputation of a body part. If the amputated part is recovered, it should be kept clean and covered, and submerged in ice-water if available. Ice should not be applied directly to the amputated part.
- Another rare, but potentially limb threatening, complication in MSK injuries is compartment syndrome. This is where there is bleeding into muscles enclosed by the fascia, which impedes circulation, causing irreversible muscle and nerve damage. Signs of compartment syndrome are pain, pallor, pulselessness, paraesthesiae, and paralysis.

In a hospital or other clinical environment

Hospital and other healthcare organizations will have local policies, protocols, or guidelines for dealing with MSK injuries, and these should always be followed.

It may be necessary to prepare the person for emergency surgery. (See also ➲ Chapter 22, Surgery and ➲ Chapter 20, Musculoskeletal conditions.)

Burns

A burn is damage to the skin by a source of heat or high energy such as fire, electricity, radiation, or chemicals. Burns can vary in severity and are classified according to the depth of the skin damaged and the amount of total body surface area involved. Types of burns include:

- Moist burns, or scald, due to steam or hot liquid.
- Dry burn due to flames or friction.
- Electrical burn from high-voltage current or lightning strike.
- Cold injuries such as frostbite, or those from liquid gases such as liquid oxygen.
- Chemical burns from a variety of compounds.
- Radiation burns from the sun, ultraviolet, or radioactive sources.

All burns with a surface area greater than the person's hand, or which are white, charred, or blistered, and involve the hands, arms, feet, legs, or genitals, need to be assessed and treated by specialist clinicians. Burns across joints also need specialist assessment and treatment, as do electrical and chemical burns.

People with large and serious burns, of any cause, will normally be treated in specialist burns or intensive care units.

First-aid treatment for burns

- For *dry, moist radiation and electrical burns*, if possible, cool the affected body part with running tap water for 10 minutes.
- In cases where the area of the burn is >5% of the body surface area, cooling techniques may result in hypothermia so should not be used.
- Never apply ice, creams, or greasy substances to a burn, as they can exacerbate skin damage.
- After cooling, apply a covering of clear cellophane wrap as a temporary dressing.
- In case of *fire burns*, if it is safe to do so, attempt to stop the burning process and remove the person from the source of the fire.
- If possible, burnt clothing and any jewellery should be carefully removed (unless it is stuck to the person).
- For burns sustained as the result of a fire, the person should also be assessed for smoke inhalation injuries. Inhalation injuries would be suspected if the person had facial burns, soot around the face, mouth, or nose, or singed hair, difficulty in breathing, sore throat, a hoarse voice, or coughing.
- Smoke inhalation should be treated urgently, as burnt airways can become swollen and obstructed very quickly.
- *Chemical burns* need special consideration as, in some instances, irrigation with water increases the damage. All manufacturers of chemical substances are required by law to provide advice on how to proceed if accidental exposure occurs. Treatment of chemical burns should always be carried out in accordance with manufacturers' advice.

- If a burn is >15% of the body surface area, then IV fluid replacement will be required.
- People with burns may also need oxygen therapy and analgesia, which can be provided by paramedics or emergency services and hospital emergency departments.
- Always observe and assess the person's general condition and the circumstances of the burn, so that concise and accurate information can be passed to emergency services if necessary.

(For details of specific clinical procedures, see ➲ *Oxford Handbook of Clinical Skills in Adult Nursing*.)

Temperature-related emergencies

Temperature-related emergencies are a result of extremes of both heat (hyperthermia) and cold (hypothermia). People most at risk of temperature-related emergencies are those who are very old or very young, people under the influence of alcohol, and those who are obese, homeless, or participating in extreme sports.

Heat stroke

Heat stroke is a serious, and potentially life-threatening, medical emergency. Although it most often occurs in tropical and sub-tropical regions, it can occur anywhere.

Heat stroke occurs when the body's temperature-regulating mechanisms fail and the person is unable to sweat. The body temperature rises rapidly, and the signs of heat stroke are:
- Red, hot, and dry skin.
- No sweating.
- High temperature >40°C.
- Abnormal breathing.
- Headache.
- Dizziness, nausea, and vomiting.
- Confusion.
- Unconsciousness.

Where someone is displaying signs of heat stroke, if it is safe to do so, they should be removed from direct sunlight or the heat source.

If possible, remove clothing and immerse in, or spray, the affected person with cool water or wrap in a wet sheet. Encourage them to drink cool fluids, avoiding alcohol.

Observe and record vital signs and LOC, and call emergency services. A person with heat stroke is likely to need assessment and treatment in hospital.

Heat exhaustion

Heat exhaustion is caused by dehydration, usually after prolonged exposure to high temperatures, with inadequate fluid replacement. Heat exhaustion is not normally as serious as heat stroke, and symptoms include:
- Facial pallor.
- Moist and sweaty skin.
- Feeling tired, lethargic, and weak.
- Headache.
- Nausea or vomiting.
- Weak rapid pulse.
- Fainting,

Where someone is displaying signs of heat exhaustion, if it is safe to do so, they should be removed to a cool place and encouraged to slowly rehydrate with cool, non-alcoholic drinks.

Heat cramps

Heat cramps are muscle pains or spasms of the legs, arms, or abdomen, most often affecting athletes. Heavy sweating during strenuous activity depletes body fluid and salts, resulting in muscular spasm.

If someone is displaying signs of heat cramp, they should stop the physical activity and rest in a cool place, drinking clear cool fluids or hypotonic sports drinks.

It is advisable to wait until several hours after the muscular spasms have subsided before engaging in further sports or physical activity.

If symptoms persist for >60 minutes, medical advice should be sought.

Hypothermia

Hypothermia is when the core body temperature falls below 35°C. It can very quickly become life-threatening and should be treated as a clinical emergency.

It is usually caused by a low ambient temperature, compounded by social and environmental conditions. Hypothermia may also be caused by accidents, prolonged immersion in cold water, and overexposure to winter weather conditions.

People at risk include those who are homeless or live in inadequate housing, people who are very old or with long-term health conditions, people with limited mobility, and those working outside. People who participate in extreme winter sports are also at risk.

Signs of hypothermia include:
- Uncontrolled shivering.
- Increased respiratory rate.
- Tiredness and lethargy.
- Cold and pale skin.
- Confusion and delirium.
- Unconsciousness.

If someone is displaying signs of hypothermia, if it is possible to do so, they should be moved into a warm environment or shelter to prevent further heat loss.
- It is important that the person is not rewarmed too quickly, as this can cause vasodilation, leading to hypovolaemic shock.
- Any wet clothing should be removed and replaced with dry clothing, blankets, towels, or coats.
- If possible, encourage the person to have warm drinks, avoiding alcohol as it dilates superficial blood vessels, risking further cooling and heat loss.
- If the person's condition deteriorates in any way or they are unconscious, emergency services should be called, as urgent medical intervention will be needed to restore body temperature.

Frostbite

Frostbite is damage to tissues caused by exposure to freezing temperatures. This occurs most often in the body's extremities, involving the fingers, toes, nose, ears, and lips.

Due to the numbing effect of extreme cold, a person with frostbite is often unaware that tissue damage is occurring. As the body warms, the affected body part becomes painful and they may have a sensation of prolonged 'pins and needles'.

Frostbite carries a risk for gangrene and often requires surgical debridement, and sometimes amputation.

• If someone is displaying signs of frostbite, they should be removed from the cold and kept warm.
• If there is no risk of further exposure to freezing temperatures, the affected area should be re-warmed in water at between 40 and 41°C. This is often very painful and will normally require large amounts of analgesia.
• As soon as is possible, medical assessment and advice should be sought.

Temperature related emergencies are often associated with high degrees of anxiety and pain, and until pre-hospital or expert help arrives, nurses should seek to allay anxiety, maintain a safe and calm environment, and, as far as possible, ensure physical comfort.

Recreational drug use

Recreational drug use is the intentional use of any psychoactive substance to alter the state of consciousness and promote feelings of euphoria, confidence, and energy.

The lifestyle often associated with regular recreational drug use, the mode of ingestion, and the substances themselves can lead to both physical and mental ill health.

In the UK, the production, supply, or use of most drugs used for nonmedicinal recreational purposes is illegal. The production, supply, and use of alcohol is legal.

Common recreational drugs

- Alcohol.
- Cannabis (weed, grass, hash, dope, pot, skunk, kush, green).
- Cocaine (charlie, crack, coke, white).
- Heroin (smack, H, brown, gear).
- Amphetamines (speed, whizz, dexies, meth).
- Ecstasy (E, MDMA, pills, mandy, or dolphins).
- Ketamine (K, Ket, vitamin K, super K, special K).
- Mephedrone (meow meow, M-smack, M-cat, drone, or bubble).
- Volatile substances (glue, paint thinners, petrol, hair spray, nail polish remover).

Some physical consequences of recreational drug use

- Liver disease.
- GI haemorrhage.
- Cardiovascular effects such as tachycardia, hypertension, MI, and stroke.
- Endocarditis.
- Barotrauma to the lungs.
- Chemical burns around the nose and mouth.
- Injury to the nasal septum.
- Increased risk of infection with IV drug use such as HIV, hepatitis, and sepsis.
- Bladder damage associated with the use of ketamine.
- Dizziness and headache.
- Psychological disturbances.
- Hallucinations.
- Paranoia.

Key nursing considerations

A person presenting to health services as a clinical emergency, who is suffering from the effects of recreational drug use, may present with cardiac, respiratory, or neurological symptoms. They may be in a state of collapse or altered LOC, and the priority is to first treat any life-threatening physical symptoms.

- People identified as having a drug-related health problem may need to be referred to the local safeguarding team, particularly if there are children involved in the family of a habitual drug user.
- Follow local procedures for notification of any criminal activity.

People threatening or attempting suicide

Suicide is the leading cause of death amongst adult males aged between 20 and 49 years of age in the UK (www.ons.gov.uk). Men, women, children, and elderly people are all vulnerable to suicidal thoughts, but people most at risk may have a history of:

- Severe depression.
- Schizophrenia.
- Bipolar disorder.
- Bereavement.
- Psychological trauma.
- Profound loss of self-esteem.
- Prolonged physical illness.
- Emotional or psychosocial problems.
- Alcohol or drug dependency.

Although suicide or attempted suicide cannot be confidently predicted, in people at risk, it may be the case that ordinary tasks become increasingly difficult, attention span decreases, and fatigue or lethargy increases.

People may develop obsessional behaviours or withdraw from social activities and relationships. They may complain of real or imagined physical illness, or suffer from chronic insomnia or early morning wakening.

Key nursing considerations

If a person is known to be a high suicide risk, they should not be left alone. All reasonable attempts to prevent self-harm and preserve life should be made.

- In the community setting, the police and ambulance service should be alerted if a person is in imminent danger.
- If a person threatening suicide is a hospital inpatient, local policies should be followed, which may include calling the police for further assistance.
- An inpatient threatening or attempting suicide will need to be urgently assessed by the mental health team and may need to be retained in hospital under a section of the Mental Health Act.
- Attempt to prevent the patient from harming themselves.
- If necessary, and without posing danger to oneself, intervene to preserve the patient's life.
- Remove any possible means of self-harm from the patient's immediate environment.
- Demonstrate understanding
- Be willing to listen.
- Remain accepting and non-judgmental.
- Establish rapport, wherever possible
- If appropriate, involve close family and friends.

(See also ➔ *Oxford Handbook of Mental Health Nursing*, second edition.)

People demonstrating psychotic behaviours

Psychotic behaviour is a symptom of an underlying illness, rather than a diagnosis, and it manifests uniquely in each person.

The two main presenting symptoms are delusions and hallucinations. Delusions refer to an unwavering belief in something that is obviously bizarre or untrue, whilst hallucinations occur when a sight, sound, smell, or touch is perceived but is not real.

Whilst psychotic behaviour is often related to mental illnesses, this is not always the case. Medical conditions such as HIV, Parkinson's disease, MS, and brain tumours can also cause psychotic behaviour, as can misuse of drugs and alcohol.

People with psychotic behaviour can pose a risk to themselves and others; therefore, a full physical and mental health assessment should be undertaken to allow the appropriate treatment to be offered.

This assessment may need to be made in an acute psychiatric unit, in which case the person will be referred to mental health services. Admission to a psychiatric facility can be made under a section of the Mental Health Act, if the person is deemed to be a danger to themselves or others.

Symptoms of psychotic behaviour may include:
- Sensory hallucinations.
- Hearing voices no one else can hear.
- Suspicion/paranoia.
- Grandiose behaviour with delusions.
- Chaotic behaviour.
- Confusion.
- Vagueness.
- Gaps in memory.
- Withdrawal.
- Aggression and/or violence.

Key nursing considerations

People displaying symptoms of psychotic behaviour will need to be fully assessed by a mental health team.
- As far as is possible, maintain a calm and safe environment.
- Remove any items or equipment that could potentially harm people.
- Use clear and direct language.
- Show receptiveness and a desire to help.
- Do not agree or disagree with the person's delusions.
- Seek cooperation for any investigations, treatments, or medicines ordered.
- Accurately record all observations of the patient's behaviour.
- Ensure timely and accurate reporting of any observations, measurements, or changes to the person's condition.
- Clearly explain all actions or interventions to the person and any family or carers present.

(See also ➔ *Oxford Handbook of Mental Health Nursing*, second edition.)

Domestic violence and sexual assault

Sexual assault and domestic violence are both criminal acts that can result in physical, emotional, or mental harm, and in extreme cases, death.

Domestic violence is often a pattern of controlling, threatening, or violent behaviours by one family member against another, which may include physical, psychological, or sexual violence.

Both women and men can be the victims of domestic violence and sexual assault. Neglect or ill treatment of elderly people is also recognized as criminal abuse. (See ➋ Chapter 9, Communicating concerns in healthcare.)

Domestic violence

Domestic violence is classified as any incident of threatening behaviour, violence, or abuse between adults who are, or have been, in a relationship together, or between family members regardless of gender or sexuality. Abusive behaviour may include:

- Coercion.
- Emotional or psychological abuse.
- Physical abuse, including neglect.
- Financial abuse.
- Sexual abuse.
- Stalking and harassment.

Sexual assault

A sexual assault is any sexual act conducted without active consent or with the use of force against someone's will. It includes rape, groping, forced kissing, or torture in a sexual manner. Most sexual crimes reported in the media involve unknown assailants, but the majority of sexual assaults are committed by a person known to the victim.

Key nursing considerations

If a person presents to health services with injuries associated with domestic violence or sexual abuse, local protocols for physical assessment and treatment of any injuries should be carried out. In addition, local safeguarding guidance must be followed.

- Safeguarding procedures may include completing a risk identification tool, with the person's consent.
- People identified as high risk should have the opportunity to have their case managed by the local multi-agency risk assessment team.
- With the person's consent, the local police service may be informed of any victims of domestic violence or sexual assault.
- It may be necessary to collect tissues or other materials which may be used as evidence in any future prosecution.
- Accurate contemporaneous notes should be made, as they may be required in any future criminal proceedings.
- Seek to allay the person's anxieties.
- Clearly explain all actions and interventions, and give accurate explanations of other likely events and investigations.
- Maintain a safe and calming environment.
- As far as is possible, ensure physical comfort.
- Provide support and engage family or friends, if appropriate.

Useful sources of further information
- NHS Getting help for domestic violence ℘ www.nhs.uk/Livewell/ abuse/Pages/domestic-violence-help.aspx
- NHS Help after rape and sexual assault ℘ www.nhs.uk/Livewell/ Sexualhealth/Pages/Sexualassault.aspx

Unexpected childbirth

Unrecognized pregnancy, whilst rare, does happen. The pregnant woman may continue to bleed monthly and carry the fetus in such a way that she shows no outward signs of pregnancy. Some women who are pregnant may be of an age to think they are experiencing the menopause.

Other women, especially those who are very young, may recognize their pregnancy but conceal it from family and friends, due to fear or denial. A lack of prenatal care increases the risk of unexpected childbirth. Other causes include:

- Inaccurate calculation of expected date of delivery.
- Premature birth.
- Rapid progress of labour.
- Involvement in an accident that stimulates the onset of labour.

Labour

- The first stage of labour is where the uterus begins regular contractions and the baby positions itself for birth. The first stage may also see the expulsion of a small 'plug' of blood and mucus, with or without the expulsion of amniotic fluid (known colloquially as the 'waters').
- The second stage is where the baby is born, and onset of the second stage will normally be indicated by the woman experiencing a strong urge to 'push'.
- The third stage is where the placenta detaches itself from the uterine wall and is expelled. During this stage, the woman is at risk of postpartum haemorrhage, which can be a life-threatening condition.

Key nursing considerations

In a situation where a woman needs help delivering a child, nurses who are not trained midwives should prioritize seeking help from a qualified midwife or the emergency services.

Until assistance arrives, the general nurse can offer comfort and support and help the woman with small practical preparations for the delivery.

In the first stage of labour, this may include helping the woman undress or change clothes, helping her position herself or to walk around, offering small physical comforts such as rubbing the small of her back, and contacting any partners, friends, or relatives she wants with her.

If there is a delay in suitably experienced help arriving, and the woman is entering the second stage of labour, then general nurses should take direction on the telephone from the emergency services.

These directions will offer guidance about what to do in relation to key aspects of childbirth, to ensure the safety of mother and baby.

- What to do when the baby's head emerges.
- Checking the umbilical cord is not wrapped around the baby's neck, and how to remove it if necessary.
- How to handle the baby and remove any mucus from the upper airway.
- What to do if the baby is not breathing.
- Wrapping the baby to maintain body temperature.
- Keeping the placenta and umbilical cord intact (there is no urgency to cut the cord, and this should be done by a suitably qualified person).
- What to do with the cord and placenta if they are delivered naturally.
- What to do if the placenta is not delivered.

(See ➔ *Oxford Handbook of Midwifery*.)

Part 4

Nursing leadership, teamwork, and collectives

Leadership

Defining leadership

There is an ongoing professional debate about the nature of effective nursing leadership. It is important that general adult nurses have an understanding of definitions and key principles of leadership, and the leadership skills and attributes which are relevant to nursing care delivery. Exploring these issues will support nurses in reflecting on their role and responsibilities, examining how, as a leader of care, they can enhance nursing practice and improve patient experience.

Leadership knowledge and skills are fundamental to safe, effective nursing care. It is widely recognized that an absence of leadership can result in distress for patients and families, 'never events', serious incidents, harm to patients and the public, and even death.

In the past, there have been official inquiries into failings of some UK healthcare organizations and services which have found absent or poor leadership responsible. The impact of failures in care provision on patients, the public, and the nursing profession is demoralizing for all concerned, and in an attempt to address this, the UK has an NHS Constitution, which explicitly states the expectations and rights of all people receiving healthcare (℅ www.england.nhs.uk).

Delivery of the standards of healthcare outlined within the NHS Constitution in based on an expectation that nurses adopt a leadership role at every point of contact with people. The constitution also places patients and shared values at the centre of all healthcare, and this position is reinforced by the NMC Code (℅ www.nmc.org.uk). The professional code envisages nurses as models of integrity and leadership.

The need for nurses to develop leadership knowledge and skills is widely acknowledged, and yet there is no clear definition or common understanding of nurse leadership. This puts nurses in the difficult position of being expected to adopt leadership roles and responsibility, but with no real clarity about which skills and attributes they are to employ.

The lack of professional consensus mirrors the wider leadership debate outside the nursing profession, in which the different theories and definitions are dependent on very different philosophical approaches and world views. Theories of leadership vary from traditional 'heroic' or 'great man' leadership styles through to relationship-based models.

Given the nature of nursing work in all environments and the importance of respectful and empathic communication skills in nursing practice, the relationship-based models of leadership are the ones likely to have most resonance for the nursing profession.

However, nurses have traditionally worked in a hierarchical culture, with decision-making seen to be the responsibility of those who hold the most status, professional authority, and organizational power. If, as part of the UK NHS Constitution, nurses are to demonstrate leadership at every point of contact with people, then this hierarchical culture in nursing will have to be challenged.

Recognition of these issues has facilitated the emergence of ideas and definitions of leadership which identify the specific nature and responsibilities of clinical leaders working within a healthcare environment. These important relationship-based processes and characteristics have been variously described as:

- Developing a culture of caring.
- Continually improving quality of care.
- Continually enhancing safety.
- Flexibility.
- Vision.
- Adaptability.
- Thinking differently.
- Open-mindedness.
- Challenging orthodoxies.
- Taking risks to lead and manage change.

Leadership and management

Within any organization, of whatever size or structure, both leaders and managers are likely to be found. However, whilst people working in managerial positions may demonstrate leadership qualities, management is a very different function to that of leadership. The concepts should not be considered as interchangeable.

> Relationship-based *leadership* focuses on the needs and development of individuals.
> *Management* focuses on controlling and monitoring the systems and structures necessary to deliver organizational goals.

Within the context of healthcare, recognition of the different, yet co-dependent, functions of managers and leaders becomes increasingly important, as healthcare becomes more complex.

The complexity of healthcare provision, with multiple health providers working towards externally determined targets and measures, requires healthcare providers to ensure there are clear systems and structures to deliver care services within the allocated resources. As a result, effective organizational structures, managerial processes, and competent managers are essential. Healthcare is provided by and for people, and therefore effective leadership for care delivery is also essential.

Nurse leaders have a role in promoting professional values and demonstrating them through their actions, for which they are accountable. They must also seek to inspire others to work to these same values and principles. Therefore, understanding and working in the domains of both management and leadership practice are key skills for nurses.

Transactional and transformational leadership

The effects of neo-liberal health and social policy, technological and pharmacological developments, and new understandings of diseases and treatments, alongside a population who have unprecedented access to sources of information about health and illness, mean that healthcare provision is in a constant state of change.

The impact of a leader's values and behaviours is recognized as a key factor in shaping care provision and, in the context of these wider political and cultural factors, means there is a need for nurse leaders to support the evolution and transformation of nursing practices. The concurrent need to deliver healthcare in line with national healthcare strategy, normally within fixed resources, also means there is a place for clinical leadership which can affect the best patient outcomes through negotiation and transaction.

These approaches to understanding leadership are described as transactional and transformational, and both have relevance for contemporary healthcare.

Transactional leadership

Transactional leadership approaches are predominantly based on traditional power relations where the leader supports practice through:
- Setting clear goals.
- Clarifying desired outcomes.
- Providing or withdrawing rewards.
- Exchanging rewards or compliments.
- Imposing sanctions.

The transactional leadership approach assumes that the followers of a leader will adopt rational decision-making when they engage in changing care behaviours and practices. It also assumes that followers accept the leader's vision and respond to rewards and sanctions.

The transactional leadership approach can be seen to clearly align with management practices which focus on systems and processes to deliver organizational goals. However, in challenging times, it is sometimes necessary for nurse leaders to adopt transactional leadership approaches in order to ensure continued safety for patients, staff, and the public.

Transformational leadership

Transformational leadership recognizes that leaders who adopt an interpersonal relational approach can gain genuine support for changes in care behaviours and practices. The core characteristics of a transformational leader are identified as the ability to:
- Evaluate the potential of team members.
- Broaden and elevate team members' personal goals.
- Develop confidence in people to perform beyond expectations.
- Inspire.
- Motivate.
- Stimulate team members to think differently about change.
- Recognize and acknowledge individual contributions.
- Recognize and acknowledge individual strengths and limitations.

Transformational leadership approaches, which can accommodate and build on constant change, are now recognized as the approach to leadership which is best suited to healthcare. Transformational leadership is applicable to nursing practice, both at team and organizational levels, and is consistent with nursing's core professional values and beliefs.

Values-based leadership

The need for effective leadership to be based on a shared set of values is well established, and for the nursing profession, this means that nurse leaders need to have clear vision and strong values, which can inspire and motivate others.

Within the values-based leadership paradigm, the successful leader should be guided by four key principles.

Self-reflection

This refers to the understanding of the self as a practitioner and a leader, having an awareness of core values and the means to reach personal potential.

Balance and perspective

Describes the process by which the leader is open to other perspectives, actively seeking out opinions that differ from their own to gain a greater understanding.

Self-confidence

This refers to a leader's understanding of their own knowledge base, including their strengths and limitations. This does not require a leader to be knowledgeable in all areas, but rather to build a team with complementary knowledge and skills.

The confidence and ability to develop a team with strengths that complement those of the leader supports a transformational approach. This facilitates teamworking to shared values, recognizing ability, and valuing individual contributions.

Humility

This requires a leader to reflect on their own professional trajectory, especially their starting position, and the path they have followed. In demonstrating humility, the values-based leader does not adopt a hierarchical approach but treats all individual team members with respect, equality, fairness, and honesty.

The principles outlined in the values-based leadership theory align closely with core nursing values and, as such, offer a framework through which nurses can develop their knowledge and skills.

NHS England (℠ www.england.nhs.uk) has established a framework for developing nurse leaders which acknowledges the importance of compassion in relation to patients, colleagues, and oneself. This provides a useful framework for nurse leadership actions which can support the delivery of high-quality care. (See also ➔ Chapter 1, Professional nursing values.)

Leadership skills and attributes

Whilst there is no universal consensus on the core skills and attributes that define a nurse leader, there is a recognition that these include:

• Integrity.
• Communication.
• Problem-solving.

These reflect the core nursing competencies of professional values, communication, and decision-making which are central to all nursing practice. So in effecting a leadership role, nurses need to utilize these core skills and attributes beyond the sphere of direct patient care and apply them to the wider organization of care within the clinical environment. The application of leadership skills and attributes can be supported by the development of personal and professional confidence.

Professional insight requires both the ability to consider one's own behaviour and an ability to critically reflect on both practice experience and formal learning. Critical reflection can also support a nurse's personal growth as a clinical leader.

Emotional intelligence

It is widely understood that effective clinical leaders have emotional intelligence. Emotional intelligence has been described as a subset of social skills that involves the ability to monitor and discriminate the feelings and emotions of the self and others.

In the language of nursing, emotional intelligence can be recognized as empathy and compassion, which influences nurse decision-making and practices. The insights and understandings central to emotional intelligence have been described as personal values and beliefs, goals, intentions, emotional responses, and behaviours.

Emotional intelligence also recognizes the feelings, behaviours, and goals of others and is able to discriminate between those of the self.

These attributes have been summarized as the four key components of emotional intelligence:

• *Self-awareness*—the recognition of one's own values and behaviours and the confidence to behave in an appropriate way.
• *Social awareness*—sensitivity to the impact of one's actions and responses to people in the wider social and environmental context.
• *Self-management*—self-regulation to harness and control actions, adaptability, trust worthiness, initiative, and drive.
• *Social skills*—active engagement with people to build relationships, bonds, and connections and to influence people.

Understanding personal strengths and areas for development as an emotionally intelligent leader is central to the development of nurse leadership roles.

The emotional labour of nursing

Whilst emotional intelligence is recognized as an important leadership quality, it is also known that managing personal reactions and emotions in the context of providing a compassionate care service can be incredibly stressful for nursing staff.

Nursing is an intense medium for emotional labour. Aspects of nurses' work often place individual practitioners and teams in circumstances of highly charged emotions—the expectation being that nurses remain in control of their own emotions, whilst empathizing and providing skilled intervention and support.

Emotionally demanding work necessitates that nurses are thoroughly supported and have opportunities to debrief stressful encounters. Hence the need for effective clinical leadership and strong, supportive teamworking.

Not being able to fully care for patients, perhaps because of lack of resources, can be equally stressful as it undermines fundamental caring values and human relational communication. This can create disturbing dissonance between an ideal, preferred professional nursing identity and the actuality of feeling that one may be complicit in compromised care standards.

A relative lack of control over how nursing work is organized can be acutely alienating, so strong clinical leadership is needed to achieve high standards of care within supportive teams.

Followership

It has long been recognized that leaders cannot function without the commitment, support, and willingness to work towards a shared vision by followers.

One of the most significant aspects of effective leadership is the ability to inspire and motivate others. The relationship between the follower and the leader is important in all leadership practice.

The collective action of a significant number of individuals has the greatest impact when leaders are able to develop a wider collective vision in which all followers can share and participate.

The UK King's Fund health think tank (www.kingsfund.org.uk) describes the role of the follower as fundamental to enabling effective delivery of healthcare. They describe different types of followers as being:

• *Compliant*: those who comply with the leader's decisions.
• *Technical*: those who rigidly adhere to established procedures and processes.
• *Responsible*: those who share collective decision-making and responsibility.
• *Mutineers*: those who rebel against the leader.
• *Chronic*: those who work to rule
• *Refuseniks*: those who do not participate or accept collective responsibility.

As followers or members of care teams, there is an obligation to work collectively to enable care to be delivered to a high standard, through respectful engagement with those people in receipt of care (see also ➲ Chapter 28, Teamwork).

The UK NHS Leadership Academy

The recognition that leadership is fundamental to healthcare has necessitated a focus on the development of knowledge and skills to support practitioners in becoming effective care leaders.

The UK NHS Leadership Academy (🏠 www.leadershipacademy.nhs.uk) works to promote better leadership, in order to provide better care, experience, and outcomes for people and clinical staff in their day-to-day work.

The model comprises nine domains, which are identified as:
- Inspiring shared purpose.
- Leading with care.
- Evaluating information.
- Connecting our service.
- Sharing the vision.
- Engaging the team.
- Holding to account.
- Developing capability.
- Influencing for results.

This interactive model facilitates self-assessment against each of the domains and allows nurses to establish their own leadership development plan. Self-assessment can be made at any point in professional experience or development. An examination of leadership within the context of different practice contexts can be useful for nurses working at all levels and in all clinical environments.

Establishment of the Leadership Academy self-assessment tool and recognition of the centrality of leadership for practice have led to a clear professional development route for all nurses. Leadership programmes can now be accessed through higher education institutions and the Leadership Academy.

Whilst not all nurses will become leaders within an organizational structure or hierarchy, through their professional values, clinical knowledge, and communication skills, all nurses have the capacity to lead values-based, well-informed, and respectful nursing practice.

Useful sources of further information

There is a large body of literature concerned with nursing management and leadership, and for those interested in exploring the topic further, a useful starting point is the *Journal of Nursing Management*. Other useful sources include:

- Followership ℘ www.kingsfund.org.uk/publications/articles/followership-nhs
- The King's Fund ℘ www.kingsfund.org.uk
- NHS Constitution ℘ www.england.nhs.uk/2013/03/nhs-constitution/
- NHS England ℘ www.england.nhs.uk
- NHS Leadership Academy ℘ www.leadershipacademy.nhs.uk
- Eisler R, Potter T. Breaking down the hierarchies. *Nurs Manag (Harrow)*. 2014;**21**:12

Teamwork

Teamwork

The importance of teamworking has been long established in healthcare, with nurses working both as part of a nursing team and as members of the wider MDT. Effective organization and delivery of healthcare services depend upon a wide range of health professionals, patients, families, and carers working together to achieve the best health outcomes and quality of life.

Whether healthcare is necessary for an acute illness episode, helping someone with a long-term health condition achieve an acceptable level of function, or supporting a person who is dying, placing people at the centre of care decisions demands effective teamworking.

Understanding the nature and characteristics of teams can help nurses to work effectively and uphold professional caring values when working with people in any healthcare setting. The RCN acknowledges that teamworking is difficult and requires commitment, hard work, and respect. The College also suggests that the essence of good teawork is how individuals communicate and understand their role as part of the team.

Effective teams are innovative and creative, have a focus on quality, and normally have lower levels of stress, all of which impacts on healthcare delivery and outcomes. Effective teamworking is therefore important not only for improving health outcomes, but also for maintaining morale and job satisfaction for nurses and other health professional staff.

Whilst teamworking is accepted as fundamental to care provision, there is an assumption that if individuals work together, they are a team. However, whilst individuals may identify themselves as part of a team, many people work within groups or pseudo-teams. Distinguishing between these concepts is important.

Features of groups and teams

Group

Within the disciplines of psychology, sociology, and organizational studies, a considerable amount of effort has been invested in understanding how collections of people behave together. In terms of working together, a group has been defined as:

- People who collaborate for mutual benefit and survival.
- A collection of people, working independently, with a common aim, and who have the ability to act in a unitary manner.

Team

Similar effort has been dedicated to understanding what differentiates a group from a team. It has been suggested that defining features of teams are:

- Common aims.
- Shared goals.
- Complementary skills.
- Complementary personal abilities.
- Mutual respect.
- Interdependence.
- Collective accountability.

The key differences between groups and teams are summarized in Table 28.1.

Pseudo-team

Pseudo-teams have also been described where there are shared characteristics of both groups and teams. Whilst there may be an apparent commitment to a common goal, individuals effectively remain independent. In pseudo-teams, members do not necessarily share common objectives and have disparate goals and permeable boundaries, and there is uncertainty about who is part of the team.

Table 28.1 Comparison of group and team characteristics

Group	Team
Workers are independent	Work to a common vision
Ownership and responsibilities are not always clear	Co-ownership of team goals
Lack of trust between members	Open and honest communication
Potential for conflict	Cooperate and aim to understand each other and resolve conflict
Cautious communication	Mutual respect and report
Decisions often made without discussion	Participatory decision-making
	Broad range of skills

Characteristics of successful teams

A successful team is characterized as one where members are committed to working well together to a common aim to achieve the best possible results.

- Recognizing that personal achievement is dependent upon the success of others.
- Working to a common aim requires all team members to be open and honest and to share the values which underpin their practice.
- Being aware of personal and professional values and beliefs.

Being confident in the values which underpin nursing practice necessitates an understanding of professional, organizational, and personal values. Professional values are defined within the NMC Code (℠ www.nmc.org.uk). Organizational values are agreed within each healthcare organization and are aligned with the UK NHS Constitution (℠ www.england.nhs.uk).

Personal values are significant in influencing how individual nurses work. Within successful nursing teams, these values are shared and developed to support practice and decision-making.

Team formation

Tuckman's seminal work on teams suggested that as individuals come together to form a team, they experience four key stages of development and may reach a fifth stage. These are described as:

- *Forming stage*—during this phase, individuals come together, behaviour is generally polite, ground rules are established, and team members begin to work to an agreed agenda.
- *Storming stage*—this phase is characterized by conflict, with personality differences becoming apparent as members develop a greater understanding of each other. The conflict may not be overtly hostile but will be present within the group.
- *Norming stage*—at this phase, the members come together, roles are established and clarified, and there is a sense of a team emerging.
- *Performing stage*—this phase is evidenced by effective structures and ways of working together. Mutual trust and respect, effective working, and high levels of morale and job satisfaction are realized.
- *Adjourning stage*—this is the phase where the team may become complacent and cease striving to improve. They may become reliant on past performance and begin to focus upon tasks.

This model of team formation assumes that all teams will need to go through the first three stages before they can begin 'performing' together. It also implies that every time there is a change in team membership, the team needs to be re-established and the three building phases repeated.

In terms of nursing work, team formation is likely to be something nurses have to deal with on a regular basis. In all areas of practice, there is constant change of team membership, with both student nurses and doctors in training being allocated to clinical areas for clinical placement experience.

Alongside these rotational staff changes, there are also likely to be irregular changes in permanent staff members and organizational and structural changes to contend with, which means many nursing and healthcare teams will be in a state of constant change.

Teamworking in healthcare

It has been established that effective teamworking in healthcare settings requires a culture which values collaborative working. This is enabled through a continual process of engagement, assessment of team effectiveness, team development, and reassessment. Establishing an effective healthcare team requires:

- Clear team identity.
- Team objectives—developed by the team in line with organizational objectives.
- Role clarity.
- Clear decision-making.
- Effective communication.
- Constructive debate.
- Inter-teamworking—recognizing interdependence between other healthcare teams and professional groups.

Building and maintaining an effective healthcare team is likely to be an ongoing process. The role of the team leader will be fundamental to successful group dynamics.

Functional teams

The functional team is founded on trust and interpersonal respect, which extends to other teams, patients, and the public. The characteristics of functional teams have been described as where all members are able to:

- Recognize weaknesses.
- Admit mistakes.
- Ask for help.
- Accept questions about their areas of responsibilities.
- Accept contributions to their areas of responsibilities.
- Give each other the benefit of the doubt before arriving at negative conclusions.
- Take risks in offering feedback and assistance.
- Appreciate each other's skills and experiences.
- Focus time and energy on important issues, rather than organizational politics.
- Offer and accept apologies without hesitation.
- Be open-minded and responsive.
- Be prepared to learn.
- Look forward to meetings and opportunities to work as a group.

A significant number of the characteristics of a functional team are aligned with the behaviours associated with quality-focused care. They also support the establishment of effective nurse/patient relationships and facilitate professional learning and development.

Dysfunctional teams

It is recognized that, for many reasons, some teams do not work effectively. In teams where there is an absence of trust or lack of respect, it is likely that conflict and ineffective working will result.

A pyramid of behaviours in dysfunctional teams have been described by Lencioni (2002) (see Figure 28.1).

In order to maintain a functional team, it is important that these behaviours are addressed, and once again leadership is crucial in restoring equilibrium and function to the team.

Particularly important for nurses are the team's characteristics in relation to accountability. Restoration of effective team functioning can be achieved through the rapid identification of problems. Once identified, it is important to address poor performance, ideally as a learning, rather than disciplinary, opportunity and avoid excessive bureaucracy.

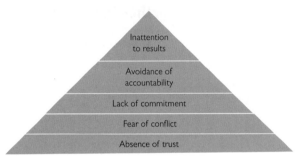

Figure 28.1 Characteristics of dysfunctional teams.

Reproduced from *The five dysfunctions of a team: a leadership fable*, Lencioni P, ISBN 9780787960759, Copyright (2002) with permission from Jossey-Bass and Wiley.

Nursing teams

Dynamic and functional nursing teams will be influenced by the quality of leadership and the sharing of values and beliefs. The level of success is indicated by:
- Lively interesting team meetings.
- Exploring the ideas of all team members.
- Solving problems quickly.
- Expressing conflicting views, without aggression or negativity towards other team members.
- Creating clarity around priorities and direction.
- Uniting in the interest of common objectives.
- Learning from mistakes.
- Taking advantage of opportunities.
- Excellent nursing practice and patient care.

Useful sources of further information

- NHS England (2014) *Working toward an effective multidisciplinary/ multiagency team* ℘ www.england.nhs.uk/wp-content/uploads/2015/ 01/mdt-dev-guid-flat-fin.pdf
- Royal College of Nursing. Developing sustainable and effective teams ℘ www.rcn.org.uk
- Whelan SA. *Creating effective teams*. Sage publications: London, 2014.
- Aston Organisation Development (team building) ℘ www.astonod.com

Professional development

Introduction

Achieving the highest standards of nursing practice necessitates an active commitment to learning and a continual and critical engagement with ideas about nursing and healthcare. The development of both individual nurses and the nursing profession requires learners and registered nurses to commit to the sharing of knowledge and experience and for all nurses to take opportunities to develop clinical and practical skills. Registered nurses also have a professional responsibility to support and guide learner nurses and colleagues, as they acquire and develop nursing values, knowledge, and skills.

Mentorship

Guiding and supporting the development of others' practice is central to professional nursing. The UK NMC Code expects all registered nurses to support students' and colleagues' learning to help them develop their professional competence and confidence.

Whilst mentorship is a concept widely employed in many professions, the concept, as it applies in the nursing profession, the role and responsibilities of the mentor can be summarised as;

Organizing and co-coordinating student learning activities in practice.

Supervising students in learning situations and providing them with constructive feedback on their achievements.

Setting and monitoring achievement of realistic learning objectives.

Assessing total student performance, including skills, attitudes, and behaviours.

Providing evidence, as required by programme providers, of student achievement or lack of achievement.

Liaising with others, practice facilitators, practice teachers, personal tutors, and programme leaders to provide feedback, identify any concerns about the student's performance, and agree remedial action as appropriate.

Providing evidence for, or making decisions about achievement of proficiency at the end of a programme of study.

The importance of the role of the mentor cannot be overstated, as it is within this role that nurses are setting the template for future nursing practice, maintaining professional standards and protecting patient and public safety.

Preceptorship

It is well understood that the transition from student to registered nurse can be very difficult, and newly qualified nurses often need a lot of personal support. Alongside these challenges, the increasing complexity of healthcare provision has led the UK NHS to recommend that a period of preceptorship represents best practice in supporting this transition.

Preceptorship has been described as a period of structured transition where the newly registered practitioner is supported by an experienced preceptor. The aim is to help develop their confidence as an autonomous professional and refine nursing skills, values, and behaviours. Preceptor support should enable newly qualified nurses to:

• Develop and apply knowledge, skills, and values gained in their pre-registration programme.
• Develop specific competences that relate to their role.
• Access support in embedding the values and expectations of the profession.
• Embrace the principles of the NHS Constitution.

The period of preceptorship is also an opportunity for the newly qualified nurse to meet their personal learning needs, reflect on practice, and receive constructive feedback. The role of the preceptor is fundamental to this process, acting as a positive role model, sharing a commitment to professional values, and demonstrating empathy with the new nurse.

The impact of preceptorship on nursing practice is not easily identifiable, although it has been suggested that preceptorship has the potential to:

• Enhance patient care and experience.
• Improve recruitment and retention of nursing staff.
• Reduce sickness absence.
• Build confident nurses.
• Increase staff job satisfaction and morale.

Where preceptorship arrangements are in place, these will be structured by the employing organization. Although an initial 12-month period is identified as normal practice, different healthcare organizations may well have other arrangements.

Preceptorship can provide a unique opportunity for both the preceptor and the newly qualified nurse to actively engage in the process of nursing decision-making and practice, and arguably support the development of excellence in nursing practice and patient care.

Revalidation

In 2016, the UK NMC introduced a new revalidation process for registered nurses and midwives. This new approach has built upon the preceding re-registration process that required nurses to evidence their learning and continuous professional development through the development and maintenance of a professional portfolio.

Significant to the newly established revalidation process is the introduction of a formal assessment of practice through the introduction of a review of reflections in practice by another registrant.

The portfolio of evidence now needs to be confirmed by the line manager or employer, ideally an NMC registrant. Revalidation is required on a 3-yearly basis, with all nurses needing to develop a portfolio of evidence which includes, as a minimum:

A record of practice hours—in order to revalidate, nurses must complete a minimum of 450 hours over the 3 years preceding the application to revalidate. These hours must be related to the nurse's area of practice.

Continuing professional development—a minimum of 35 hours of learning activity must be completed, of which a minimum of 20 must be learning with others. Learning with others is important, as it enables the sharing of knowledge, learning from others, and having an opportunity to challenge and question practice.

Practice-related feedback—five pieces of feedback relevant to a nurse's domain of practice are required. The inclusion of feedback, both positive and negative, is important in focusing on other people's perspectives and learning from others' experiences of nursing work.

Reflective accounts—the inclusion of reflective accounts supports a critical engagement with practice, identifying learning, and opportunities to improve personal practice.

Reflective discussion—this requires the nurse to discuss their five reflective accounts with another registrant. The process enables the reflections on practice to be validated, but importantly it provides an opportunity for nurses to have a professional conversation in relation to their practice and how they uphold the NMC Code in their everyday work.

Professional indemnity arrangements—this is usually met by nurses' employing organizations if they are working for NHS organizations; however, if nurses are working within independent organizations, they must provide evidence that professional indemnity arrangements are in place.

A health and character declaration.

Confirmation—this final part of the process is to verify the information collated for the portfolio.

To support this revalidation process, all UK-registered nurses are encouraged to register with the NMC online. Online registration enables the registrant to not only receive updates on NMC policy, but also to be provided with reminders of the revalidation process. The revalidation process is completed online, with key documentation and extensive guidance provided by the NMC (⅏ www.nmc.org.uk).

Nursing career development

Although many nurses have personal ambition that does not extend beyond direct patient care, there are now myriad opportunities for nurses to develop their individual careers in many different directions, all of which make an important contribution.

- In the *clinical* arena, in any sector of the service, opportunities can include promotion, advanced practice roles, and specialist nursing roles, all of which maintain a level of direct contact with patients and families.
- There are also multiple opportunities for nurses to progress to formal *leadership and management* roles such as ward managers, community matrons, and directors of nursing services.
- In addition, nurses can pursue *research* activities, either working as a nurse member of a medical, multi-professional, or sociological research team. They can also pursue independent nursing research through PhD studies or funded research projects.
- There are also opportunities for nurses to contribute to nurse *education and scholarship* at many different levels such as clinical practice tutors, clinical demonstrators, and nurse lecturers.

Whichever route individual nurses choose to pursue their personal professional development and career ambitions, it is most likely that they will need to undertake further academic study. This may be at Bachelors level (level 6 studies) or Masters level (level 7 studies), and may be in the form of certificated study days or workshops, short specialist courses, or full programmes of study.

Undertaking further academic study can be challenging for nurses working in full-time clinical or other roles, but for both personal and professional development, critical engagement with nursing ideas and knowledge will ultimately be of benefit to the ideals and values of the profession.

The majority of academic programmes of study will be designed to foster key transferable skills, develop knowledge, and critical engagement. This will require professional nurses to have the independent learning ability required to advance nursing knowledge, skills, and understanding.

Examples of knowledge and skills relevant to developing nursing practice and careers include, but are not limited to:

- Understanding and critical awareness of a complex body of knowledge informed by the latest evidence in nursing.
- Knowledge and understanding of the contextual issues which impact on nurses and their practice.
- Critical understanding of the global socio-economic and political factors which impact on nursing.
- Knowledge of the contribution and scope of nursing in healthcare.
- Understanding of how the boundaries of nursing knowledge are advanced through research and scholarship.

Skills in the application of knowledge to practice, whether clinical, leadership, research, or education.

Skills in communicating complex information in any circumstances.

Ability to utilize information and communication technology skills in furthering professional knowledge and expertise.

Skills in reflecting critically on learning, for oneself, colleagues, and nurses in training.

Useful sources of further information

- Department of Health (2010) *Preceptorship framework for newly registered nurses, midwives and allied health professionals* ℜ http://webarchive.nationalarchives.gov.uk/+/http://www.dh.gov.uk/en/Publicationsandstatistics/Publications/PublicationsPolicyAndGuidance/DH_114073
- NHS Employers. *Preceptorships for newly qualified staff* ℜ www.nhsemployers.org/your-workforce/plan/education-and-training/preceptorships-for-newly-qualified-staff
- NMC. *Standards to support learning and assessment in practice* ℜ www.nmc.org.uk/globalassets/sitedocuments/standards/nmc-standards-to-support-learning-assessment.pdf
- NMC. Revalidation ℜ http://revalidation.nmc.org.uk

Chapter 30

Nursing collectivism

Introduction

In ever changing social and political cultures, it is important that nurses are able to work together and support each other in upholding the core values which are important to the profession. Different forms of collective organizations are available for nurses, including professional organizations and trade unions. Despite notional and philosophical differences, the workplace practices of the representative organizations tend to be similar, and nurses can accrue particular benefits from membership of a collective. Local organizing strength is often the best predictor of which organization nurses will join, and ultimately collective strength requires mass membership. Professional bodies and trade unions are involved in substantial efforts to maintain strong representation of nurses, and an ultimate goal is the democratization of healthcare workplaces.

Representative organizations for nurses

There are two main forms of collective membership organizations for nurses in the UK, which are professional associations and trade unions.

The main professional association is the Royal College of Nursing (RCN), the structure of which is modelled on medical royal colleges. The Royal College of Midwives (RCM) similarly represents midwives. Professional associations serve a representative function for nurses, with a focus on professional role and identity.

A number of trade unions also represent nurses, the biggest being Unison, the public service union. Unite, the large general union, also represents nurses and includes the Mental Health Nurses Association (MHNA) and the Community Practitioners & Health Visitors Association (CPHVA). Because of its organizational powers and bargaining experience, Unison often takes the lead in national nursing pay negotiations and the provision of evidence to the NHS Pay Review Body. The trade unions are affiliated to the Trades Union Congress (TUC) and the Labour Party, and they prioritize workplace rights and terms and conditions of employment.

The professional bodies and trade unions are all concerned with employment relations and professional interests and operate across these boundaries. The major difference between the trade unions and professional associations is that the unions are more thoroughly integrated into a broader labour movement and have a more diverse membership base, organizing occupational groups beyond nursing. The professional associations eschew political affiliations and only recruit nurses to their membership. For most of its history, the RCN was only concerned with registered nurses but has changed its rules to allow healthcare assistants to be members. Hence distinctions between professional associations and trade unions are increasingly blurred.

All of these representative organizations are committed to working together in alliances, and typically they also seek to work in partnership with NHS employers.

Benefits of membership

Trade unions and professional associations often offer a package of benefits as incentives to recruitment of members. Arguably, for nurses, the major incentive of this sort is professional indemnity insurance. Both Unison and the RCN offer student nurses substantially cut-price membership for the period of their pre-registration training, with a view to recruiting them as full members on registration and their taking up employment. The RCN also produces journals, notably the *Nursing Standard*, and organizes various annual conferences for practitioners and academics.

Unison and Unite also operate professional services, with Unite producing the *Mental Health Nursing* and *Community Practitioner* journals that are distributed to members. Unison operates a National Nursing and Midwifery Occupational Group, staffed by professional officers who provide advice and produce guidance on professional matters relating to employment relations.

All of the respective representative organizations offer packages of member benefits. These typically include special deals on car and home insurance, and holiday and other shopping discounts. More importantly, the benefits of membership are essentially a contingency on which to rely if trouble occurs within the workplace. These benefits can include:

• Support, advice, and help at work.
• Help with grievances or disciplinary matters.
• Legal help—often extending beyond the workplace to include assistance with family legal problems or making wills.
• Covering the costs of registering a claim at an employment tribunal.
• Assistance in securing compensation for injury or accident at work.

Unions and professional associations are structured to deliver their work through a mixture of paid officers and volunteer representatives, the latter often referred to as 'reps', 'stewards', or 'activists'.

Individual nurses often join the organization that is best organized within their immediate workplace, and it is this level of organization that will be most useful if the member experiences difficulties in their employment which requires representation or support.

All representative organizations offer to support members should they wish to action grievances, escalate concerns about patient welfare, or if they find themselves subject to managerial censure or discipline or in circumstances of organizational change leading to insecure employment.

UK NHS pay and other terms and conditions of employment are negotiated centrally and subject to the deliberations of an independent Pay Review Body. Increasingly, however, the restructuring of the NHS into semi-autonomous Trusts and the different strategic direction and financial settlements within the devolved nations of the UK have created pressures for local negotiation and bargaining over terms and conditions and pay. In these circumstances, it is vital that nurses have access to well-organized local representation of their interests.

Indemnity insurance

The major representative organizations offer their nurse and midwifery members substantial indemnity insurance. This is insurance cover for risks to third parties, such as patients, due to nursing practices, mistakes, or errors of judgement that result in harm. The indemnity insurance on offer from trade unions and professional associations explicitly excludes independent practitioners, such as independent midwives, who are more vulnerable to litigation.

In the UK, by common law, the NHS Employer is subject to vicarious liability, meaning the NHS has to cover damages due to employees' actions. NHS employees are therefore unlikely to be sued as individuals, as persons seeking to pursue a legal claim will usually be advised to sue the NHS Trust.

However, as the NHS becomes increasingly commercialized and fragmented, and citizens become more litigious, there may be an increase in occasions where individual nurses are taken to court and sued for damages.

The operating context of collective organizations

Following the global banking crisis of 2008, the wider political economy is now dominated by neo-liberalism and associated austerity policies. In UK health and social care services, this has led to enormous cost-cutting pressures and increasing encroachment of market forces and privatization into the NHS.

These factors have contributed to a health workforce crisis and an acute shortage of nurses at the same time as austerity policies attempt to restrain pay and dilute other terms and conditions of employment. In addition to this, nursing itself is subject to public criticism following various public enquiries into failures of care services.

These conditions make for turbulent employment relations and put partnership working under strain. When employment relations are stressed or rigid impositions, such as pay restraint, are placed upon negotiations, representative organizations seek to marshal their collective strength behind bargaining aims. This can involve forms of industrial action, up to and including strike action.

Until recently, the RCN famously operated a no-strike rule, because of concerns over potential detriment to patient care. Although this has now been rescinded, the RCN remains largely opposed to strike action.

Nursing unions across the world, however, have successfully used strike action to further a range of demands without compromising patient care. Many examples of nursing industrial action have targeted the defence of services, rather than employment or workforce issues.

Upholding professional values and escalating concerns

Nurses have an important professional role responsibility in advocacy and safeguarding, particularly on behalf of vulnerable patients (℗ www.nmc. org.uk). This can place nurses at the forefront of raising or escalating concerns over the safety of patients or colleagues.

Most good employers will have a policy to protect nurses or other staff who feel professionally obliged to highlight concerns in this way. Local policy and practices should involve recognition of professional values and responsibilities, together with a clear organizational process by which concerns can be brought to the attention of the relevant managers, and a pathway for escalation as necessary.

Where concerns are not addressed within an organization, the ultimate stage of escalation is reporting bad practice or service failings in the public domain. This practice is commonly referred to as 'whistle-blowing' and should normally only be considered if internal processes and procedures for raising concerns have been exhausted.

Whilst it will sometimes take considerable courage to uphold professional nursing values and pursue a legitimate concern, nurses should also be aware of their vulnerability. They can be subject to disciplinary action if the employer takes a view that due process has not been followed. Because of this, it is imperative that nurses who wish to raise or escalate concerns seek the support of their representative organization.

The NMC provides guidance in the *Code of Practice* and *Raising and escalating concerns: guidance for nurses and midwives* (℗ www.nmc.org.uk). Unison also offers guidance for nurses and other healthcare workers facing such circumstances in the *Duty of care handbook* and *Speaking up, speaking out* (℗ www.unison.org.uk). (See also ➍ Chapter 9, Communicating concerns in healthcare.)

Activism and organizing

Most nursing collective organizations recognize the importance of recruiting members and getting people more actively involved once they are members. The particular social and relational ways in which people are persuaded to join and become more active in representative groups is known as 'organizing'.

Representative organizations, such as trade unions or professional associations, are more powerful when they are able to demonstrate collective strength. This requires a number of things:

- A strong base, ideally with a representative in each workplace or team.
- Recruitment of as many staff as possible into membership.
- Commitment amongst the membership to the aims of the collective organization.
- Establishment of close social ties between members, activists, and officers.
- Active involvement in systems of internal democracy.
- Solidarity and respectful working relations between different representative organizations.
- Interests and connections to groups outside of the workplace who have an interest in healthcare work.

In any workplace, the membership density is the proportion of all staff eligible to be in a staff-side organization who actually are a member of one. However, many people do not see the immediate benefit of being in a union. To some extent, there is an effect where non-members can get some of the benefits of membership without paying subscription fees if the collective is fairly successful locally or nationally. Ultimately, however, dilution of collective strength weakens everybody's position.

Alliances with patient organizations

The efforts of professional bodies and unions to become better organized in the UK health sector have been fairly successful in maintaining membership figures in the face of service cuts and job losses.

However, it is also recognized that the defence of UK health services needs to work with patients and the public. Engaging in alliances with members of the public and organized patient groups can help professional bodies and trade unions become mutually, cooperatively, and reciprocally involved in communities, rather than solely focused on workplace concerns.

Engaging the public in nursing and healthcare campaigns can also help the nursing profession by fostering understanding about nursing work. Greater understanding may make it less likely that individual nurses, or nursing in general, are blamed for apparent failures of care and compassion.

Democratizing the workplace

All of the various representative organizations open to nurse membership are organized democratically. Various local, regional, and national meetings and delegate conferences decide policy and strategic direction of the collective.

Important issues such as leadership and executive positions and key policy issues are often decided by full-membership postal ballots. UK employment law requires that votes for industrial action are delivered by independent postal ballot. All of this voting means that unions and professional associations are amongst the most democratic organizations in contemporary society. However, internal democracy can always be strengthened, largely by increasing the level of participation of the membership.

Although nursing collectives are democratically organized, it is perhaps surprising that the majority of healthcare workplaces are most often operated by hierarchical managerial command structures.

It is not outside the bounds of imagination that nurses, other healthcare workers, their collective organizations, patients, ex-patients, carers, and the public at large could find creative ways to have dialogue and deliberation that would actually help organize healthcare work and make service provider organizations more democratically accountable.

The desirability of more democratic involvement in organizational decisions and planning is also implicated in calls for more horizontal, distributed approaches to leadership. It may actually prove to be the case that democracy at work is most suited to public health services where the ultimate goals of high-quality care are not in dispute.

Useful sources of further information

- Royal College of Nursing ✎ www.rcn.org.uk/
- Unite, the union ✎ www.unitetheunion.org/
- Unison, the public service union ✎ www.unison.org.uk/

Chapter 31

Patient and public involvement in healthcare

Introduction

The impulse for patient and public involvement (PPI) in health services reflects wider societal and policy concerns with citizenship and democratic participation. A consumerist turn in health policy has opened the door to advances in involvement initiatives, with nurses often playing a lead role.

These involvement practices have developed in the interlinked areas of nursing practice, research, and education. Effective involvement is predicated upon emancipatory values and, as such, involvement practices are concerned with prevailing power relations. The actual form that involvement takes can be thorough, systematic, and empowering or partial, tokenistic, and subsumed under oppressive governance systems.

Ultimately, involvement poses key questions for professional nursing identity, allowing for a re-imagining of professionalism that is essentially democratized and cooperative.

Defining patient and public involvement (PPI)

Public involvement in UK health services has a long history, which pre-dates the foundation of the NHS. In recent times, there have been efforts to distinguish between different forms and contexts of public involvement, such as noting the difference between patients being involved at the level of individual care encounters, sharing in decision-making about treatment, and more strategic involvement in planning and organizing healthcare services.

The concept of patient and public involvement raises important questions concerning who exactly is being involved and what language is used to best describe or identify participants. Policy guidance often refers to service user involvement, and occasionally consumer involvement as practical synonyms for PPI.

Involvement practices quite often seek to include family carers, and the PPI label can be understood to include carers, as well as patients and the wider public. There is a need, however, to distinguish between the different sets of interests and needs of these people. Sometimes an individual patient's interests and treatment choices can conflict with the wishes of their family members.

The vocabulary of involvement is also important and sometimes contentious.

- The term *patient* is well understood in a clinical context and by lay people, however, it has been criticized for the implications of passivity and deference to an assumed professional authority.
- *Service user* has come into fashion as a replacement for patient, but this term can also be criticized, especially in some settings such as mental health, where personal choice to use services can be limited.
- *Consumer* also has some currency and is widely used across North America and Australia but can be unacceptable to people who are concerned about the apparent commodification of healthcare.

As such, there is no perfect lexicon for referring to involvement practices and, to some extent, endlessly debating the most appropriate terminology is best avoided. It is more important to establish the practices that maximize involvement of diverse individuals, to allow for the genuine and authentic expression of views and wishes and for these to be respectfully acted upon.

Involvement practices can be organized at a range of different levels:

- Involvement at the level of patient care.
- Involvement in planning, service development, and organizing services.
- Involvement in nurse education.
- Involvement in health research.
- Involvement in policy formulation.
- The UK NHS England has the Patients and Information Directorate, which also runs surveys and consultations targeting the public.

Rationale for involvement

Despite a growing interest in a range of involvement practices, not everyone is willingly engaged and there remains a need to persuade people of the value of PPI. Reasoning in support of involvement initiatives includes:

- Policy mandates.
- Expression of institutional values and organizational identity.
- A business case—involvement practices can improve organizational efficiency and effectiveness.
- Improved outcomes—particular forms of involvement lead to improved quality of care, better research, and enhanced experience of learning.
- Increased service user satisfaction—authentic involvement lends to better appreciation of services.
- Workforce fulfilment—working in alliance with people is more implicitly rewarding for nurses and healthcare staff.

In addition, the prevailing social and political climate reinforces the case for patients and the public to have an authentic voice in all aspects of health services.

Involvement in context

Practice

In the field of healthcare practice, there are a number of ways that involvement is enacted. Direct, face-to-face encounters can be organized democratically, with the approach to delivery of care negotiated from as equal a basis as is possible to achieve in the circumstances.

Case reviews and care team meetings can also be democratized, offering people a full role and putting them at the centre of shared decision-making. When there are differences of opinion between patients and care teams, or between different members of the team, then nurses can take on the role of advocate, to ensure that individuals' voices are heard and attended to in decisions over care and treatment.

In certain contexts, such as when a person lacks capacity to make decisions, is subject to the Mental Health Act, or apparently makes choices against a clinical view of best interest, there will be a need for independent advocacy.

Health services can seek patient feedback to support quality improvements and involvement practices. Certain service developments, typically within the voluntary sector, are run by and for people, without professional direction.

Research

There has been a significant growth in involvement in health research. These initiatives are based on an assumption that involving people who use health services in clinical research projects results in the framing of more appropriate research questions and leads to better-quality findings.

Patients and the public can be involved at all stages of the research process, but projects that show comprehensive levels of involvement are unusual. Some research methodologies are implicitly and, by design, better suited to involvement, and there is debate about whether research that is led by service will produce the most relevant findings.

Some research centres employ researchers who have significant personal experience of health service use, making a virtue of this in the conduct of their research.

The NIHR has organized a number of clinical research networks to involve the public in research communities and contribute to strategic planning for research. These notably include the cancer research network (ℜ www.nihr.ac.uk/nihr-in-your-area/cancer/).

NIHR also funds the INVOLVE network to support public involvement in research across health, public health, and social care sectors (ℜ www.invo.org.uk).

NICE (ℜ www.nice.org.uk) endeavours to involve service users within the various working groups who define clinical guidelines from evidence reviews.

Education

Critical pedagogies emphasize democratic learning relationships and are suited to supporting involvement practices. In recent times, the education of nurses and other healthcare practitioners has been greatly enhanced by involvement of patients and the public in curriculum design and delivery.

Exposure to people's narratives is a powerful form of learning that arguably helps student nurses to develop empathy and become skilled in negotiating the emotional labour of caring.

Strategy

Various forums and networks have been established to facilitate unit level, service level, or organizational level involvement in strategic decision-making or service planning.

At the level of wards or care teams, these can take the form of simple meetings, at which fairly basic decisions are taken to enhance the way work is organized and treatment is scheduled or to decide matters such as decor, menus, or visiting arrangements.

Higher up the organization, members of the public may be involved in the strategic decision-making of directorate management teams or Trust Boards, and it has been suggested that NHS Foundation Trust status should be aligned with such goals.

Healthcare organizations committed to involvement practices can demonstrate more or less authentic levels of commitment through democratization. Models of asset-based community engagement and development can bring in diverse community voices and help shape local services.

Values for involvement

Key values for supporting and engaging in involvement initiatives are covered in numerous sets of guidance and explicit commitments made by healthcare organizations such as NHS Trusts. These values are similar to the required conditions for effective deliberative democracy and are consistent with key nursing values.

- *Ensuring empowerment*—involves a commitment to allowing everyone's voice to be heard. In reality, it is very challenging to think of giving power to another, but a crucial first step is attentive listening to others' points of view, however unsettling or even upsetting this may be.
- *Respect*—mutual regard and appreciation, valuing people as individuals, and acknowledging their goals and aspirations.
- *Treating people with dignity and kindness*—speaks clearly of commitment to providing compassionate care. Such compassion needs to frame dialogue and discussions in the context of involvement and include care for each other.
- *Embracing diversity and celebrating difference*—respect across difference, including differences of opinion or views over *best interest*, is crucial to effective involvement.
- *Openness*—a commitment to honesty and open communication, and is linked to a duty of candour.
- *Togetherness*—relates to a commitment to *cooperation and alliances*, working with partners and communities for mutual benefit.

Barriers to effective involvement

The main barriers to meaningful public involvement are co-option and incorporation threats. These are the many means by which patient and public voices can become diluted or muted by becoming too close to the systems of power they wish to influence or change.

This often occurs through the establishment of friendly relationships with healthcare staff and managers to the point where it feels uncomfortable to challenge the status quo. At the same time, it is also healthily friendly relations that can drive the most effective involvement. As a result, care needs to be taken over appropriate boundaries.

Within NHS organizations, there is also a need to incorporate PPI values in leadership and ensure they are embedded in human resource policies and practices.

Without deliberate design or purpose, involvement practices can fail because of external pressures on resources that constrain staff time or motivation to commit to high-quality relationships. These factors include staffing levels, agency staff, job security, workload, and workplace environments. Where health organizations have not yet perfected involvement practices, there is a risk that involvement may not be adequately valued or supported, resulting in tokenism or co-opted forms.

Co-production and shared decision-making

The notion of shared decision-making is emphasized within current policy that works with a concept of co-production. In co-production, care is the result of democratized working alliances between staff and patients. Good involvement practices open up possibilities to renegotiate what it means to be a professional nurse.

- Nurses and their collective organizations can be central to supporting involvement, particularly as they comprise the major part of the healthcare workforce and have the most contact with patients and the public.
- At the level of individual patient encounters and relationships, nurses are well placed to bring into play effective interpersonal skills and nursing values to support involvement. The most relevant aspect of the nursing role is their ability to devote time to discuss care and treatment with patients and their families, ensuring they are fully informed and have real opportunity to gain influence. A crucial frontline nursing skill is active listening.
- Nurses can also play an important role in holding their employing organizations to account for the extent and quality of involvement practices. There should be clarity about:
  - The nature of communications, both internal and external to the organization.
  - Mechanisms for capturing patient, user, and carer experiences.
  - Opportunities for involvement—with regard to explicit PPI processes and more general membership.
  - The volunteering strategy.
  - Connection with the wider community.
  - Relationships with the voluntary and community sectors, NHS partners, and the Local Authority.

Self-organized groups and community activism

Commentators on health services and communities have noted that people who engage in involvement practices are often also connected to a range of other community groups and activities. Patient and public interests can be voiced within self-organized groups or social movements which include:

- Advocacy.
- Popular protest.
- Alliances with staff groups.

Social movements arise when particular interests are not served by usual democratic channels. As such, they are often organized around identity or single-issue politics, with such movements including rights-based appeals around particular health conditions or disability. Radical and critical groups can pose quite unsettling questions or make challenging demands on services and practitioners.

Shared characteristics between involved service users and social movement actors include:

- Motivation and sustaining enthusiasm.
- Identity issues.
- Activism.
- Making meaning out of action.
- Inclusive forms of organization.
- Emotional nature of involvement.
- Relationships, connections, and wider community networks.

Democratizing care and clinical leadership

Democratization represented by involvement practices has resonance with contemporary thinking about NHS leadership. This involves models of relational and non-hierarchical leadership.

In embedding PPI in the organizational culture of healthcare, clinical leadership has a crucial role, alongside staff agency. Leadership provides endorsement of, and support to, innovation and development, whilst staff agency is responsive to patients and the public at the interface of care.

Transformative change in healthcare requires wholesale involvement of the workforce, and lasting change needs to be owned by individuals and teams. (See also ➔ Chapter 27, Leadership and ➔ Chapter 28 Teamwork.)

In democratizing care, true participation has to be organized, which demands an intensely relational approach, well suited to nursing skills and values. The effects of empowerment through PPI would benefit patients, members of the public, and staff, and has the potential to lead to better healthcare and more rewarding work.

Useful sources of further information

- NHS INVOLVE ✍ www.invo.org.uk
- National Institute for Health and Care Excellence ✍ www.nice.org.uk
- James Lind Alliance ✍ www.jla.nihr.ac.uk
- Care Opinion ✍ www.careopinion.org.uk
- People Matters Network ✍ www.peoplemattersnetwork.com
- National Survivor User Network ✍ www.nsun.org.uk

Appendix 1: MUST screening process

See Figure A1.1.

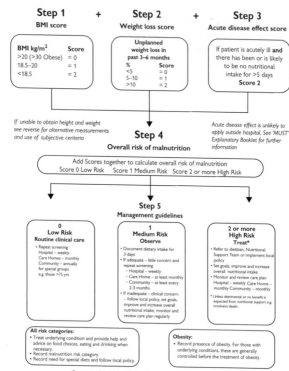

Figure A1.1 The Malnutrition Universal Screening Tool.

The 'Malnutrition Universal Screening Tool' ('MUST') is reproduced here with the kind permission of BAPEN (British Association for Parenteral and Enteral Nutrition). For further information on 'MUST' see ℘ www.bapen.org.uk'.

Appendix 2: Risk assessment tool for VTE

See Figure A2.1.

RISK ASSESSMENT FOR VENOUS THROMBOEMBOLISM (VTE)

All patients should be risk assessed on admission to hospital. Patients should be reassessed within 24 hours of admission and whenever the clinical situation changes.

STEP ONE

Assess all patients admitted to hospital for level of mobility (tick one box). All surgical patients, and all medical patients with significantly reduced mobility, should be considered for further risk assessment.

STEP TWO

Review the patient-related factors shown on the assessment sheet against **thrombosis** risk, ticking each box that applies (more than one box can be ticked).

Any tick for thrombosis risk should prompt thromboprophylaxis according to NICE guidance.

The risk factors identified are not exhaustive. Clinicians may consider additional risks in individual patients and offer thromboprophylaxis as appropriate.

STEP THREE

Review the patient-related factors shown against **bleeding risk** and tick each box that applies (more than one box can be ticked).

Any tick should prompt clinical staff to consider if bleeding risk is sufficient to preclude pharmacological intervention.

Guidance on thromboprophylaxis is available at:

National Institute for Health and Clinical Excellence (2010) Venous thromboembolism: reducing the risk of venous thromboembolism (deep vein thrombosis and pulmonary embolism) in patients admitted to hospital. NICE clinical guideline 92. London: National Institute for Health and Clinical Excellence.

http://www.nice.org.uk/guidance/CG92

This document has been authorised by the Department of Health
Gateway reference no: 10278

(DH) Department of Health

1

Figure A2.1 Risk assessment for venous thromboembolism (VTE).

RISK ASSESSMENT FOR VENOUS THROMBOEMBOLISM (VTE)

Mobility – all patients (tick one box)	Tick		Tick		Tick
Surgical patient		Medical patient expected to have ongoing reduced mobility relative to normal state		Medical patient NOT expected to have significantly reduced mobility relative to normal state	
Assess for thrombosis and bleeding risk below				**Risk assessment now complete**	

Thrombosis risk			
Patient related	**Tick**	**Admission related**	**Tick**
Active cancer or cancer treatment		Significantly reduced mobility for 3 days or more	
Age > 60		Hip or knee replacement	
Dehydration		Hip fracture	
Known thrombophilias		Total anaesthetic + surgical time > 90 minutes	
Obesity (BMI >30 kg/m²)		Surgery involving pelvis or lower limb with a total anaesthetic + surgical time > 60 minutes	
One or more significant medical comorbidities (eg heart disease;metabolic,endocrine or respiratory pathologies;acute infectious diseases; inflammatory conditions)		Acute surgical admission with inflammatory or intra-abdominal condition	
Personal history or first-degree relative with a history of VTE		Critical care admission	
Use of hormone replacement therapy		Surgery with significant reduction in mobility	
Use of oestrogen-containing contraceptive therapy			
Varicose veins with phlebitis			
Pregnancy or < 6 weeks post partum (see NICE guidance for specific risk factors)			

Bleeding risk			
Patient related	**Tick**	**Admission related**	**Tick**
Active bleeding		Neurosurgery, spinal surgery or eye surgery	
Acquired bleeding disorders (such as acute liver failure)		Other procedure with high bleeding risk	
Concurrent use of anticoagulants known to increase the risk of bleeding (such as warfarin with INR >2)		Lumbar puncture/epidural/spinal anaesthesia expected within the next 12 hours	
Acute stroke		Lumbar puncture/epidural/spinal anaesthesia within the previous 4 hours	
Thrombocytopaenia (platelets< 75x10⁹/l)			
Uncontrolled systolic hypertension (230/120 mmHg or higher)			
Untreated inherited bleeding disorders (such as haemophilia and von Willebrand's disease)			

© Crown copyright 2010
301292 1p March 10

2

Figure A2.1 (Continued)

Appendix 3: Height and weight conversions

To convert a person's height from inches to centimetres, multiply the number of inches by 2.54. To convert a patient's height from centimetres to inches, multiply the number of centimetres by 0.394. See Tables A3.1 and A3.2.

Table A3.1 Approximate height conversions

Imperial (feet and inches)	Inches	Metric (cm)
4'8"	56	142
4'9"	57	144.5
4'10"	58	147
4'11"	59	150
5'	60	152.5
5'1"	61	155
5'2"	62	157.5
5'3"	63	160
5'4"	64	162.5
5'5"	65	165
5'6"	66	167.5
5'7"	67	170
5'8"	68	172.5
5'9"	69	175
5'10"	70	177.5
5'11"	71	180
6'	72	183
6'1"	73	185.5
6'2"	74	188
6'3"	75	190.5

Table A3.2 Approximate weight conversions

kg	st	lb	kg	st	lb	kg	st	lb	kg	st	lb
0.5		1	44	6	13	83	13	1	122	19	3
1		2	45	7	1	84	13	3	123	19	6
1.5		3	46	7	3	85	13	6	124	19	7
2		4	47	7	6	86	13	7	125	19	10
2.5		6	48	7	8	87	13	10	126	19	11
3		7	49	7	10	88	13	11	127	20	0
3.5		8	50	7	13	89	14	0	128	20	1
4		9	51	8	0	90	14	3	129	20	5
4.5		10	52	8	3	91	14	4	130	20	7
5		11	53	8	4	92	14	7	131	20	8
5.5		12	54	8	7	93	14	8	132	20	11
6		13	55	8	10	94	14	11	133	20	13
			56	8	11	95	14	13	134	21	1
10	1	8	57	9	0	96	15	1	135	21	3
15	2	6	58	9	1	97	15	4	136	21	6
20	3	1	59	9	4	98	15	6	137	21	8
21	3	4	60	9	6	99	15	8	138	21	10
22	3	7	61	9	8	100	15	10	139	21	13
23	3	8	62	9	11	101	15	13	140	22	0
24	3	11	63	9	13	102	16	1	141	22	3
25	3	13	64	10	1	103	16	3	142	22	5
26	4	1	65	10	3	104	16	6	143	22	7
27	4	3	66	10	6	105	16	7	144	22	10
28	4	6	67	10	7	106	16	10	145	22	11
29	4	8	68	10	10	107	16	11	146	23	0
30	4	10	69	10	13	108	17	0	147	23	1
31	4	13	70	11	0	109	17	3	148	23	5
32	5	0	71	11	3	110	17	5	149	23	6
33	5	3	72	11	4	111	17	7	150	23	8
34	5	6	73	11	7	112	17	8	151	23	11
35	5	7	74	11	8	113	17	11	152	23	13
36	5	10	75	11	11	114	17	13	153	24	1
37	5	11	76	12	0	115	18	1	154	24	3
38	6	0	77	12	1	116	18	5	155	24	6
39	6	1	78	12	5	117	18	6	156	24	7
40	6	3	79	12	6	118	18	8	157	24	10
41	6	7	80	12	8	119	18	10	158	24	13
42	6	8	81	12	10	120	18	13	159	25	0
43	6	11	82	12	13	121	19	0	160	25	3

Index